Essential Medical Genetics

Edward S. Tobias
BSc MBChB PhD FRCP
Professor of Medical Genetics
University of Glasgow
and Honorary Consultant in Medical Genetics
West of Scotland Regional Genetics Service
Institute of Medical Genetics
Glasgow

Michael Connor
MD, DSc, FRCP
Professor of Medical Genetics
University of Glasgow
and Director of the West of Scotland
Regional Genetics Service
Institute of Medical Genetics
Glasgow

Malcolm Ferguson-Smith
MBChB, FRCPath, FRCP, FRSE, FRS
Emeritus Professor of Pathology
University of Cambridge
and formerly Director of the East Anglia Regional Genetics Service
Addenbrookes Hospital
Cambridge

Sixth edition

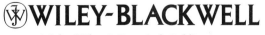
WILEY-BLACKWELL
A John Wiley & Sons, Ltd., Publication

D0898692

This edition first published 2011, © 2011 by Edward S. Tobias, Michael Connor and Malcolm Ferguson-Smith
Previous editions © 1984, 1987, 1991, 1993, 1997 by Blackwell Science Ltd.

Blackwell Publishing was acquired by John Wiley & Sons in February 2001. Blackwell's publishing program has been merged with Wiley's global Scientific, Technical and Medical business to form Wiley-Blackwell.

Registered office: John Wiley & Sons Ltd, The Atrium, Southern Gate, Chichester, West Sussex, PO19 8SQ, UK

Editorial offices: 9600 Garsington Road, Oxford, OX4 2DQ, UK
The Atrium, Southern Gate, Chichester, West Sussex, PO19 8SQ, UK
111 River Street, Hoboken, NJ 07030-5774, USA

For details of our global editorial offices, for customer services and for information about how to apply for permission to reuse the copyright material in this book please see our website at www.wiley.com/wiley-blackwell

Library of Congress Cataloguing-in-Publication Data
Tobias, Edward.
    Essential medical genetics / Edward Tobias, Michael Connor, Malcolm Ferguson-Smith.
– 6th ed.
        p. ; cm.
    Rev. ed. of : Essential medical genetics / Michael Connor, Malcolm Ferguson-Smith. 5th ed. 1997.
    Includes bibliographical references and index.
    ISBN 978-1-4051-6974-5 (pbk. : alk. paper)   1. Medical genetics.   I. Connor, J. M. (James Michael), 1951- II. Ferguson-Smith, M. A. (Malcolm Andrew)   III. Connor, J. M. (James Michael), 1951- Essential medical genetics.   IV. Title.
    [DNLM: 1. Genetics, Medical. QZ 50]
    RB155.C66 2011
    616′.042–dc22
                                2010031705

ISBN: 9781405169745

A catalogue record for this book is available from the British Library.
Set in 10/12 pt and Adobe Garamond by Toppan Best-set Premedia Limited

Printed in Singapore by C.O.S. Printers Pte Ltd

5 2016

Contents

Companion website
This book has a companion website:

www.wiley.com/go/tobias

with:
- Regularly updated links to genetic databases and analysis tools
- Updated information relating to the book's content
- Additional self-assessment questions and answers
- Figures from the book in Powerpoint format

Preface

This book has been written for those to whom an understanding of modern medical genetics is important in their current or future practice as clinicians, scientists, counsellors and teachers. It is based on the authors' personal experience in both clinical and laboratory aspects of busy regional genetics services over a period of many years. This period has seen the emergence of modern cytogenetics and molecular genetics alongside the development of medical genetics from a purely academic discipline into a clinical specialty of relevance to every branch of medicine. As in our undergraduate and postgraduate education programmes, we emphasize the central role of the chromosome and the human genome in understanding the molecular mechanisms involved in the pathogenesis of genetic disease. Within the term genetic disease, we include not only the classic Mendelian and chromosomal disorders but also the commoner disorders of adulthood with a genetic predisposition and somatic cell genetic disorders, such as cancer.

For this sixth edition, the text has been extensively updated throughout. The structure of the book has, where appropriate, been reorganised, in order to provide a clear description of the essential principles of the scientific basis and clinical application of modern medical genetics. Where appropriate, we have included descriptions of genetic conditions that have been carefully selected as examples of the important principles being described. Since the last edition of this book, several important and exciting new advances have been made in the field of medical genetics, and we have incorporated information about them into the book. Such advances include, for example, the completion of the sequencing of the human genome (with the generation of huge quantities of publicly accessible data), the identification of new classes of RNA molecules, the development of a number of invaluable new molecular genetic and cytogenetic laboratory techniques, the further development of preimplantation genetic diagnosis, and improved methods for antenatal and neonatal screening.

A very significant additional advance has been the development and enormous expansion of many invaluable online clinical and molecular genetic databases. These databases have greatly facilitated the medical genetics work of most clinicians and scientists. The optimal use of several important databases is, however, in many cases far from straightforward. Consequently, retrieving specific information or data from them can take a great deal of time and effort for users who do not access them frequently. The final chapter of this book is therefore devoted to providing guidance on the most efficient use of these databases, together with clear illustrated advice explaining how to find different types of information via the internet as quickly as possible. It is hoped that this guidance, which to our knowledge is currently unavailable elsewhere, will make this process much more straightforward for the reader.

We have also provided an accompanying website (accessed via www.wiley.com/go/tobias) that we will regularly update in order to provide the reader with a way of easily accessing the very latest clinical and molecular genetic information relating to the thousands of genetic conditions, in addition to patient information and support organizations, the identified genes, and gene-testing laboratories worldwide. The links are grouped on the website in a very similar manner to the way in which they are categorised within the final chapter of this book, in order to make it as easy as possible for readers to find relevant information quickly.

Although we have made every effort to ensure that the information contained within this book is accurate at the time of going to press, we look to the continued generosity of our readers in helping to correct any misconceptions or omissions. We would be happy to receive any comments, or recommendations for improvements, at essentialmedgen@gmail.com.

The role of genetic counselling, prenatal diagnosis, carrier detection and other forms of genetic screening in the prevention of genetic disease is now well established and this is reflected in the increasing provision of genetic services throughout the world. It is hoped that our book will be useful to those in training for this important task.

E.S.T, J.M.C. and M.A.F-S.

Acknowledgements

We wish to thank all of the many people who have influenced the production of this book. These include, particularly, our colleagues and students at the Institute of Medical Genetics in Glasgow and at the Cambridge University Centre for Medical Genetics. We also wish to acknowledge the invaluable contributions made by Professor Carolyn Brown (Life Sciences Centre, Vancouver, Canada), Professor Mark Jobling (University of Leicester, UK) and Dr Zofia Esden-Tempska (Medical University of Gdansk, Poland).

The authors are indebted to the editorial and production team at Wiley-Blackwell, including Martin Sugden, Hayley Salter, Laura Murphy, Elizabeth Bishop and Elizabeth Johnston, in addition to the freelance project manager, Anne Bassett.

E.S.T. would like to express his enormous gratitude to his wife, family and friends for their continuous support and understanding while he worked on the manuscript.

We are most obliged to Professor Tom Ellenberger (Washington University School of Medicine, St Louis, Missouri, USA) for his generous permission to use the front cover image, which depicts the interaction between human DNA ligase I and DNA.

We are very grateful to the patients and their families, and to the following, for permission to reproduce these figures:

Fig. 4.2: Alexander Fletcher;
Fig. 4.4: Joån Lavinha;
Figs. 4.5, 4.8 and 4.9: Gillian Stevens;
Figs. 4.6 and 4.7: Maria Jackson and Leah Marks;
Fig. 4.10: Jim Kelly;
Figs. 4.11 and 7.22: Jayne Duncan;
Fig. 4.12, 13.5 and 16.2: Alexander Cooke;
Fig. 4.14: Julia El-Sayed Moustafa;
Fig. 4.15: Paul Debenham (Cellmark Diagnostics);
Figs 5.2–5.5, 6.17b, 7.6, 7.8, and 9.2: Elizabeth Boyd;
Fig. 5.8: Nigel Carter;
Fig. 5.13: The Editor, *Birth Defects Original Article Series*;
Fig. 5.14: The Editior, *Annales de Génetique*;
Fig. 5.15: Peter Pearson;
Figs 6.2, 6.3, 6.9 and 7.9: The Editor, *Excerpta Medica*;
Figs 6.8 and 7.4(d): Anne Chandley;

Fig. 6.16: John Tolmie;
Fig. 6.18c: Lionel Willatt;
Figs 7.4(b) and 7.4(c): The Editor, *Journal of Medical Genetics*;
Fig. 7.15: Maj Hulten and N. Saadallah;
Figs 7.16 and 7.17: The Editor, *Cytogenetics and Cell Genetics*;
Fig. 8.6: Brenda Gibson;
Figs 8.12 and 18.4: Douglas Wilcox;
Figs. 7.2, 7.21 and 7.32: Catherine McConnell;
Fig. 7.19: Aspasia Divane;
Fig. 7.20: Diana Johnson and BMJ Publishing Group Ltd.;
Fig. 7.30: Evelyn Schröck and Thomas Ried;
Figs. 11.4 and 11.5: Gary Stix and Nature Publishing Group;
Fig. 12.4, 15.5 and 18.20: Margo Whiteford;
Figs. 12.8 and 7.23–26: Norma Morrison;
Figs. 13.7 and 13.8: Janet Stewart;
Fig. 13.10: Springer, Heidelberg;
Fig. 14.1 and 14.2: Inga Prokopenko and Elsevier;
Fig. 14.3: Bart Dermaut and Elsevier;
Fig. 15.7: Peter Cackett and Nature Publishing Group;
Fig. 16.5: Bernhard Horsthemke, Joseph Wagstaff and American Journal of Medical genetics;
Figs. 17.1–17.4: Jenny Crossley and David Aitken;
Fig. 17.5: Joan Mackenzie and Arlene Brown;
Fig. 18.16: WE Tidyman, KA Rauen and Cambridge Journals;
Fig. 18.22: Marie-France Portnoi and Elsevier; and
Figs. 19.45–19.48: Michael Baraitser.

We would also like to thank the curators of the following websites for permission to reproduce screenshots: National Center for Biotechnology Information (NCBI), Ensembl (Wellcome Trust Sanger Institute), GeneCards (Weizmann Institute of Science), University of California Santa Cruz (UCSC) Genome Browser, UK Genetic Testing Network (UKGTN), European Directory of DNA Diagnostic Laboratories (EDDNAL), Primer3Plus, RCSB Protein Data Bank (PDB) and The Phenomizer.

The authors and publisher have made every effort to seek the permission of all copyright holders for the reproduction of copyright material. If any have been overlooked inadvertently, the publisher will be pleased to make the necessary amendments at the earliest opportunity.

How to get the best out of your textbook

Welcome to the new edition of *Essential Medical Genetics*. Over the next two pages you will be shown how to make the most of the learning features included in the textbook.

An interactive textbook ▶

For the first time, your textbook gives you free access to a Wiley Desktop Edition – a digital, interactive version of this textbook. Your Wiley Desktop Edition allows you to:

Search: Save time by finding terms and topics instantly in your book, your notes, even your whole library (once you've downloaded more textbooks)

Note and Highlight: Colour code highlights and make digital notes right in the text so you can find them quickly and easily

Organize: Keep books, notes and class materials organized in folders inside the application

Share: Exchange notes and highlights with friends, classmates and study groups

Upgrade: Your textbook can be transferred when you need to change or upgrade computers

Link: Link directly from the page of your interactive textbook to all of the material contained on the companion website.

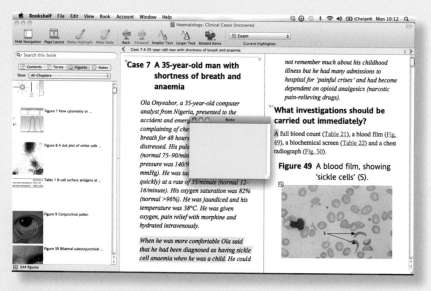

Simply find your unique Wiley Desktop Edition product code and carefully scratch away the top coating on the label on the front cover of this textbook and visit:

http://www.vitalsource.com/software/bookshelf/downloads/ to get started.

A companion website ▶

Your textbook is also accompanied by a FREE companion website that contains:

- Regularly updated links to genetic databases and analysis tools
- Updated information relating to the book's content
- Additional self-assessment questions and answers
- Figures from the book in Powerpoint format.

Log on to **www.wiley.com/go/tobias** to find out more.

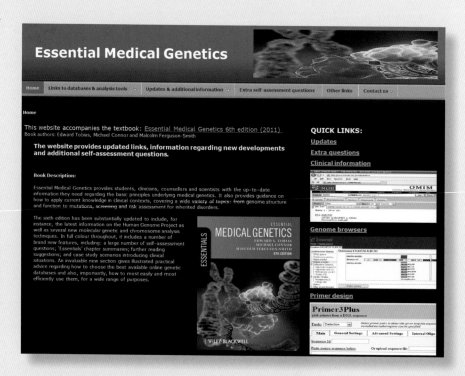

Features contained within your textbook

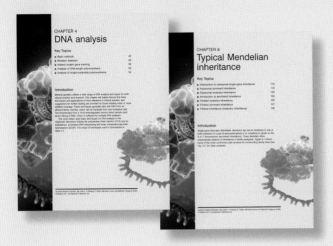

◀ Every chapter has its own chapter-opening page that offers a list of key topics contained within the chapter.

Throughout your textbook you will find this icon which points you to the online databases and resources found on the companion website. You can also access the website by clicking on this icon in your Desktop Edition.

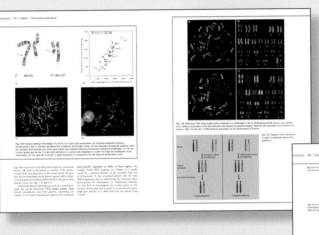

◀ Your textbook is full of useful photographs, illustrations and tables. The Desktop Edition version of your textbook will allow you to copy and paste any photograph or illustration into assignments, presentations and your own notes.

▼

SUMMARY

- Multifactorial inheritance implies a contribution of both genetic and environmental factors.
- Twin concordance and family correlation studies can provide support for the multifactorial inheritance of a trait. The observed frequencies in relatives provide the empiric risks upon which genetic counselling for multifactorial disorders is based.
- Multifactorial traits that are continuous (such as height) have a continuously graded distribution, while those that are discontinuous (i.e. with individuals being either affected or unaffected) are present only when a certain threshold of genetic factors is reached.

- For twins, placental membranes that are monochorionic indicate monozygosity, whereas dichorionic membranes represent either monozygous or dizygous twins. Zygosity is determined most reliably by DNA fingerprinting.
- Monozygotic twins are identical genetically (i.e. at the DNA level), whereas dizygotic twins exhibit the same degree of genetic similarity as siblings.
- Genome-wide analyses of the genetic determinants of multifactorial traits may now be undertaken by association studies of the frequencies of each of hundreds of thousands of SNPs in cases and controls.

▲

Every chapter ends with a summary which can be used for both study and revision purposes.

We hope you enjoy using your new textbook. Good luck with your studies!

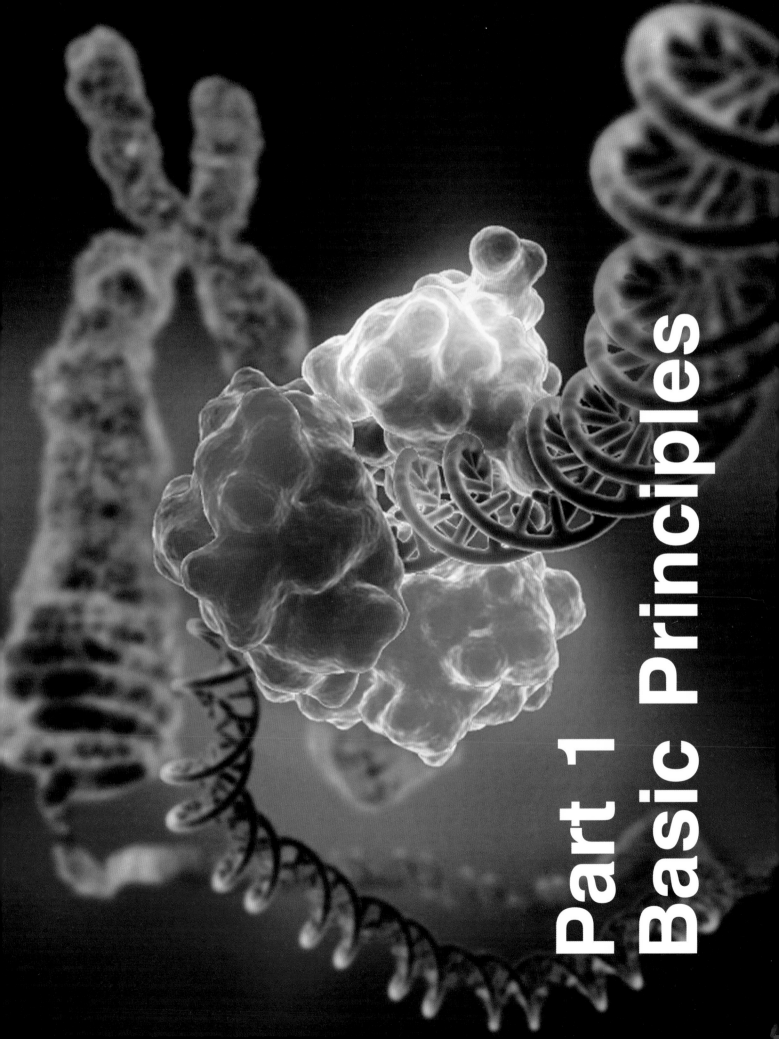

Part 1
Basic Principles

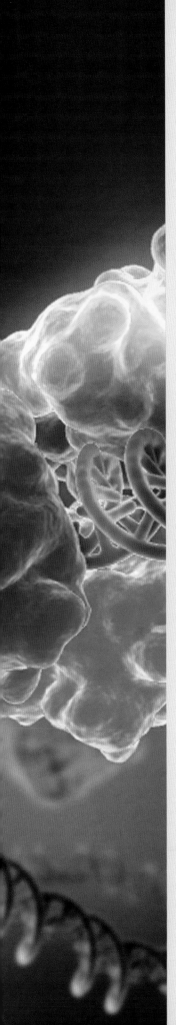

CHAPTER 1
Medical genetics in perspective

Key Topics

Introduction

Medical genetics is the science of human biological variation as it relates to health and disease. Although people have long been aware that individuals differ, that children tend to resemble their parents and that certain diseases tend to run in families, the scientific basis for these observations was only discovered during the past 140 years. The clinical applications of this knowledge are even more recent, with most progress confined to the past 50 years (see Table 1.1). In particular, the rapid sequencing of the entire human genome, completed in 2003, has greatly accelerated the process of gene mapping for genetic conditions and a vast quantity of valuable and continuously updated information has become readily accessible via the internet (as described in detail in Part 3 and on this book's accompanying website at www.wiley.com/go/tobias).

Essential Medical Genetics, 6th edition. © Edward S. Tobias, Michael Connor and Malcolm Ferguson-Smith.
Published 2011 by Blackwell Published Ltd.

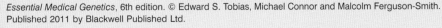

Table 1.1 Some important landmarks in the development of medical genetics

Year	Landmark	Key figure(s)
1839	Cell theory	Schleiden and Schwann
1859	Theory of evolution	Darwin
1865	Particulate inheritance	Mendel
1882	Chromosomes observed	Flemming
1902	Biochemical variation	Garrod
1903	Chromosomes carry genes	Sutton, Boveri
1910	First US genetic clinic	Davenport
1911	First human gene assignment	Wilson
1944	Role of DNA	Avery
1953	DNA structure	Watson, Crick, Franklin and Wilkins
1956	Amino acid sequence of sickle haemoglobin (HbS)	Ingram
1956	46 chromosomes in humans	Tjio and Levan
1959	First human chromosomal abnormality	Lejeune
1960	Prenatal sexing	Riis and Fuchs
1960	Chromosome analysis on blood	Moorhead
1961	Biochemical screening	Guthrie
1961	X chromosome inactivation	Lyon
1961	Genetic code	Nirenberg
1964	Antenatal ultrasound	Donald
1966	First prenatal chromosomal analysis	Breg and Steel
1966	First print edition of Mendelian Inheritance in Man (MIM)	McKusick
1967	First autosomal assignment	Weiss and Green
1970	Prevention of Rhesus isoimmunisation	Clarke
1970	Chromosome banding	Caspersson and Zech
1975	DNA sequencing	Sanger, Maxam and Gilbert
1976	First DNA diagnosis	Kan
1977	First human gene cloned	Shine
1977	Somatostatin made by genetic engineering	Itakura
1979	*In vitro* fertilisation	Edwards and Steptoe
1979	Insulin produced by genetic engineering	Goeddel
1982	First genetic engineering product marketed (Humulin)	Many contributors
1985	DNA fingerprinting	Jeffreys
1986	Polymerase chain reaction (PCR)	Mullis
1987	Linkage map of human chromosomes developed	Many contributors
1987	Online Mendelian Inheritance in Man (OMIM) first available	McKusick
1990	First treatment by supplementation gene therapy	Rosenberg, Anderson, Blaese
1990	First version of London Dysmorphology Database	Baraitser and Winter
1990	First clinical use of preimplantation genetic diagnosis (PGD)	Handyside, Winston and others
1991	First version of London Neurogenetics Database	Baraitser and Winter
1993	First physical map of the human genome	Many contributors

Year	Landmark	Key figure(s)
Table 1.1 *continued*		
2000	First draft of the human genome sequence	Many contributors
2003	Completion of human genome sequencing (99.999%)	HGSC and Celera
2006	Preimplantation genetic haplotyping (PGH) announced	Renwick, Abbs and others
2007	Human genome SNP map (3.1 million SNPs) reported	International HapMap Consortium
2007	Completion of DNA sequencing of personal genomes	Watson and Venter
2008	Launch of project to sequence the genomes of over 1000 individuals from 20 different populations worldwide	International 1000 Genomes Project
2010	Publication of catalogue of human genetic variation (believed to be 95% complete)	International 1000 Genomes Project

HGSC: Human Genome Sequencing Consortium; OMIM: Online Mendelian Inheritance in Man; SNP: single nucleotide polymorphism.

Scientific basis of medical genetics

Mendel's contribution

Prior to Mendel, parental characteristics were believed to blend in the offspring. While this was acceptable for continuous traits such as height or skin pigmentation, it was clearly difficult to account for the family patterns of discontinuous traits such as haemophilia or albinism. Mendel studied clearly defined pairs of contrasting characters in the offspring of the garden pea (*Pisum sativum*). These peas were, for example, either round or wrinkled and were either yellow or green. Pure-bred strains for each of these characteristics were available but when cross-bred (the first filial or F_1 progeny) were all round or yellow. If F_1 progeny were bred then each characteristic was re-observed in a ratio of approximately 3 round to 1 wrinkled or 3 yellow to 1 green (in the second filial or F_2 progeny). Mendel concluded that inheritance of these characteristics must be particulate with pairs of hereditary elements (now called genes). In these two examples, one characteristic (or trait) was dominant to the other (i.e. all the F_1 showed it). The fact that both characteristics were observed in the F_2 progeny entailed *segregation of each pair of genes with one member to one gamete and one to another gamete* (Mendel's first law).

Figures 1.1 and 1.2 illustrate these experiments with upper-case letters used for the dominant characteristic and lower-case letters used for the masked (or recessive) characteristic. If both members of the pair of genes are identical, this is termed homozygous (for the dominant or recessive trait), whereas a heterozygote has one gene of each type.

In his next series of experiments Mendel crossed pure-bred strains with two characteristics, e.g. pure-bred round/yellow with pure-bred wrinkled/green. The F_1 generation showed only the two dominant characteristics – in this case round/yellow. The F_2 showed four combinations: the original two, namely round/yellow and wrinkled/green, in a ratio of approximately 9:1 and two new combinations – wrinkled/yellow and round/green in a ratio of approximately 3:3 (Fig. 1.3).

In these experiments, there was thus no tendency for the genes arising from one parent to stay together in the offspring. In other words, *members of different gene pairs assort to gametes independently of one another* (Mendel's second law).

Although Mendel presented and published his work in 1865, after cultivating and studying around 28,000 pea plants, the significance of his discoveries was not realised until the early 1900s when three plant breeders, De Vries, Correns and Tschermak, confirmed his findings.

Chromosomal basis of inheritance

In 1839, Schleiden and Schwann established the concept of cells as the fundamental living units. Hereditary transmission through the sperm and egg was known by 1860, and in 1868, Haeckel, noting that the sperm was largely nuclear material, postulated that the nucleus was responsible for heredity. Flemming identified chromosomes within the nucleus in 1882, and in 1903 Sutton and Boveri independently realised that the behaviour of chromosomes during the production of gametes paralleled the behaviour of Mendel's hereditary elements. Thus, the chromosomes were discovered to carry the genes. However, at that time, although the chromosomes were known to consist of protein and nucleic acid, it was not clear which component was the hereditary material.

Chemical basis of inheritance

Pneumococci are of two genetically distinct strains: rough or non-encapsulated (non-virulent) and smooth or encapsulated (virulent). In 1928, Griffith added heat-killed smooth bacteria to live rough bacteria and found that some of the rough pneumococci were transformed to the smooth, virulent type. Avery, MacLeod and McCarty repeated this experiment in 1944 and showed that nucleic acid was the transforming agent. Thus, nucleic acid was shown to carry hereditary information. This stimulated intense interest in the composition of nucleic acids,

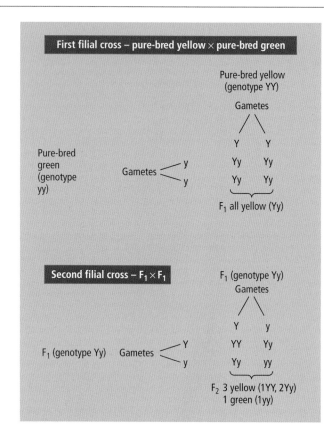

Fig. 1.1 Example of Mendel's breeding experiments for a single trait (yellow or green peas).

Fig. 1.2 Example of Mendel's breeding experiments for a single trait (round or wrinkled peas).

Fig. 1.3 Example of Mendel's breeding experiments for two traits (yellow or green and round or wrinkled peas).

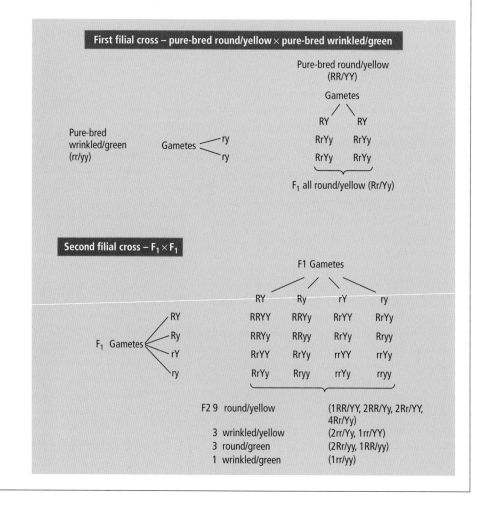

which culminated in the discovery, by Watson, Crick, Franklin and Wilkins, of the double-helical structure for deoxyribonucleic acid (DNA) in 1953.

Chromosomal disorders

By 1890, it was known that one human chromosome (the X chromosome) did not always have a partner, and in 1905 Wilson and Stevens extended this observation by establishing the pattern of human sex chromosomes. At this time, it was believed that there were 47 chromosomes, including one X chromosome, in each male somatic cell and 48 chromosomes, including two X chromosomes, in each female cell. In 1923, the small Y chromosome was identified, and both sexes were thought to have 48 chromosomes. Tjio and Levan refuted this in 1956 when they showed the normal human chromosome number to be 46. In 1959, the first chromosomal disease in humans, trisomy 21, was discovered by Lejeune and colleagues, and by 1970, over 20 different human chromosomal disorders were known. The development of chromosomal banding in 1970 markedly increased the ability to resolve small chromosomal aberrations, and so by 1990 more than 600 different chromosome abnormalities had been described, in addition to many normal variants. This number has increased further with the development of improved techniques including various fluorescence *in situ* hybridisation (FISH) methods and comparative genomic hybridisation (CGH). In fact, the increased resolution of the more recently developed techniques such as array CGH (see Chapter 7), has led to greater difficulties in differentiating between the increasingly numerous normal and abnormal chromosomal variants. This, in turn, has necessitated the development of international databases of such submicroscopic variants such as DECIPHER (Fig. 1.4), based at the Sanger Institute (http://decipher.sanger.ac.uk/), and the Database of Genomic Variants at Toronto (http://projects.tcag.ca/variation).

Mitochondrial disorders

Mitochondria have their own chromosomes and these are passed on from a mother to all of her children but not from the father. These chromosomes are different in several respects from their nuclear counterparts. For instance, they contain only 37 genes, a high and variable number of DNA copies per cell, very little non-coding DNA and no introns (see Chapter 5). Mutations in genes on these mitochondrial chromosomes can cause disease and this was first shown in 1988 for a maternally inherited type of blindness (Leber optic neuropathy). Since then, it has been shown that many different mitochondrial mutations, including point mutations, deletions and duplications, alone or in combination, can result in a variety of different disorders. Moreover, the relationship between genotype and phenotype is not straightforward, in part due to heteroplasmy, the tendency for a mitochondrial mutation to be present in only a proportion of the cell's mitochondrial genome copies (see Chapter 10).

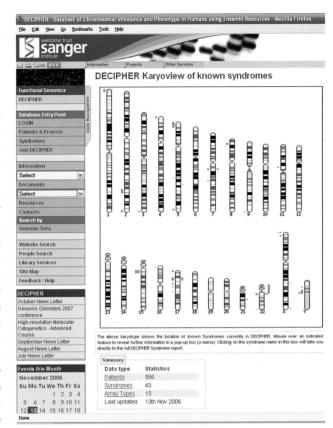

Fig. 1.4 Diagram displayed on the DECIPHER website (at http://decipher.sanger.ac.uk/syndromes) indicating chromosomal loci associated with known clinical syndromes. Reproduced with permission from the Wellcome Trust Sanger Institute. Flicek et al. (2010) Nucleic Acids Res 38 (Database issue):D557–62.

Single-gene disorders

In 1902, Garrod presented his studies on alkaptonuria, a rare condition in which patients have urine that darkens on standing and arthritis. He found three of 11 sets of parents of affected patients to be blood relatives and, in collaboration with Bateson, proposed that this was a Mendelian recessive trait with affected persons homozygous for the underactive gene. This was the first disease to be interpreted as a single-gene trait. Garrod also conceived the idea that patients with alkaptonuria and other inborn errors of metabolism really represented one extreme of human biochemical variation and that other less clinically significant variations were to be expected.

There followed numerous descriptions of distinct human single-gene traits and at the present time more than 7,000 human single-gene traits are known (Table 1.2). In 1949, Pauling suspected an abnormal haemoglobin to be the cause of sickle-cell anaemia, and this was confirmed by Ingram in 1956, who found an altered haemoglobin polypeptide sequence. This was the first demonstration in any organism that a mutation in a structural gene could produce an altered amino acid sequence. In 1959, only two abnormal haemoglobins were known; now the number exceeds 450. In 1948, Gibson

Table 1.2 Human genes and single-gene traits (see McKusick, 2007, and the OMIM database)

	1966	1975	1986	1994	2010
Autosomal dominant	837	1,218	2,201	4,458	19,007 (6,469)
Autosomal recessive	531	947	1,420	1,730	autosomal*
X-linked	119	171	286	412	1,131 (515)
Y-linked	–	–	–	19	59 (11)
Mitochondrial	–	–	–	59	65 (30)
Total	1,487	2,336	3,907	6,678	20,262 (7,025)

*The distinction between autosomal dominant and autosomal recessive traits was not maintained in the Mendelian Inheritance in Man (MIM) catalogue after May 1994 for several reasons. These included: the distinction being only relative (with, for instance, a deficiency state in an otherwise 'autosomal recessive' condition being detectable in a heterozygote with a sufficiently sensitive detection system); and for several conditions, the occurrence of both autosomal dominant and recessive forms that result from the same gene, depending on which specific mutations are present. Figures correct on 22 November 2010. In parenthesis are the total numbers of OMIM entries that have phenotypic information.

demonstrated the first enzyme defect in an autosomal recessive condition (NADH-dependent methaemoglobin reductase in methaemoglobinaemia). The specific biochemical abnormalities in over 400 inborn errors of metabolism have now been determined, but the polypeptide product is still unknown in many human single-gene disorders. Study of these rare, and not so rare, single-gene disorders has provided valuable insights into normal physiological mechanisms; for example, our knowledge of the normal metabolic pathways has been derived largely from the study of inborn errors of metabolism.

Huge progress has been made in the assignment of genes to individual chromosomes, in mapping the genes' precise locations and, more recently, in identifying their entire nucleotide sequences. The first human gene assignment was made by Wilson, who identified the X-linked trait for colour blindness in 1911 and assigned the gene to the X chromosome. Other X-linked traits rapidly followed, while the first autosomal gene to be assigned was thymidine kinase to chromosome 17 in 1967. By 1987, a complete linkage map of all human chromosomes had been developed and this was followed in 1993 by the first physical map. These were essential steps towards the final goal of the Human Genome Project. The Human Genome Project, initiated in 1990, aimed to map and sequence all human genes by the year 2005. Rapid technological advances, particularly the development of high-throughput automated fluorescence-based DNA sequencing (see Chapter 4), in addition to competition between the publicly funded (International Human Gene Sequencing Consortium) and private company (Celera) schemes, led to the early completion of the human genome sequence in 2003 (see Chapter 2). This sequence information, together with an enormous body of associated data, has been made publicly available via internet databases. The information available includes associations with human diseases, gene mapping data, cross-species comparisons, expression patterns and predicted protein features (Fig. 1.5). These and other valuable databases are described in Part 3, and a user's guide is provided online (at www.wiley.com/go/tobias).

Multifactorial (part-genetic) disorders

Galton studied continuous human characteristics such as intelligence and physique, which did not seem to conform to Mendel's laws of inheritance, and an intense debate ensued, with the supporters of Mendel on the one hand and those of Galton on the other. Finally, a statistician, Fisher, reconciled the two sides by showing that such inheritance could be explained by multiple pairs of genes, each with a small but additive effect. Discontinuous traits with multifactorial inheritance, such as congenital malformations, were explained by introducing the concept of a threshold effect for the disorder: manifestation only occurred when the combined genetic and environmental liability passed the threshold. Many human characteristics are determined in this fashion. Usually factors in the environment interact with the genetic background.

Although the genetic contribution to multifactorial disorders is now well accepted, the number and nature of the genes involved and their mechanisms of interaction between each other and environmental factors are largely unknown. This is the current focus of a great deal of research and progress has been made in identifying the genetic contribution for several of these conditions including insulin-dependent diabetes mellitus, rheumatoid arthritis, dementia due to Alzheimer's disease, premature vascular disease, schizophrenia, Parkinson disease, atopic dermatitis and asthma.

Somatic cell genetic (cumulative genetic) disorders

All cancers result from the accumulation of genetic mutations. Usually these mutations only occur after conception and are thus confined to certain somatic cells, but in a small but clinically important proportion, an initial key mutation is inherited. Boveri first advanced the idea that chromosomal changes caused cancer, and early support for this idea came from the demonstration in 1973 of a specific chromosomal translocation (the Philadelphia chromosome) in a type of leukaemia. Subsequently, a large number of both specific and non-specific chromosomal changes have been found in a wide variety of cancers. In turn,

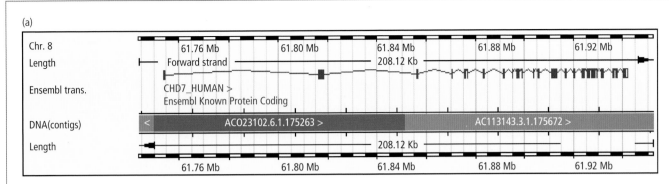

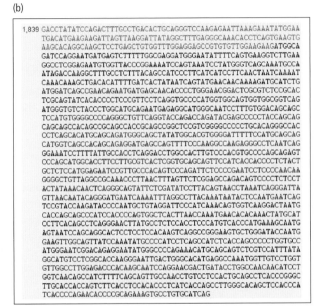

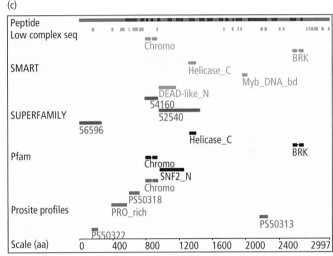

Fig. 1.5 (a) Transcript structure of the 38-exon CHARGE association gene, *CHD7*, on human chromosome 8. (b) DNA sequence of the first coding exon (containing the start codon). The DNA sequence displayed in purple is the untranslated region of this exon, immediately preceding the ATG start codon. (c) Protein features of CHD7, as predicted by the different computer programs (e.g. SMART) shown on the left. Reproduced with permission from the Ensembl database at the Wellcome Trust Sanger Institute. Flicek et al. (2010) Ensembl's 10th year. Nucleic Acids Res 38 (Database issue):D557–62. See Chapter 19.

these changes were clues to specific genes that were key determinants of progression to cancer. Many of these genes have now been cloned and this has resulted in an improved understanding of the molecular basis of cancer and provided the clinician with a means of detection of presymptomatic carriers of cancer-predisposing genes. In addition, it is now recognised that changes in the DNA sequence occurring within somatic cells play an important role in ageing and in certain mosaic disorders such as McCune–Albright syndrome, which results from postzygotic somatic activating mutations in the *GNAS1* gene. They also may be responsible for the exacerbation of symptoms with age in some inherited disorders such as myotonic dystrophy, in which there is somatic expansion of the inherited mutation (see Chapter 16), and mitochondrial disorders (see Chapter 10).

Clinical applications of medical genetics

Genetically determined disease has become an increasingly important part of ill health in the community now that most

infections can be controlled and now that modern medical and nursing care can save many affected infants who previously would have succumbed shortly after birth. This has led to an increased demand for informed genetic counselling and for screening tests both for carrier detection and to identify pregnancies at risk.

Genetic assessment and management

Davenport began to give genetic advice as early as 1910 in the USA, and the first British genetic counselling clinic was established in 1946 at Great Ormond Street, London. Public demand has since caused a proliferation of genetic counselling centres so that there are now more than 40 in the UK and more than 450 in the USA. The scope for genetic counselling has, in fact, in recent years expanded dramatically with the increasingly available data on human genetic disorders (e.g. their mechanism of inheritance in addition to their associated genes and markers) and the increasing availability of mutation analysis. Clinical geneticists play an increasingly important role in the clinical assessment and genetic testing of patients with genetic conditions and their at-risk relatives. Furthermore, geneticists are now much more involved in the management of patient follow-up, often coordinating several other specialties and initiating patient participation in multicentre clinical studies. These include trials of clinical screening methods and of new therapeutic strategies.

In addition to an accurate assessment of the risks in a family, the clinical geneticist also needs to discuss reproductive options. Important advances in this respect have been made with regard to prenatal diagnosis with the option of selective termination, and this has been a major factor in increasing the demand for genetic counselling. Prenatal diagnosis and now, in certain cases, preimplantation diagnosis (see below), offer reassurance for couples at high risk of serious genetic disorders and allow many couples, who were previously deterred by the risk, the possibility of having healthy children.

Genetic amniocentesis was first attempted in 1966 and the first prenatally detected chromosome abnormality was trisomy 21 in 1969. Chromosome analysis following amniocentesis is now a routine component of obstetric care, and over 200 different types of abnormality have been detected. Amniocentesis or earlier chorionic villus sampling can also be used to detect biochemical alterations in inborn errors of metabolism. This was first used in 1968 for a pregnancy at risk of Lesch–Nyhan syndrome and has since been used for successful prenatal diagnosis in over 150 inborn errors of metabolism. Prenatal diagnosis can also be performed by DNA analysis of fetal samples. This approach was first used in 1976 for a pregnancy at risk of α-thalassaemia and has now been used in over 200 single-gene disorders, and for many of these, including cystic fibrosis, the fragile X syndrome and Duchenne muscular dystrophy, it has become the main method of prenatal diagnosis.

Preimplantation diagnosis (PGD), first used clinically (for sex determination) in 1990, is a more recently established technique that permits the testing of embryos at a very early stage following *in vitro* fertilisation (IVF), prior to implantation in the uterus. In this procedure, a single cell or blastomere is removed by suction, apparently harmlessly, from the embryo. This is usually carried out at the five- to ten-cell stage, at approximately 3 days post-fertilisation. Using the polymerase chain reaction (PCR) or FISH, it is then possible to determine the fetal sex in cases of sex-linked disease or to detect a specific mutation or chromosomal abnormality (also see Chapter 12).

A more recent extension of the PGD technology is the technique known as preimplantation genetic haplotyping (PGH), which was announced in 2006 (see Renwick *et al.*, 2006 in Further reading). In this technique, as in PGD, a cell is extracted from an embryo following IVF. In PGH, however, the DNA undergoes testing for a set of DNA markers closely linked to the disease gene without requiring the prior identification of the precise causative mutation. This can be performed by carrying out simultaneous or multiplex PCRs of several DNA markers, using fluorescence to detect and differentiate the products. The possible future possibilities and likely limita-

tions of PGD are discussed in an interesting opinion article published very recently in *Nature* (see Handyside, 2010).

The prenatal tests that detect chromosomal, biochemical or DNA alterations cannot, however, detect many of the major congenital malformations. The alternative approach of fetal visualisation has been necessary for these. High-resolution ultrasound scanning was first used to make a diagnosis of fetal abnormality (anencephaly) in 1972 and since then over 400 different types of abnormality have been detected. The clinical benefits of the more recently developed three-dimensional ultrasound techniques over standard two-dimensional ultrasound fetal imaging are not yet clear and three-dimensional ultrasound is not currently in routine clinical use during pregnancy in the UK.

Treatment and prevention of genetic disease

A great deal of research has been undertaken into the possibility of effective treatment of genetic diseases. In 1990, the first attempts at human supplementation gene therapy for a single-gene disorder (adenosine deaminase deficiency) were performed. Since then, different gene therapy methods have been devised, depending on the nature of the mutation, and several hundred gene therapy trials are now underway. Unfortunately, the development of a safe, effective, non-immunogenic, well-regulated system that permits the efficient delivery of the therapeutic DNA to sufficient numbers of target cells continues to present a significant challenge.

Although cures for genetic diseases continue to remain elusive, there are now many genetic conditions for which a precise diagnosis leads to significant benefits in terms of clinical management. In some conditions, for example, the almost complete prevention or reversal of the phenotypic effects of a genotype is achievable. This is the case, for instance, with regular venesection for haemochromatosis, with dietary treatment of phenylketonuria (PKU) and medium-chain acyl-CoA dehydrogenase (MCAD) deficiency and with modern enzyme replacement therapy for Gaucher's disease and Fabry's disease. In other cases, appropriate surveillance for clinical complications to permit their early treatment can be instituted. For example, as described in more detail in Chapter 13, screening can permit the early removal of pre-cancerous neoplastic lesions in hereditary cancer syndromes such as familial adenomatous polyposis (FAP), MYH polyposis, hereditary non-polyposis colorectal cancer (HNPCC) and familial breast cancer. In addition, in many other familial conditions, a genetic diagnosis facilitates the detection and early treatment of other complications such as diabetes and heart block in myotonic dystrophy; scoliosis, optic glioma and hypertension in neurofibromatosis type 1 (NF1); and aortic dilatation in Marfan syndrome. Moreover, as mentioned above, following their genetic diagnosis, patients are increasingly enrolled by clinical geneticists in large multicentre trials of new clinical screening and therapeutic methods. Such trials currently include, for instance, biochemical and ultrasound ovarian screening for women at high risk of developing ovarian cancer and the Mirena intra-uterine device for women with mismatch repair gene mutations who are at risk of endometrial cancer.

The majority of couples are not aware that they are at risk of having offspring with a genetic condition until they have an affected child. This has led to an increased emphasis on prenatal screening, for example by fetal ultrasound examination and by measurement of maternal serum α-fetoprotein and other analytes to detect pregnancies at increased risk of neural tube defects and chromosomal abnormalities. For example, the efficiency of prenatal screening has increased to a point where approximately 85–90% of cases of fetal Down syndrome can

be detected by 10–13 weeks' gestation for a false positive rate of 3.5%. Maternal age alone is no longer a suitable indication for prenatal diagnosis and far fewer amniocenteses are now required (see Chapter 17). Neonatal screening was introduced in 1961 for PKU and other conditions where early diagnosis and therapy will permit normal development, such as congenital hypothyroidism. More recently, neonatal screening for cystic fibrosis has been introduced, and it is likely that in the future there will be continued development of population screening, as well as prenatal, neonatal and preconceptional screening, which should lead to a reduced frequency of several genetic diseases.

SUMMARY

- The scientific basis of medical genetics began to be elucidated in 1865 when Mendel published his laws of segregation and independent assortment. These were confirmed around 40 years later.
- Chromosomes were identified in 1882, the hereditary information was shown in 1944 to consist of nucleic acid and the double-helical structure of DNA was discovered in 1953.
- The first single-gene trait, alkaptonuria, was identified in 1902 as a Mendelian recessive condition. Numerous other genes associated with Mendelian traits have been discovered since.
- Extremely rapid advances have been made in gene mapping and automated sequencing, facilitating the

early completion of the human genome sequence in 2003.
- Prenatal diagnosis and screening are important adjuncts to genetic counselling as they allow couples at risk of fetal abnormality the confidence to plan for future healthy children.
- PGD is an IVF-based technique that can permit the detection of genetic abnormalities in certain cases, before implantation of an embryo.
- An enormous quantity of human molecular genetic information is now freely available on the internet. Ways of accessing this information are presented in Chapter 19 and online at (www.wiley.com/go/tobias).

FURTHER READING

Bejjani BA, Shaffer LG (2006) Targeted array CGH. *J Mol Diagn* **8**:537–9.

Handyside A (2010) Let parents decide. *Nature* **464**:978–9.

McKusick VA (2007) Mendelian Inheritance in Man and its online version, OMIM. *Am J Hum Genet* **80**:588–604.

Ogilvie CM, Braude PR, Scriven PN (2005) Preimplantation genetic diagnosis – an overview. *J Histochem Cytochem* **53**:255–60.

Renwick PJ, Trussler J, Ostad-Saffari E, Fassihi H, Black C, Braude P, Ogilvie CM, Abbs S (2006) Proof of principle and first cases using preimplantation genetic haplotyping – a paradigm shift for embryo diagnosis. *Reprod Biomed Online* **13**:110–9.

WEBSITES

European Society for Human Reproduction and Embryology (ESHRE):
http://www.eshre.com

Human Fertilisation and Embryology Authority (HFEA):
http://www.hfea.gov.uk

OMIM (Online Mendelian Inheritance in Man):
http://www.ncbi.nlm.nih.gov/omim/

Preimplantation Genetics Diagnosis International Society (PGDIS), which is monitoring PGD activity worldwide:
http://www.pgdis.org/

Self-assessment

1. Which of the following is not a typical feature of mitochondrial inheritance?
A. Maternal transmission
B. Heteroplasmy
C. More introns in mitochondrial genes than in nuclear genes
D. The presence of fewer than 40 genes in the mitochondrial genome
E. Lack of a straightforward genotype–phenotype relationship

2. In preimplantation genetic diagnosis (PGD), which of the following does not take place?
A. *In vitro* fertilisation
B. Testing of each of the cells of the embryo for the specific mutation
C. Fetal sex determination of embryos in sex-linked disease
D. The use of the polymerase chain reaction (PCR) to detect a specific mutation or haplotype
E. The use of fluorescence *in situ* hybridisation (FISH) to detect an unbalanced chromosome abnormality

3. Which one of the following conditions is not usually regarded as multifactorial?
A. Rheumatoid arthritis
B. Insulin-dependent diabetes mellitus
C. McCune–Albright syndrome
D. Asthma
E. Parkinson disease

4. Which of the following is not useful in connection with the following genetic conditions?
A. Venesection for iron overload in haemochromatosis
B. Regular blood pressure check in neurofibromatosis type 1 (NF1)
C. Neonatal screening for hypothyroidism and phenylketonuria (PKU)
D. Dietary treatment for PKU
E. Enzyme replacement therapy for familial adenomatous polyposis (FAP)

5. Which of the following pairings between individuals and a genetics landmark is incorrect?
A. Mendel and the independent assortment of different gene pairs to gametes
B. Flemming and the identification of chromosomes within the nucleus
C. The discovery of the helical structure of DNA and Watson, Crick, Franklin and Wilkins
D. The first identification of a chromosomal abnormality and Jeffreys
E. PCR and Mullis

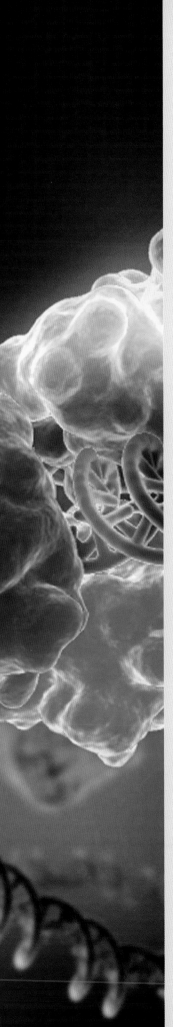

CHAPTER 2
The human genome

Key Topics

Introduction

Our knowledge and understanding of the structure and function of the human genome have been vastly augmented by the data generated by the Human Genome Project, completed in 2003. Although, prior to this achievement, the general location of many genes on the chromosomes and their positions relative to each other had been determined (i.e. by 'gene mapping'), the full nucleotide sequence of the chromosomes elucidated by the Human Genome Project provided far more detailed and reliable information. How this was achieved, the insights gained from the data and the uncertainties that remain are outlined within this chapter.

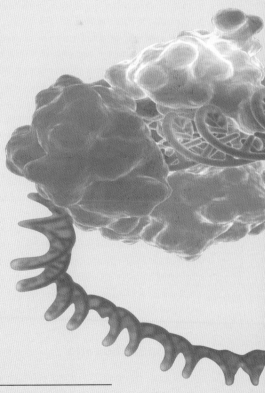

Essential Medical Genetics, 6th edition. © Edward S. Tobias, Michael Connor and Malcolm Ferguson-Smith.
Published 2011 by Blackwell Published Ltd.

Structure and organisation of the genome

The human nuclear genome contains approximately 3280 million base pairs (bp). In contrast, the much smaller mitochondrial genome (discussed in Chapter 10), which was sequenced in 1981, contains only 16,569 bp and 37 genes. The size of the coding region of a human gene contained in the nucleus is approximately 1000–3500 bp, and there are currently only 30,073 identified genes (21,598 protein-encoding genes and 8,475 RNA genes – see the Ensembl website in Further reading for the latest update. In fact, only 1.1% of the genome is actually protein-coding DNA. Another 4% at least, is, however, also important, consisting of gene-regulatory sequences and RNA genes. A large proportion of the non-coding DNA, around 20% of the genome, consists of introns and untranslated regions of genes in addition to other non-coding gene-related sequences such as pseudogenes. The majority of the non-coding DNA, however, around 75% of the genome, is extragenic, and much of this DNA (55% of the genome) consists of repeated sequences. The majority of this repetitive sequence is derived from transposable elements or transposons, sequences that insert additional copies of themselves randomly throughout the genome and constituting around 45% of the total DNA. These repetitive sequences permit, through the process of recombination (crossing over between two homologous DNA molecules), the rearrangement of parts of the genome, over time modifying the properties of existing genes and even creating new genes. Intriguingly, the proportion of repetitive sequence within the human genome (>50%) is significantly higher than in other organisms, with the corresponding figure being only 3% in the fly and 7% in the worm.

The genes are now known to be clustered in randomly distributed areas within the genome with long regions of non-coding DNA between these gene-dense regions. In general, the gene-rich areas tend to have a higher guanine and cytosine (G + C) content than the gene-poor regions and they tend to appear negative or pale on Giemsa chromosome staining (see Chapter 5).

The clustering of genes encoding structural proteins in part reflects ancestral small duplications with subsequent divergence of function, facilitating evolution by natural selection where the resulting new gene can provide a selective advantage. In this process, some genes become non-functional gene copies termed pseudogenes (e.g. those within the β-globin cluster), some retain similar functions (e.g. the red–green colour vision genes) and some develop novel functions as a result of small sequence changes or exon shuffling. In contrast, the loci for genes of sequential steps in a metabolic pathway tend to be scattered, as are the loci for subunits of complex proteins and the loci for mitochondrial and soluble forms of the same enzyme.

Gene identification

In the past, if a gene's protein product was known, the gene could be cloned by functional cloning. The protein was isolated and the partial sequence of its amino acids determined. This then allowed the synthesis of a corresponding series of oligonucleotide probes based on the genetic code (see Table 3.2) which could be used to identify the complementary gene from a DNA library.

If the gene's protein product was unknown, the gene could be cloned by positional cloning. The first step was to chromosomally map the gene and then to identify candidate genes from that region. The correct candidate was identified by mutational analysis in patients with the disease trait. This procedure has now been greatly facilitated by the availability of accurate mapping and sequence data resulting from the Human Genome Project.

Recently, many genes have been identified by the automated DNA sequencing of the genome as part of the Human Genome Project followed by gene prediction analyses in which genes are recognised by the computerised detection of typical gene features such as transcriptional and translational initiation and termination sequences. The probable functions of these genes can often also be predicted, by automated homology searches in which similarities are found between the sequences of newly identified genes and those of genes, proteins or protein domains already listed in the databases. Nevertheless, the functions and disease associations of many recently identified genes remain to be ascertained.

The Human Genome Project

How it was carried out

The Human Genome Project was commenced in 1990, with the aims of identifying and sequencing all the genes in the human genome within 15 years and making the data publicly available. It was initially coordinated by the US Department of Energy (directed by Ari Patrinos) and the US National Institutes of Health (directed by Francis Collins). The Wellcome Trust Sanger Institute at Hinxton in the UK also became a major partner, ultimately sequencing around one-third of the genome (chromosomes 1, 6, 9, 10, 11, 13, 20, 22 and X), under the direction of Sir John Sulston (Nobel laureate, 2002). In fact, a Human Genome Sequencing Consortium comprising a total of 16 institutions in the USA, Europe, China and Japan was required to carry out the enormous sequencing task. In addition, three institutions provided the necessary complex computational analysis: the National Center for Biotechnology Information (NCBI) at the National Institutes of Health, USA; the European Bioinformatics Institute (EBI) in Cambridge, UK; and the University of California, Santa Cruz (UCSC), USA. The strategy used was a 'hierarchical shotgun method' in which the regions of chromosomes submitted for fragmentation ('shotgunning') and sequencing were large stretches of DNA whose location in the genome had already been determined and which were contained in so-called bacterial artificial chromosomes (BACs).

In September 1999, Craig Venter's private company, Celera, also began to sequence the genome, but using a different strategy known as the 'whole genome shotgun approach'. This involved initially breaking up the entire genome (rather than BAC clone inserts) into millions of small fragments, sequencing these pieces in no particular order and subsequently reassembling the chromosome sequence by a massive computer analysis on the basis of sequence overlaps. Although the whole shotgun method did not necessitate the prior construction of a map of large fragments covering the genome, there were other challenges in the assembly phase. The public and private projects both used similar fluorescence-based automated sequencing technology, based on the dideoxy sequencing strategy originally devised by the double Nobel laureate Fred Sanger and colleagues, many years previously (see Chapter 4). The even faster recent sequencing technologies now provide the opportunity to compare many individual human genomes and to determine the extent and significance of genetic variation among people and between different ethnic groups (see the review by Tucker *et al.*, 2009, in Further reading).

Total gene numbers

The number of genes on each chromosome varies greatly, with the largest chromosome, chromosome 1, containing the most (2706 genes) and the Y chromosome the fewest (104 genes). The precise total number of genes varies according to the methods used to identify sequences as genes and by the subtypes of genes that are included in the totals. For instance, as mentioned above, in addition to at least 21,598 protein-coding genes, there are at least 8,475 genes that code for RNA molecules but do not encode polypeptides. These RNA genes currently include at least 727 ribosomal RNA (rRNA) and 131 transfer RNA (tRNA) genes. A surprising number of other RNA genes are also now known to be present, although, due to the difficulty in precisely identifying these genes within the genome, the total number is probably still not completely determined.

Recently described RNA gene classes

While their physiological roles are not yet as clearly understood as those of messenger RNAs (mRNAs), rRNAs and tRNAs, a number of intriguing additional RNA molecules are generally believed to be involved in the regulation of gene expression. They include, for instance, at least 903 small cytoplasmic RNA (scRNA) genes, 1048 microRNA genes and 2019 genes that encode small nuclear RNAs (snRNAs) (see Table 2.1). The snRNAs include RNAs that participate in splicing and a subclass of 1173 small nucleolar RNA (snoRNA) genes. These snRNAs are now known to direct the formation and chemical modification (by methylation and pseudouridylation) of other RNAs such as precursor rRNAs. Remarkably, many snoRNAs are processed from the spliced-out introns of other genes rather than being transcribed from separate genes (see Kiss, 2006, in Further reading). In contrast, small cytoplasmic RNAs are usually found in association with cytoplasmic proteins in complexes termed small cytoplasmic ribonucleoproteins (scRNPs), of which an example is the so-called signal recognition particle. MicroRNAs (termed miRNAs in 2001) are short single-stranded RNA molecules of 21–23 nucleotides that regulate the expression of other genes by binding to mRNAs (particularly the 3' untranslated region, or 3' UTR, in humans) and causing the degradation of the latter or blocking their translation into proteins. In recent years, there has been enormous scientific interest in these molecules, which do not encode proteins themselves, and a large number of reports of miRNA expression profiles (patterns) or 'signatures' that may be characteristic of specific tissues. In this respect, the tissues that have been particularly frequently studied are those that have been affected by

Table 2.1 Types of RNA

Type	Location	Comments
Messenger RNA (mRNA)	Nucleus and cytoplasm	Variable size, base sequence complementary to transcribed DNA strand, about 4% of total cellular RNA, half-life 7–24 h
Transfer RNA (tRNA)	Cytoplasm	Hairpin-loop shape, 49 cytoplasmic (and 22 mitochondrial) types, amino acid specific, about 10% of total cellular RNA with tens to hundreds of copies of the genes for each tRNA species
Ribosomal RNA (rRNA)	Ribosomes	40–50% of total cellular RNA, synthesised and stored in the nucleolus and nucleoli
Heterogeneous RNA (hnRNA)	Nucleus	High-molecular-weight mRNA precursors; 40–50% of total cellular RNA
Small nuclear RNA (snRNA)	Nucleus	Several types (e.g. U1–U12), involved mainly in RNA splicing
Small nucleolar RNA (snoRNA)	Nucleolus	At least 340 types, involved in chemical modification of rRNA molecules
Small cytoplasmic RNA (scRNA)	Cytoplasm	Form complexes (e.g. signal recognition particle) with cytoplasmic proteins
MicroRNAs (miRNA)	Cytoplasm	Very small (21–23 nucleotides) antisense regulators of other genes. Formed from a long precursor hairpin RNA by the enzyme DICER. Bind to mRNAs and can prevent their translation or induce their degradation. At least 1048 human miRNAs recognised.

conditions such as cancer of various types. It is believed that such miRNA profiles (like mRNA profiles) could serve, in the future, as useful biomarkers of specific phenotypes and may thus be able to provide improved diagnostic and prognostic information to clinicians. Furthermore, the possible pharmacological targeting of specific miRNAs is now being explored (see review by Ferracin *et al.*, 2010, in Further reading).

Uses of the Human Genome Project data and ways of accessing it

An important benefit of the Human Genome Project is the ability to use the electronically compiled genome data to identify genes of interest at particular locations in the genome. This could include, for instance, those genes located around an identified translocation breakpoint, within a microdeletion or microduplication region (e.g. following array comparative genomic

hybridisation or aCGH), or those residing at a locus resulting from a linkage study. Such a locus may be defined as a cytogenetic band. Alternatively, it may be a region spanned by a specific probe (such as a recombinant plasmid BAC probe), delineated by known DNA markers (such as microsatellites, see Chapter 3), or defined by precise nucleotide positions as counted from the end of the short arm of the chromosome. Accessing the genome data can be achieved by using one of the well-established genome browsers, such as Ensembl (Figs 2.1 and 2.2) or UCSC (Fig. 2.3), further details of which are given in Chapter 19 (and updated web-links are provided online at www.wiley.com/go/tobias). The genome databases can also be interrogated using BLAST (Basic Local Alignment Search Tool), which will find the site in the genome of any entered stretch of DNA (or protein) sequence. Detailed information about the sequence is available, such as its precise chromosome location, whether it is within an exon or intron or part of a repeat, if it is part of a known gene or gene

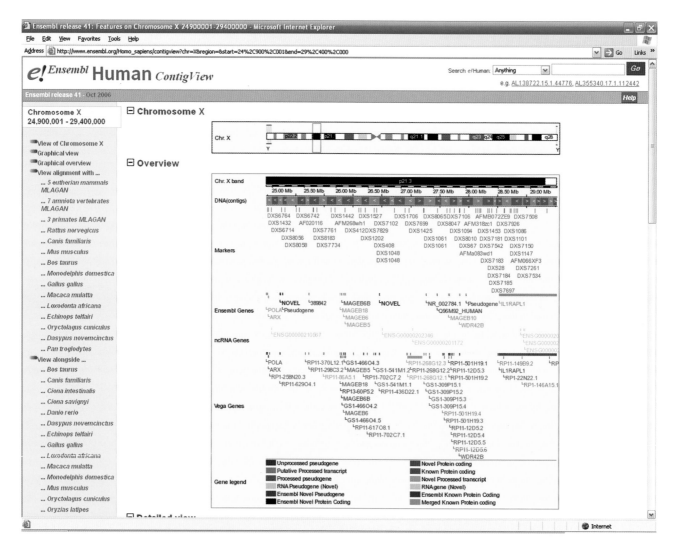

Fig. 2.1 A *Homo sapiens* genome browser display page at Ensembl. This can be reached via the search page at http://www. ensembl.org/Homo_sapiens/index.html. The same region as that shown in the UCSC genome browser example in Fig. 2.3 is displayed. This can be revealed by typing the nucleotide boundaries of the region directly into the sequence position boxes in the *H. sapiens* browser window, shown in Fig. 2.2. Reproduced with permission from the Wellcome Trust Sanger Institute. Flicek et al. (2010) Ensembl's 10th year. Nucleic Acids Res 38 (Database issue):D557–62.

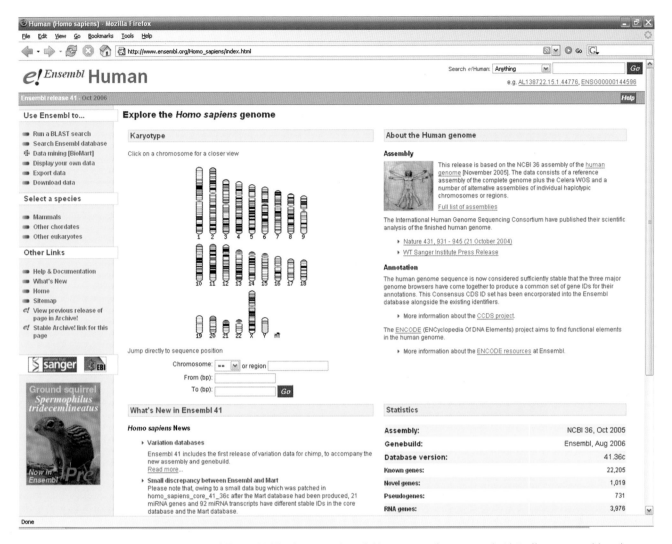

Fig. 2.2 The *H. sapiens* browser window of Ensembl. The latest version of this page can be accessed at http://www.ensembl.org/Homo_sapiens/index.html. Reproduced with permission from the Wellcome Trust Sanger Institute. Flicek et al. (2010) Ensembl's 10th year. Nucleic Acids Res 38 (Database issue):D557–62.

family and whether or not it is conserved in other organisms (see chapter 19 and the accompanying website for further details).

There are many clinical applications of the genome data. For instance it is often helpful to use the DNA sequence of a particular gene to act as an initial reference sequence when carrying out mutation screening, and in order to identify the intron/exon boundaries, regulatory elements and untranslated regions of a gene. The data also permit the rapid identification of genetic markers within or adjacent to genes of interest for human family linkage studies. Moreover, a searchable database of DNA reference sequences is invaluable when designing an oligonucleotide PCR primer that will anneal to a sequence of interest without binding to any other sequence in the genome. Databases (discussed in Chapter 19) also exist that provide continuously updated information regarding gene-related human disease information together with the publications that reported all of these findings.

There are many other uses of the data, including several research-related applications. For instance, the databases facili-

tate the rapid identification of previously unknown members of recognised gene families, the expression patterns in different stages of embryonic development and in different tissues, and studies of inter-individual sequence variation, including single nucleotide polymorphisms, or SNPs. In addition, cross-species comparisons of gene sequences can be made, allowing identification of evolutionarily conserved, functionally important regions of a gene or protein.

Remaining uncertainties

Despite the abundance of data resulting from the sequencing of the human genome (in addition to that of several other organisms) and from the complex post-sequencing analyses that are currently underway, there remain several areas of uncertainty. These include, firstly, the total gene count. Much of the uncertainty relating to the precise total number of functional genes is a result of the necessary extensive use of *in silico* sequence comparisons and analyses by complex gene

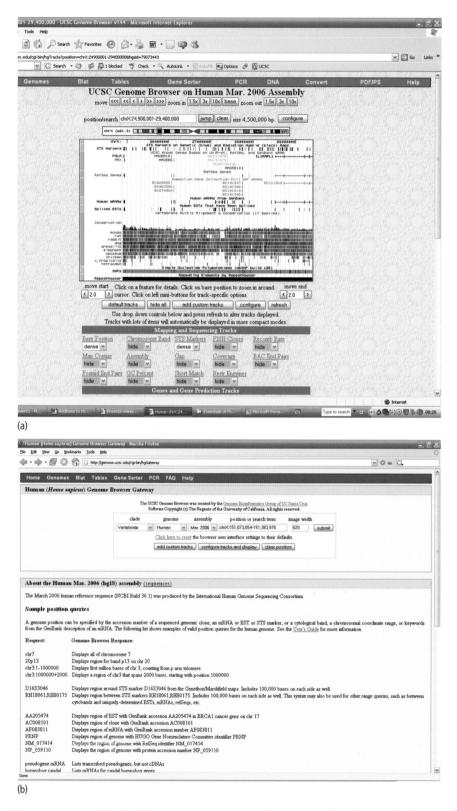

Fig. 2.3 The human data search page of the UCSC genome browser. The window shows the display of all identified genes within a specific chromosomal band. In (a), the genes located within Xp21.3 are shown, after opening the UCSC Genome Browser at http://genome.ucsc.edu/cgi-bin/hgGateway, typing the cytogenetic band name into the 'position or search term' and pressing 'submit' (b). Alternatively, a precise region could have been defined by the flanking nucleotide positions (counted from the telomere of the p arm) or by specific genetic markers. Kent et al. (2002) The human genome browser at UCSC. Genome Res.12(6):996–1006.

prediction computer programs to identify many of the genes rather than the use of experimental testing of gene function in laboratories. Moreover, the identification of some types of genes within the DNA sequence, especially the RNA genes, which do not possess certain standard sequence motifs (such as start and stop codons) that are usually present in polypeptide-encoding genes, is particularly challenging.

Much additional uncertainty relates to the precise functions of several classes of DNA sequence in humans. The functions of many protein-encoding genes and their products continue to be clarified, as do those of the more recently identified RNA gene classes such as snoRNAs. In addition, the functions, quantity and distribution of the various regions of non-coding DNA, such as long-range transcriptional regulatory sequences, are not yet completely determined. Crucially, much also remains to be learned with regard to the interplay of genes and their products during development and with environmental factors. In particular, the detailed mechanisms of gene expression regulation and coordination are still not fully elucidated.

In relation to human disease, there is an enormous body of work that remains to be undertaken in order to identify the genes that are responsible for many single-gene disorders and, in particular, those that play a role in the aetiology of multi-factorial conditions. Those human genes and genetic disorders that have already been identified are catalogued in the Online Mendelian Inheritance in Man (OMIM) database (see http://www.ncbi.nlm.nih.gov/sites/entrez?db=omim). An already vast and continuously expanding SNP database is now accessible online at http://www.ncbi.nlm.nih.gov/projects/SNP/. In time, an increasing volume of data will become available regarding such genetic polymorphisms, which underlie not only the susceptibility of different individuals to such diseases but also, to a large extent, the varied and previously unpredictable responses of different patients to pharmacological agents.

Genetics, or pharmacogenetics, in fact, can affect not only the way a drug is absorbed, metabolised and excreted (pharmacokinetics) by the body but also the physiological effects of a drug, such as receptor-binding (pharmacodynamics). The inter-individual variation in drug response is often due to significant variation in the rates of drug metabolism (often related to polymorphisms in cytochrome P450 enzymes such as CYP2D6 or CYP2C9) and, in certain individuals, can result in unexpected and serious toxicity (see Tarantino *et al.*, 2009, in Further reading, for example). Other well-known examples of genetically determined drug sensitivity are the responses to isoniazid (determined by *N*-acetyltransferase activity and *NAT2* gene polymorphisms), malignant hyperthermia following exposure to halothane (in those with an *RYR1* mutation), abnormal sensitivity to suxamethonium/succinylcholine (determined by homozygous *CHE1* mutations) and sensitivity to the anti-malarial drug primaquine as a result of glucose-6-phosphate dehydrogenase deficiency. The term pharmacogenomics refers to the incorporation, into this field of pharmacogenetics, of additional information from the Human Genome Project, especially in relation to the increasing number of recognised genetic polymorphisms mentioned above.

While the full analysis of the genome is a very significant challenge, an additional challenge is to understand the complexity of the entire protein complement ('proteome') in a cell, tissue or biological fluid. A major area of research, known as proteomics, now aims to determine the way in which the vast number of proteins (at least 500,000) are generated from less than 25,000 protein-coding genes (including alternative splicing patterns and the many post-translational modification processes) and to reveal the complex ways in which these proteins interact with each other. In addition, the ongoing study of disease-related qualitative and quantitative changes in tissue and biological fluid proteomes will hopefully identify useful biomarkers of particular conditions such as bile duct cancer (see Bonney *et al.*, 2008, in Further reading).

In contrast, the relatively recently developed 'metabolomics' is the study of the small molecule metabolites such as metabolic substrates, intermediates and end-products as well as lipids, small peptides, vitamins and cofactors. It involves techniques such as mass spectrometry or nuclear magnetic resonance spectroscopy (see Claudino *et al.*, 2007, in Further reading) and provides an indication of total cell biochemical activity. In time, in combination with proteomics, genomics and transcriptomics (the study of actively transcribed genes in a given cell type by the determination of mRNA expression levels), it may eventually contribute to a more complete understanding of cell physiology and pathology.

SUMMARY

- The human nuclear genome contains approximately 3280 million bp but only around 1.1% of this represents protein-coding DNA.
- Gene-rich areas tend to have a higher G + C content and to appear pale on Giemsa chromosome staining.
- The mitochondrial genome contains just 16,568 bp with only 37 genes, but, unlike the nuclear genome, it contains no introns.
- Many nuclear genes have been identified in recent years as a result of the Human Genome Project, although the precise functions of many of the corresponding proteins have not yet been determined.
- In addition to polypeptide-encoding genes, over 8,000 genes have been discovered that code for various types of RNA molecules (such as miRNAs) that regulate gene expression
- Data generated by the Human Genome Project is publicly accessible via web browsers such as Ensembl (http://www.ensembl.org) and UCSC (http://genome.ucsc.edu/cgi-bin/hgGateway). A user's guide

is provided in Chapter 19 and updated web-links are provided online at www.wiley.com/go/tobias.
■ Remaining uncertainties include: the functions of many genes, proteins and regions of non-coding DNA; the complex mechanisms by which genes and their products interact and are regulated; and the identification of many genes involved in human conditions, particularly multifactorial disorders.

FURTHER READING

Bonney GK, Craven RA, Prasad R, Melcher AF, Selby PJ, Banks RE (2008) Circulating markers of biliary malignancy: opportunities in proteomics? *Lancet Oncol* **9**:149–58.

Claudino WM, Quattrone A, Biganzoli L, Pestrin M, Bertini I, Di Leo A (2007) Metabolomics: available results, current research projects in breast cancer, and future applications. *J Clin Oncol* **25**:2840–6.

Ferracin M, Veronese A, Negrini M (2010) Micromarkers: miRNAs in cancer diagnosis and prognosis. *Expert Rev Mol Diagn* **10**:297–308.

Kiss, T (2006) SnoRNP biogenesis meets pre-mRNA splicing. *Molecular Cell* **23**:775–6.

Strachan T, Read AP (2010) *Human Molecular Genetics*, 4th edition. Garland Science: London.

Tarantino G, Di Minno MN, Capone D (2009) Drug-induced liver injury: is it somehow foreseeable? *World J Gastroenterol* **15**:2817–33.

Tucker T, Marra M, Friedman JM (2009) Massively parallel sequencing: the next big thing in genetic medicine. *Am J Hum Genet* **85**:142–54.

WEBSITES

1000 Genomes: A Deep Catalog of Human Genetic Variation:
http://www.1000genomes.org/

C. elegans genome page within Ensembl:
http://www.ensembl.org/Caenorhabditis_elegans/index.html

Homo sapiens Genome (ENSEMBL):
http://www.ensembl.org/Homo_sapiens/index.html

NCBI MapViewer Build Statistics:
http://www.ncbi.nlm.nih.gov/mapview/stats/BuildList.cgi?type=org#Homosapiens

NCBI SNP database homepage:
http://www.ncbi.nlm.nih.gov/projects/SNP/

Online Mendelian Inheritance in Man (OMIM) – database of human genes and genetic disorders:
http://www.ncbi.nlm.nih.gov/sites/entrez?db=omim

University of California Santa Cruz (UCSC) Genome Browser Gateway:
http://genome.ucsc.edu/cgi-bin/hgGateway

US Dept of Energy Human Genome Project Information:
http://www.ornl.gov/sci/techresources/Human_Genome/home.shtml

Wellcome Trust Sanger Institute web site for human genetics and bioinformatics:
http://www.sanger.ac.uk/

Self-assessment

1–6. Which of the following statements are true?

1. The human genome contains approximately 3 million base pairs

2. Pale Giemsa staining chromosomal regions tend to have a higher G + C content and to be relatively gene-rich

3. Around 50% of the human genome codes for proteins

4. Some RNA molecules are transcribed from DNA and can regulate the expression of other genes

5. The genome was sequenced using a radioactively labelled DNA sequencing method

6. The number of genes per autosome increases with chromosome number from chromosome 1 to 22, with chromosome 1 containing the fewest

7. Which one of the following is not true of human RNA molecules?

A. They may undergo splicing

B. They can function in the splicing process

C. They are present in the nucleus but not in the cytoplasm

D. They can form functional complexes with proteins

E. They are generally single-stranded

CHAPTER 3
Nucleic acid structure and function

Key Topics

Introduction

In this chapter, the structure and function of DNA and RNA will be described, together with the different stages involved in the production of products (which are usually proteins) from coding DNA sequences and the mechanisms by which this gene expression is regulated. In addition, the different types of DNA length mutations and point mutations are discussed, together with their various effects on protein function and the recent guidelines for the naming of mutations.

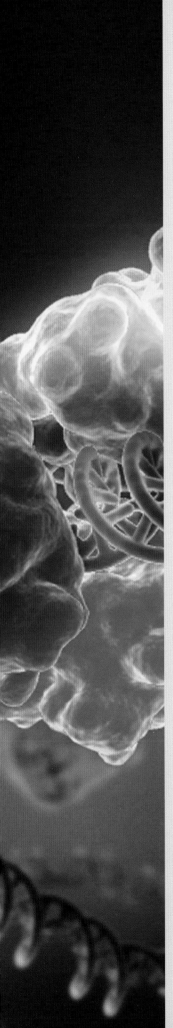

Essential Medical Genetics, 6th edition. © Edward S. Tobias, Michael Connor and Malcolm Ferguson-Smith.
Published 2011 by Blackwell Published Ltd.

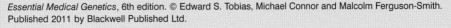

Nucleic acid structure

In humans, as in other organisms, nucleic acid is the carrier of genetic information and has a structure that is ideally suited to this function. There are two main types of nucleic acid, DNA (deoxyribonucleic acid) and RNA (ribonucleic acid), which each consist of a sugar–phosphate backbone with projecting nitrogenous bases (Fig. 3.1). The nitrogenous bases are of two types, purines and pyrimidines. In DNA, there are two purine bases, adenine (A) and guanine (G), and two pyrimidine bases, thymine (T) and cytosine (C). RNA also contains A, G and C, but contains uracil (U) in place of T. In DNA, the sugar is deoxyribose, whereas in RNA it is ribose (Fig. 3.2). The nitrogenous bases are attached to the 1′ (one prime) position of each sugar, and the phosphate links 3′ and 5′ hydroxyl groups. Each unit of purine or pyrimidine base together with the attached sugar and phosphate group(s) is called a nucleotide.

A molecule of DNA is composed of two nucleotide chains, which are coiled clockwise around one another to form a double helix with 10 nucleotides per complete turn of DNA (Fig. 3.3). The two chains run in opposite directions (i.e. 5′ to 3′ for one and 3′ to 5′ for the other) and are held together by hydrogen bonds between A in one chain and T in the other or between G and C. This base pairing is very specific, although rarely erroneous combinations may occur. As A:T and G:C pairing is obligatory, the parallel strands must be complementary to one another. Thus, if one strand reads 5′-ATGC-3′, the complementary strand must read 5′-GCAT-3′ (not 5′-TACG-3′). Hence, the ratio of A to T is 1:1 and of G to C is likewise 1:1 (Chargaff's rule). Wide variation exists in the (A + T):(G + C) ratio. Higher plants and animals tend to have an excess of A + T and in humans the ratio is 1.4:1.

The unit of length of DNA is the base pair (bp) with 1000 bp in a kilobase (kb) and 1,000,000 bp in a megabase (Mb). The total length of DNA in a half (haploid) set of human chromosomes is approximately 3280 Mb (3.28×10^9 bp) and, as the distance between base pairs in the DNA helix is 0.34 nm (Fig. 3.3), the total length of haploid DNA if extended, per cell, would be 1 m.

At present, there are approximately 21,600 protein-coding genes present in human DNA. Each protein-coding gene usually possesses only one copy in the haploid genome (well-known exceptions being the α-globin genes, histone genes and ubiquitin genes) and the average gene size is 53.6 kb with an average intergenic distance of 60–70 kb. The majority of the genome is non-coding and repetitive and has no proven function. Repetitive DNA is subdivided into tandem (multiple adjacent) repeats (satellite DNA) and interspersed (single) repeats (Table 3.1).

Tandem repeats are subdivided according to their length. Microsatellite repeat arrays are under 1 kb in length and the most common repeat motifs are A, CA, AAAN (where N is any nucleotide), AAN and AG. The arrays of CA motifs commonly have 10–60 repeats (with corresponding lengths of 20–120 bp) (Fig. 3.4) and are found approximately every 36 kb. The repeat number on corresponding chromosomes commonly differs and these common genetic differences or polymorphisms can be used to track the inheritance of that region of each chromosome (see Chapters 4 and 11).

Minisatellite repeat arrays are usually 1–30 kb in length and have longer repeat motifs than the microsatellite repeats. They again show marked variation in repeat number, and the single-copy minisatellites can be useful for gene tracking. As minisatellites are generally located close to the telomeres, however, they are less useful than microsatellites for genome-wide linkage analyses. Owing to their hypervariable sequences and the ease of detecting large numbers of them simultaneously (by using hybridisation to a common core sequence that they contain), the multilocus minisatellites provide an individual-specific pattern of bands that has been invaluable for forensic identification (see, for example, Fig. 4.15). Macrosatellite repeats are larger still and may be many megabases in length. They are found at the ends (telomeres) of the chromosomal arms and in the central chromosomal constriction (the centromere; see Chapter 5). Length variation is common and accounts for visible differences in the size of chromosomal centromeric regions (e.g. Fig. 5.11).

In contrast, interspersed repeats usually occur as single copies and these are subdivided according to length. Short interspersed repeats (SINES) are under 500 bp and the commonest type is the Alu repeat. Alu repeats are about 300 bp

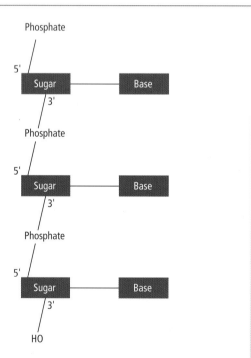

Fig. 3.1 Diagram of nucleic acid structure. The 5′ phosphate end is at the top and the 3′ hydroxyl group is at the bottom of the molecule.

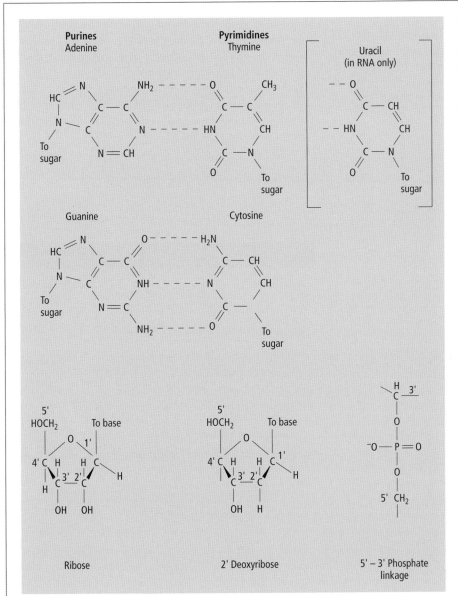

Fig. 3.2 Chemical structure of purines, pyrimidines, ribose, deoxyribose and the 5′ to 3′ phosphate linkage. The hydrogen bonds betwe en adenine and thymine (or uracil) and between guanine and cytosine are indicated.

long, possess a relatively high GC content, and contain a cutting site for the restriction enzyme *Alu*I. They are very common (constituting 11% of all human DNA), are specific to humans and other higher primates and occur every 5–10 kb. Long interspersed repeats (LINES) vary from 500 bp to 10 kb (often 6–8 kb) in length and include three families, which in total constitute about 20% of the human genome. The most common is the LINE-1 (L1) element, which, like other LINES, possesses structural similarities to retroviruses. L1 has the capacity to replicate itself (via reverse transcription, i.e. making a DNA copy from an RNA intermediate) and insert a copy at a new location in the genome. This retrotransposition may disrupt a gene at the new location and cause a genetic disorder (e.g. in some patients with haemophilia).

Single-copy and repeat DNA are double-stranded, whereas RNA is single-stranded and subdivided into several types (see Table 2.1). Ribosomal RNAs (rRNAs) are synthesised directly on DNA templates that occur as multiple clustered copies (the nucleolus organiser regions on the short arms of chromosomes 13–15, 21 and 22, and on chromosome 1). The rRNAs are synthesised as large precursors in the nucleolus and then enzymatically cleaved. Transfer RNAs (tRNAs) are also synthesised directly on a DNA template and, although 61 different types might be expected (Table 3.2), surprisingly only 49 are found, as some tRNAs can bind to more than one mRNA codon. This results from relaxed base-pairing ('wobble') at the third-base position of the codons. The DNA templates for tRNAs tend to occur as multiple copies, which may be clustered or dispersed.

Nucleic acid function

Nucleic acids have two major functions: the direction of protein synthesis and transmission of this information from one generation to the next. Proteins, whether structural components, enzymes, carrier molecules, hormones or receptors, are all composed of a series of amino acids. Twenty major amino acids are known, and the sequence of these determines the form and function of the resulting protein. All proteins are encoded by DNA, and the unit of DNA that contains the protein-coding sequence (together with the introns and the neighbouring untranslated regulatory sequences) is, by definition, its gene. Genes vary greatly in size from small genes like the globins and medium-sized genes of 15–45 kb to enormous genes such as dystrophin (Table 3.3).

Each set of three DNA base pairs (called a triplet or codon) codes for an amino acid. As each base in the triplet may be any of the four types of nucleotide (A, G, C or T), this results

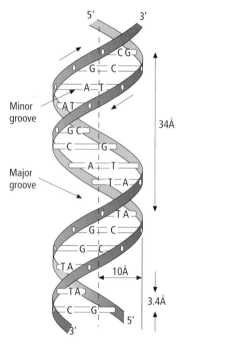

Fig. 3.3 Diagram of a DNA double helix.

Table 3.1 Proportions of different types of nuclear DNA	
Type of DNA	**Approximate percentage of total DNA**
Single copy	45
Repetitive DNA	55
Tandem repeats	(10)
Microsatellites	
Minisatellites	
Macrosatellites	
Interspersed repeats	(45)
Short interspersed repeats (SINES)	
Long interspersed repeats (LINES)	
Other transposable elements	

Genomic chr6:

```
tgtgtgctgt  ggaattcagg  atacttgggc  attgcctact  atgatactag  31708998
tgactccact  atccacttca  tgccagatgc  cccagaccac  gagagcctca  31709048
AGCTTCTCCA  GAGAGGTGGG  GATGGAACCA  TGAATTCCTC  TGCTCTCTGG  31709098
GATTGCAgat  gtgtTAcACA  CACACACACA  CACACACACA  CACACACACA  31709148
CACACACACA  CATATTTTTT  TTTTCTAgAc  AGAgTCTTGC  TCTGTTACCC  31709198
AGGCTcAAGT  GCAGTGGCGC  AATCTTGGCT  CACTGCAGCC  TCCACCTCCT  31709248
GGGtTCAAGC  AATTCTCCTG  ACTCAACCTC  CCGAGTAGCT  gggactacag  31709298
gcgtgtgcca  ccacacccag  ctagtttttt  gtgtgtgttt  ttagcacaga  31709348
cggtgtttca  ccatgttggc  cagggtggtc  tcaaactcct
```

Fig. 3.4 Sequence of a CA microsatellite DNA marker (named AFMB044XE9 or D6S1615; shown in coloured upper case letters) and its flanking DNA (shown in black lower case letters) from the UCSC (University of California, Santa Cruz) database (see Chapter 19). The (CA)n repeat itself can be seen within the genomic sequence shown on lines 4 and 5. The blue letters represent computer-predicted putative splice sites (probably erroneous) and the lower case letters on lines 4 and 5 represent bases that are present in the latest database version but were absent in a different version.

Table 3.2 The genetic code with codons shown as messenger RNA (5′ → 3′)
The corresponding DNA codons are complementary.

First base	Second base				Third base
	U	C	A	G	
U	UUU Phe	UCU Ser	UAU Tyr	UGU Cys	U
	UUC Phe	UCC Ser	UAC Tyr	UGC Cys	C
	UUA Leu	UCA Ser	UAA Stop	UGA Stop	A
	UUG Leu	UCG Ser	UAG Stop	UGG Trp	G
C	CUU Leu	CCU Pro	CAU His	CGU Arg	U
	CUC Leu	CCC Pro	CAC His	CGC Arg	C
	CUA Leu	CCA Pro	CAA Gln	CGA Arg	A
	CUG Leu	CCG Pro	CAG Gln	CGG Arg	G
A	AUU Ile	ACU Thr	AAU Asn	AGU Ser	U
	AUC Ile	ACC Thr	AAC Asn	AGC Ser	C
	AUA Ile	ACA Thr	AAA Lys	AGA Arg	A
	*AUG Met	ACG Thr	AAG Lys	AGG Arg	G
G	GUU Val	GCU Ala	GAU Asp	GGU Gly	U
	GUC Val	GCC Ala	GAC Asp	GGC Gly	C
	GUA Val	GCA Ala	GAA Glu	GGA Gly	A
	GUG Val	GCG Ala	GAG Glu	GGG Gly	G

Abbreviations for amino acids (three-letter code, with one-letter code in parentheses):

Ala	Alanine (A)	Leu	Leucine (L)
Arg	Arginine (R)	Lys	Lysine (K)
Asn	Asparagine (N)	Met	Methionine (M)
Asp	Aspartic acid (D)	Phe	Phenylalanine (F)
Cys	Cysteine (C)	Pro	Proline (P)
Gln	Glutamine (Q)	Ser	Serine (S)
Glu	Glutamic acid (E)	Thr	Threonine (T)
Gly	Glycine (G)	Trp	Tryptophan (W)
His	Histidine (H)	Tyr	Tyrosine (Y)
Ile	Isoleucine (I)	Val	Valine (V)

Stop: chain terminator (X).
*Start codon for protein synthesis.

in 4^3 or 64 possible combinations or codons. The codons for each amino acid are given in Table 3.2, and it is important to note that, by convention, each codon is shown in terms of the messenger RNA (mRNA). The corresponding DNA sequence from which the mRNA is actually transcribed will be complementary. For example, the mRNA sequence 5′-AUG-3′ is the codon for methionine and is transcribed from the complementary DNA ('antisense' strand) template 5′-CAT-3′. However, it is the sequence of the 'sense' strand (i.e. containing the AUG or ATG in the mRNA or DNA, respectively) that is usually published or used as a reference.

All amino acids except methionine and tryptophan are encoded by more than one codon: hence, the code is said to be degenerate. Three of the 64 codons designate the termination of a message and these are called stop codons (UAA,

UGA and UAG), and one codon, AUG (which also codes for methionine), acts as a start signal for protein synthesis. With a few possible exceptions, this code is identical in all species. The genetic code used for the synthesis of proteins that are encoded by the mitochondrial genome is, however, different.

The first stage in protein synthesis is transcription. The two strands of DNA separate in the area of the gene to be transcribed. One strand (the template strand – this strand is consistent for a given gene but varies from one gene to another, depending upon the gene's orientation) functions as a template and is read in the 3′ to 5′ direction by the enzyme RNA polymerase II, with the mRNA being synthesised in the 5′ to 3′ direction (Fig. 3.5). Transcription proceeds at about 30 nucleotides per second until the transcription terminator is

Table 3.3 Examples of genes and their protein products

Protein	Approximate number of amino acids in protein	Approximate gene size (bp)	Number of coding regions in each gene
Insulin	51	1,430	3
α-Globin	141	850	3
β-Globin	146	1,600	3
Hypoxanthine-guanine phosphoribosyl transferase	217	44,000	9
α₁ Antitrypsin	394	10,000	5
Phenylalanine hydroxylase	451	90,000	13
Glucose-6-phosphate dehydrogenase	515	18,000	13
Low-density-lipoprotein receptor	839	45,000	18
Cystic fibrosis transmembrane regulator protein	1,480	230,000	27
Coagulation factor VIII	2,332	189,000	26
Dystrophin	3,685	2,225,000	79
Titin	34,350	305,000	363

No.	Exon / Intron	Chr	Strand	Start	End	Start Phase	End Phase	Length	Sequence
	5' upstream sequence								...................tgtggagccacaccctagggttggccaatctactcccagg agcagggagggcaggagccagggctgggcataaaagtcagggcagagccatctattgctt
1	ENSE00001326797	11	-1	5,204,736	5,204,877	-	2	142	ACATTTGCTTCTGACACAACTGTGTTCACTAGCAACCTCAAACAGACACCATGGTGCATC TGACTCCTGAGGAGAAGTCTGCCGTTACTGCCCTGTGGGGCAAGGTGAACGTGGATGAAG TTGGTGGTGAGGCCCTGGGCAG
	Intron 1-2	11	-1	5,204,606	5,204,735			130	gttggtatcaaggttacaagacaggtttaaggagaccaatagaaactgggcatgtggaga cagagaagactcttgggtttctgataggcactgactctctctgcctattggtctattttc ccacccttag
2	ENSE00001057381	11	-1	5,204,383	5,204,605	2	0	223	GCTGCTGGTGGTCTACCCTTGGACCCAGAGGTTCTTTGAGTCCTTTGGGGATCTGTCCAC TCCTGATGCTGTTATGGGCAACCCTAAGGTGAAGGCTCATGGCAAGAAAGTGCTCGGTGC CTTTAGTGATGGCCTGGCTCACCTGGACAACCTCAAGGGCACCTTTGCCACACTGAGTGA GCTGCACTGTGACAAGCTGCACGTGGATCCTGAGAACTTCAGG
	Intron 2-3	11	-1	5,203,533	5,204,382			850	gtgagtctatgggacgcttgatgttttctttcccccttcttttctatggttaagttcatgt cataggaagggataagtaacagggtacagtttagaatgggaaacagacgaatgattgca tcagtgtggaagtctcaggatcgtttttagttttcttttatttgctgttcataacaattgtt ttcttttgtttaattcttgctttctttttttttttcttcctcgcaattttttactattatact taatgccttaacattgtgtataacaaaaggaaatatctctgagatacattaagtaactta aaaaaaaacttttacacagtctgcctagtacattactatttggaatatatgtgtgcttatt tgcatattcataatctccctactttatttttcttttattttttaattgatacataatcatta tacatatttatgggttaaagtgtaatgtttttaatatgtgtacacatattgaccaaatcag ggtaattttgcatttgtaattttaaaaaatgcttttcttcttttttaatatactttttttgttt atcttatttctaataacttttccctaatctctttctttcagggcaataatgatacaatgtat catgcctcttttgcaccattctaaagaataacagtgataattttctgggttaaggcaatagc aatatctctgcatataaatatttctgcatataaattgtaactgatgtaagagggtttcata ttgctaatagcagctacaatccagctaccattctgcttttatttttatggttgggataagg ctggattattctgagtccaagctaggccctttgctaatcatgttcatacctcttatctt cctcccacag
3	ENSE00001111247	11	-1	5,203,272	5,203,532	0	-	261	CTCCTGGGCAACGTGCTGGTCTGTGTGCTGGCCCATCACTTTGGCAAAGAATTCACCCCA CCAGTGCAGGCTGCCTATCAGAAAGTGGTGGCTGGTGTGGCTAATGCCCTGGCCCACAAG TATCACTAAGCTCGCTTTCTTGCTGTCCAATTTCTATTAAAGGTTCCTTTGTTCCCTAAG TCCAACTACTAAACTGGGGGATATTATGAAGGGCCTTGAGCATCTGGATTCTGCCTAATA AAAAACATTTATTTTCATTGC
	3' downstream sequence								aatgatgtatttaaattatttctgaatattttactaaaaagggaatgtgggaggtcagtg catttaaaacataaagaaatgaagagctagttcaaacctt...................

Fig. 3.5 Genomic nucleotide sequence of the human β-globin gene. The sequence of the primary gene transcript is shown in the 5' to 3' direction, with T in place of U. The 5' and 3' untranslated regions (UTRs) are represented in purple and the untranscribed upstream and downstream sequences are displayed in green. Letters shown in capitals, black or blue represent sequences corresponding to the mature mRNA, coding sequence and two introns, respectively. The CCAAT box within the promoter is highlighted in blue. From the exon display of transcript ENST00000335295 in Ensembl release 44 at http://www.ensembl.org as discussed in Chapter 19.

reached. After some processing and modification (described below), the mRNA molecule diffuses to the cytoplasm and the DNA strands reassociate.

The next stage of protein synthesis occurs in the cytoplasm and is called translation. Each mRNA molecule becomes attached to one or more ribosomes. As the ribosome moves along the mRNA from the 5′ to the 3′ end, each codon is recognised by a matching complementary tRNA, which contributes its amino acid to the end of a new growing protein chain until a stop codon (UAA, UGA or UAG) is reached.

Proteins are encoded by genes containing, on average, approximately 10 exons, each around 300 bp in size. Human genes, however, tend to be much larger than would be expected from the encoded protein's amino acid sequence alone (Table 3.3). This excess is mainly due to the presence of intervening sequences, but also to the 5′ and 3′ flanking sequences. The vast majority of genes consist of alternating coding segments for mature mRNA, or exons, and non-coding segments of <30 bp to over 1 Mbp, called intervening sequences or introns, whose function is largely unknown (Fig. 3.5). The initial mRNA (heterogeneous RNA or hnRNA) is a transcript of the gene that includes not only the exons, but also the intervening sequences and some flanking sequences. Prior to its entry into the cytoplasm, however, the segments corresponding to the intervening sequences are removed by splicing (Fig. 3.6). Thus, the initial mRNA may be several fold longer than the definitive mRNA. The sequences around the intron/exon junctions serve as recognition sites for splicing proteins, and characteristically an intron begins with GT (the 5′ donor site) and ends with AG (the 3′ acceptor site). Mutations in the bases adjacent to the exon/intron boundaries interfere with mRNA splicing and can cause genetic disease.

The mRNA 5′ end is protected or 'capped' (with a methyl guanylate residue), and the 5′ untranslated region (5′ UTR) extends downstream from this cap site to the beginning of the protein-coding sequence. At the other end, the 3′ untranslated region (3′ UTR) extends from the protein translation stop codon to the poly(A) tail. This tail of 100–200 adenylate (i.e. AMP) residues is not encoded in the DNA but is added enzymatically to aid cytoplasmic transport and, possibly, mRNA stability.

Many proteins are not in their final form after ribosomal translation. The subsequent post-translational alterations include the formation of disulphide bonds, hydroxylation, glycosylation, proteolytic cleavage and phosphorylation (Fig. 3.7). Each step in the production of the final protein is important, as many proteins are highly dependent for function upon their exact three-dimensional shape (or 'tertiary structure'), which in turn is determined by their amino acid sequence and post-translational modifications. In general, acidic (e.g. Asp, Glu) and basic (e.g. Lys, Arg, His) amino acids are found on the surface of a folded protein, with hydrophobic amino acids (e.g. Ala, Val, Leu) internally orientated. The effect of an amino acid substitution thus not only depends upon its relationship to the active site of the protein but also upon the change in charge or hydrophobicity and hence the degree of consequent disruption to the protein's tertiary structure.

The DNA sequence of a gene allows prediction of the mRNA and protein amino acid sequence and often the general function and intracellular location of the protein. It cannot, however, reliably predict the patterns of alternative splicing, the post-translational modifications, the three-dimensional (i.e. tertiary) structure of the protein, its precise functions or its expression patterns. To determine these characteristics, other investigations are required. For instance, to investigate gene expression, RNA analysis may be carried out by reverse transcription PCR, microarray analysis or, more rarely, Northern blotting. Protein size and abundance can be determined by the antibody-based technique known as Western blotting. Alternatively, to visualise the intracellular location of a protein, immunofluorescence microscopy can be undertaken using a fluorescent antibody that binds specifically to that protein. Finally, to determine the protein's three-dimensional structure, X-ray crystallography or nuclear magnetic resonance spectroscopy may be used.

Gene regulation

All nucleated cells of an individual have an identical genome, yet at any one time in many cell types only a small fraction of the total genes are being expressed at a significant level and the relative pattern of expression needs to vary widely, not only for the initial differentiation of cells and tissues, but also to meet fluctuating demands for the synthesis of different proteins in each cell. These demands may change, for instance in development, during which the degree of expression of several genes can vary according to the precise location of the cell and also with time. Areas of DNA flanking each gene play an important role in regulating transcription and hence synthesis of each protein (Fig. 3.8). Immediately upstream of the gene is the promoter, which is involved in the binding of RNA polymerase II to the DNA template strand. Promoters for RNA polymerase II are usually several hundred nucleotides long and often contain a consensus sequence 5′-TATAAA-3′ (the TATA box). This sequence, usually located around 25 bp upstream of the transcriptional start site, binds, via the so-called TATA-binding protein (TBP) subunit of TFIID, to a series of *general transcription factors* (e.g. TFIIA, TFIIB, TFIID, TFIIE, TFIIF, TFIIH), which are relatively abundant proteins used to initiate the transcription of nearly all mRNAs. Basal transcriptional efficiency is commonly aided by the presence of other upstream short consensus regulatory sequences within the promoter region. These often include multiple copies of the so-called GC box, which binds the ubiquitous transcription factor SpI, and the CAAT box, which is typically located 75 bp upstream of the transcriptional start site and binds the transcription factors CTF and CBF.

Fig. 3.6 Diagram of transcription, mRNA processing and translation. By convention, the 5′ end of the mRNA molecule is placed to the left.

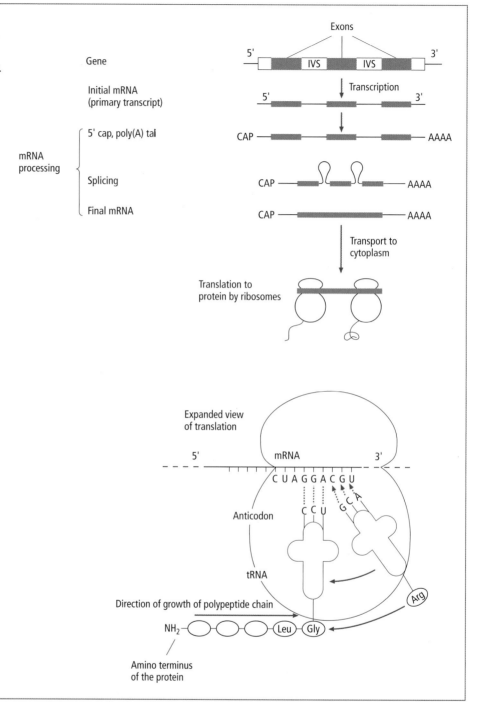

The activity of many promoters is modulated (increased or decreased) by one or more enhancers. Enhancers are generally short (less than 20–30 bp) sequences that bind *specific (i.e. tissue-restricted) transcription factors*. Most enhancers function whether on the coding or non-coding strand of DNA and can be located, in either orientation, up to several kilobases from their target promoter. Most enhancers are active only in specific cell types and thus play a central role in regulating tissue specificity of gene expression. Silencers are similar sequence elements that, in contrast, inhibit transcription of the associated gene. The large number of specific transcription factors and their interaction at individual enhancers allows complex patterns of gene activation in response to particular circumstances including tissue differentiation and physiological (or pathological) receptor signalling. Interactions between the proteins bound to enhancers and those bound to the promoter sequences are probably permitted by the intervening DNA forming long loops.

About 80% of genes are only expressed at specific times and places (e.g. insulin in the pancreatic islet β-cells). The other

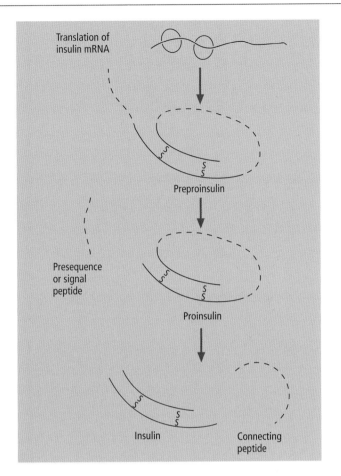

Fig. 3.7 Post-translational modification of insulin.

20%, which are called housekeeping genes, are expressed in all tissues, generally fulfil basic metabolic needs and account for 90% or more of the genes expressed in any particular cell type. The majority of housekeeping genes and about 40% of tissue-specific genes have CpG islands near their 5′ ends. The CpG islands are about 1 kb in length and contain a high proportion of 5′-CG-3′ dinucleotide pairs (indicated as C, p for phosphate, G, to distinguish them from G hydrogen bonded to C in opposite DNA strands). Generally, cytosine residues in CpG dinucleotides are methylated, but in CpG islands associated with active neighbouring gene expression, there is usually a lack of methylation.

Although the bulk of regulation probably occurs at the transcriptional level, regulation of a gene's activity may also occur later with, for example, (i) alteration of the rate of protein translation or degradation, or (ii) alternative splicing of the mRNA to produce different gene products (e.g. calcitonin or calcitonin gene-related neuropeptide).

Mutations within a gene's regulatory sequences can occur and may result in no gene product (e.g. some patients with β-thalassaemia), abnormal persistence of a fetal gene product (e.g. hereditary persistence of α-fetoprotein or haemoglobin F) or anomalous patterns of gene expression (e.g. ectopic expression of creatine kinase).

DNA replication

Accurate replication of DNA must occur with each cell division. The two strands separate at a number of points (with up to 100 of these 'origins of replication' per chromosome) and each strand serves as a template upon which the missing partner can be reconstructed by base pairing with free nucleotides (Fig. 3.9). These nucleotides are brought together by the action of the DNA-dependent DNA polymerases alpha and delta (c.f. gamma for mitochondrial DNA) and are hydrogen-bonded to

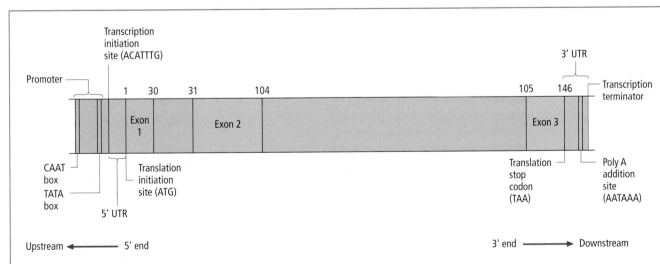

Fig. 3.8 The human β-globin gene, indicating some of the adjacent sequences involved in the regulation of transcription. The leader (5′ UTR) and trailer (3′ UTR) sequences are also shown.

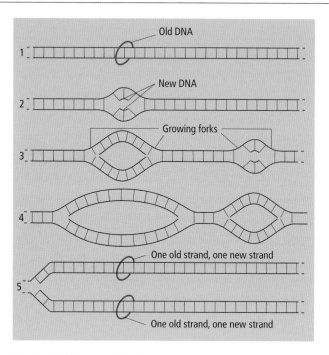

Fig. 3.9 Initiation of replication.

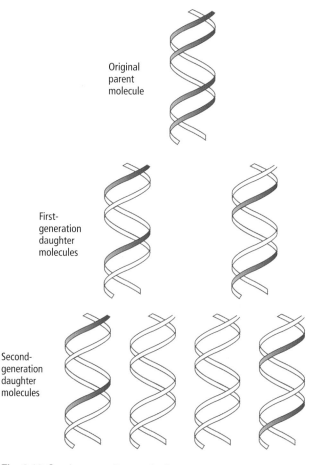

Fig. 3.10 Semiconservative replication.

the template strand. Replication proceeds in both directions from each initiation point until the two new strands of DNA are complete. This method of replication is called semi-conservative, as one strand of each new DNA duplex molecule has been conserved (Fig. 3.10). This can be shown very effectively by growing cells through two cell divisions in culture medium containing bromodeoxyuridine (BrdU), an analogue of thymine. New growing strands incorporate BrdU, so that at the end of two divisions each chromosome has only one original strand lacking BrdU. The strands can thus be stained differentially, giving the chromosomes a harlequin appearance. Each chromosome will contain one dark (containing the original strand) and one light chromatid, as the strands that incorporate the BrdU stain less intensely (Fig. 3.11).

Mutation types, effects and nomenclature

Mutations of DNA are broadly divisible into length mutations with gain or loss of genetic material, and point mutations with alteration of the genetic code but no overall gain or loss of genetic material.

Length mutations

Length mutations include deletions, duplications, insertions and trinucleotide repeat amplifications. Deletions of DNA can range from a single nucleotide to many megabases (and then be visible as a chromosomal deletion). Larger deletions can arise from chromosomal breakage, as a result of a parental chromosome rearrangement (see Chapter 7) or from unequal crossing-over between homologous gene sequences or flanking repeat sequences (see Shaw and Lupski, 2004, in Further reading). Small deletions (often 1–5 nucleotides) commonly result from slipped mispairing, and this is favoured by the presence of direct repeats of two bases or more and by runs of the same nucleotide. The spontaneous rate of chromosomal breakage is markedly increased by ionising radiation and by some mutagenic chemicals. Unequal crossing-over is especially likely to occur in areas with duplicated genes of similar sequence. This is exemplified by studies on the genes responsible for colour vision. There are three separate genes for each of the cone pigments blue (on chromosome 7), red and green (near the tip of the long arm of the X chromosome). There is a single red gene on each X chromosome and one to three

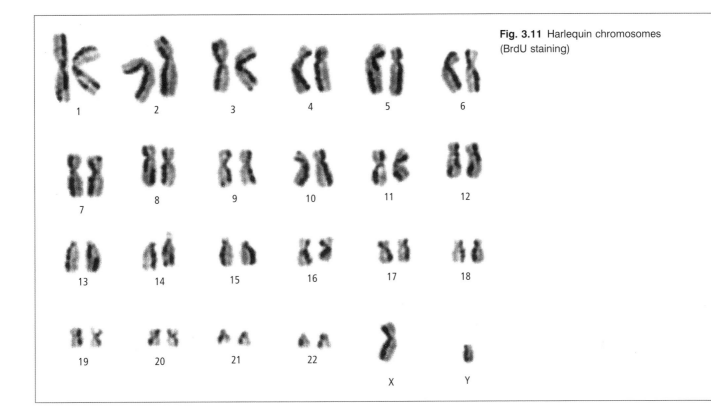

Fig. 3.11 Harlequin chromosomes (BrdU staining)

copies of the green genes. The red and green genes have 96% sequence homology, and unequal crossing-over in this area can result in loss of gene function for one type or hybrid genes that produce pigments of altered function (Fig. 3.12).

Large deletions remove many adjacent genes (contiguous gene disorders) and these should be suspected if, for instance, a boy has several X-linked disorders or if a patient with a single-gene disorder has an unexplained mental handicap and/or unexplained congenital malformations. Removal of all of a gene directly prevents transcription from that allele but smaller deletions that are not exactly 3 (or a multiple of 3) bp in length can be equally serious by altering the reading frame (frameshift mutations, Table 3.4). Large deletions are particularly common in Duchenne muscular dystrophy, α-thalassaemia and steroid sulphatase deficiency. They are also common in DiGeorge, Prader–Willi, Angelman, Williams and Smith–Magenis syndromes.

Duplications of a chromosomal region can also disrupt the reading frame. In addition, in some patients with single-gene disorders, the gene has been disrupted by insertion of a repeat element from a distant site or by a short insertion (often one nucleotide) after slipped mispairing.

Another mechanism of length (or point) mutation is gene conversion whereby one allele is converted to another. This may occur at mitosis or meiosis during the process of recombination. In normal recombination between chromosomes or chromatids (see Chapter 5), the products contain all of the original sections of DNA but in an altered configuration. In contrast, when gene conversion occurs, the product lacks one of the original sections of chromosome and this results in a 3:1 allele ratio for the involved region in contrast to the expected 2:2 ratio (Fig. 3.13).

An important type of length mutation is trinucleotide repeat amplification. About 10% of the genome is composed of tandem repeats, which are mostly stably inherited. These include repeats of trinucleotides, which may occur within or between genes. Some of these trinucleotide repeats become unstable if longer than a critical number of repeat elements and, if associated with a gene, this can result in a single-gene disorder. The faulty gene is identified by a trinucleotide repeat that is longer than normal, and the instability of long repeats means that different members of the same family can show different repeat lengths and corresponding clinical variation in disease severity. This is exemplified by myotonic dystrophy type 1, which is an adult-onset type of muscular dystrophy. The CTG repeat normally occurs 5–35 times, but in affected patients there is an expansion ranging from 50 to over 1000 repeats (Fig. 3.14). There are now over 20 known disorders that have been found to be associated with expansion of a trinucleotide repeat. The mechanism of expansion can involve unequal recombination or DNA polymerase slippage.

Much research has been carried out on the CAG trinucleotide repeat expansions that encode polyglutamine stretches, associated with, for example, Huntington disease (a cause of dementia) and spinocerebellar ataxia (SCA) types 1, 2, 3, 6, 7 and 17. In addition, some congenital malformation syndromes

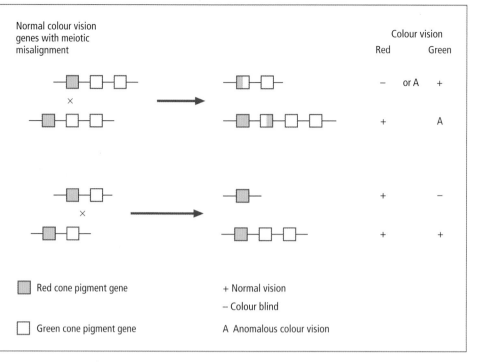

Fig. 3.12 Unequal recombination in the colour vision gene cluster resulting in loss of genes or creation of fused hybrid genes with altered action spectrums.

Table 3.4 Examples of DNA mutation			
DNA base sequence	**mRNA sequence**	**Amino acid sequence**	**Comment**
GTT AAG GCT GCT	GUU AAG GCU GCU	Val-Lys-Ala-Ala	Normal sequence
GTT AAA GCT GCT	GUU AAA GCU GCU	Val-Lys-Ala-Ala	Point mutation with unchanged amino acid sequence
GTT GAG GCT GCT	GUU GAG GCU GCU	Val-Glu-Ala-Ala	Point mutation with amino acid substitution (missense mutation)
GTT TAG GCT GCT	GUU UAG GCU GCU	Val-Stop	Point mutation with premature chain termination (nonsense mutation)
GTT AGG CTG CT	GUU AGG CUG CU	Val-Arg-Leu	Base deletion with frameshift (frameshift mutation)
GTT AAA GGC TGC	GUU AAA GGC UGC	Val-Lys-Gly-Cys	Base insertion with frameshift (frameshift mutation)

can result from shorter expansions of a GCG trinucleotide repeat that encodes an alanine tract, usually within transcription factor genes. It is also now known that repeats of sequences other than trinucleotides can result in human disease. For instance, an intronic pentanucleotide repeat is responsible for SCA-10, an enormous expansion of an intronic tetranucleotide repeat (up to 11,000 units) in the *ZNF9* gene causes myotonic dystrophy type 2, a repeat of 12 bp just upstream of the *CSTB* gene causes an autosomal recessive progressive myoclonic epilepsy and an expansion of an intronic 45 bp repeat is associated with Usher syndrome type 1C (a genetic cause of deafness and visual loss).

Point mutations

In a point mutation, a single nucleotide base is replaced by a different nucleotide base (termed transitions if the change is purine to purine or pyrimidine to pyrimidine, i.e. A $\leftrightarrow$ G, or T $\leftrightarrow$ C, or transversions if purine to pyrimidine or vice versa, i.e. G $\leftrightarrow$ C or A $\leftrightarrow$ T). This leads, in 25% of instances, to no change in the amino acid encoded for that triplet (i.e. silent mutations) due to degeneracy of the code (Table 3.2), in 70% of cases to the substitution of a different amino acid (missense mutations) and in 5% to the production of a termination codon (nonsense mutations) (Table 3.4).

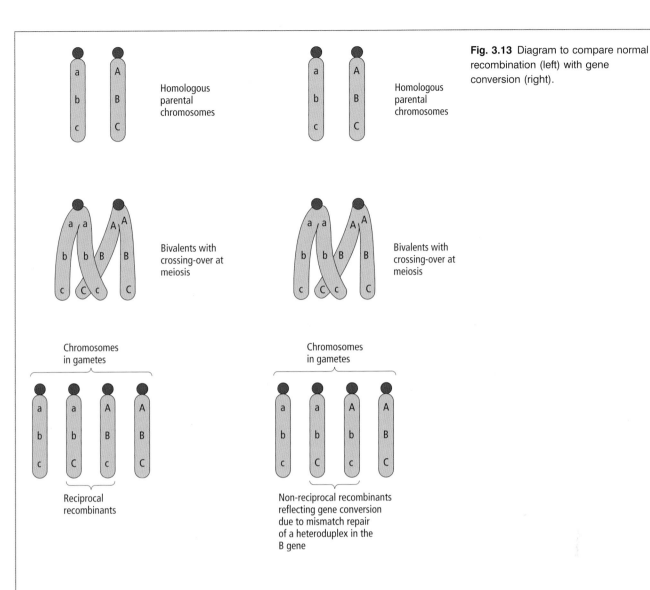

Fig. 3.13 Diagram to compare normal recombination (left) with gene conversion (right).

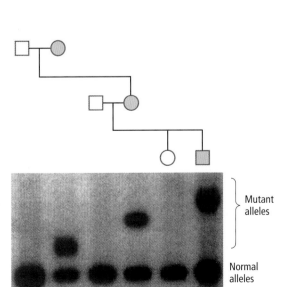

Fig. 3.14 DNA analysis of a family with myotonic dystrophy. Note the instability of the larger mutant allele, represented by the upper band, with decreasing mobility through the electrophoresis gel (from top to bottom) in successive generations.

Fig. 3.15 Examples of DNA repair mechanisms. Note that in nucleotide excision repair (NER), the exonucleases remove a stretch of nucleotides, including the altered bases. In base excision repair (BER), in contrast, only the altered base (and its sugar phosphate) is removed.

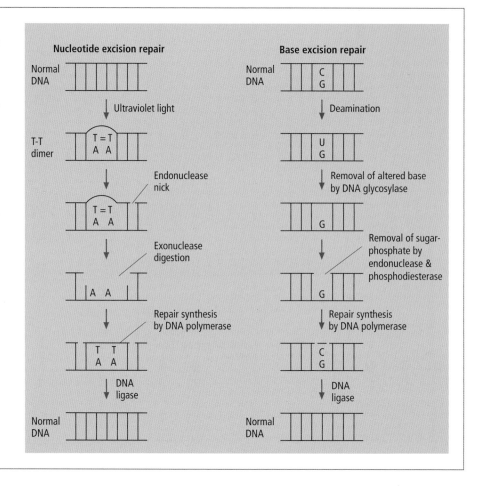

Single nucleotide substitutions are a common type of human mutation and their frequency reflects the fidelity of DNA replication and the efficiency of subsequent error-correction mechanisms. Most are spontaneous and unexplained with a mutation rate in the order of one base substitution for every 10^9 to 10^{10} bases replicated. This rate is markedly increased by exposure to mutagenic chemicals (e.g. deamination by hydroxylamine or alkylation by nitrogen mustard) in proportion to the concentration of the chemical and the duration of exposure. Ultraviolet (UV) light can also cause mutations including pyrimidine dimers in which pairs of adjacent pyrimidine bases become linked. Defence mechanisms exist to identify and repair such damage (Fig. 3.15) and patients with inherited deficiencies of key components of these pathways rapidly accumulate mutations and develop premature cancer. For instance, a deficiency in the nucleotide excision repair pathway, which normally corrects UV-induced pyrimidine dimers, can result in the cancer-predisposing condition xeroderma pigmentosum (Fig 3.16). Another example is the more recently identified *MutYH*-associated polyposis of the bowel, an autosomal recessive condition that results from a deficiency of a DNA glycosylase that normally (by base excision repair) removes adenines that have been misincorporated into DNA. This misincorporation can occur as a result of pairing with an

8-oxoG residue, a stable product of oxidative DNA damage. A separate multistep DNA mismatch repair process is involved in error correction at the time of DNA replication and patients with inherited deficiencies of components of this pathway are also prone to premature cancer, particularly of the colon (see Chapter 13).

These repair mechanisms cannot recognise one particular type of point mutation, as follows, and, as a consequence, this mutation is overrepresented amongst point mutations that cause single-gene disorders. For instance, it accounts for nearly one-half of all point mutations in unrelated patients with haemophilia. Deamination of cytosine produces uracil, which is recognised and removed by the base excision repair pathway (Fig. 3.15). However, cytosine, when it occurs in conjunction with guanine as a 5'-CpG-3' dinucleotides, is generally methylated at the 5' position and deamination of methylated cytosine results in thymine (Fig. 3.2). In turn, this substitution of C by T results in substitution of G by A on the complementary strand and neither of these changes can be recognised by the repair mechanisms. This results in an overall tendency to lose methylated CpG dinucleotides (their frequency is 1 in 50–100 compared with a random dinucleotide frequency of 1 in 16) and an overrepresentation of C to T transitions amongst point mutations (they account for 35–50% of all point mutations). Non-methylated

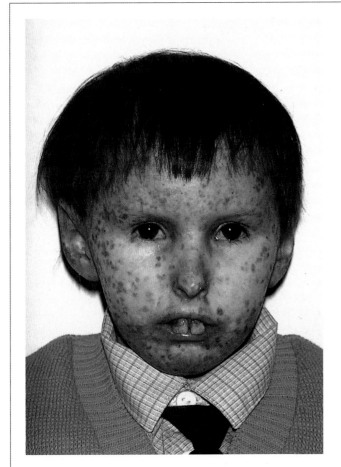

Fig. 3.16 Patient with xeroderma pigmentosum showing multiple ultraviolet-induced skin tumours

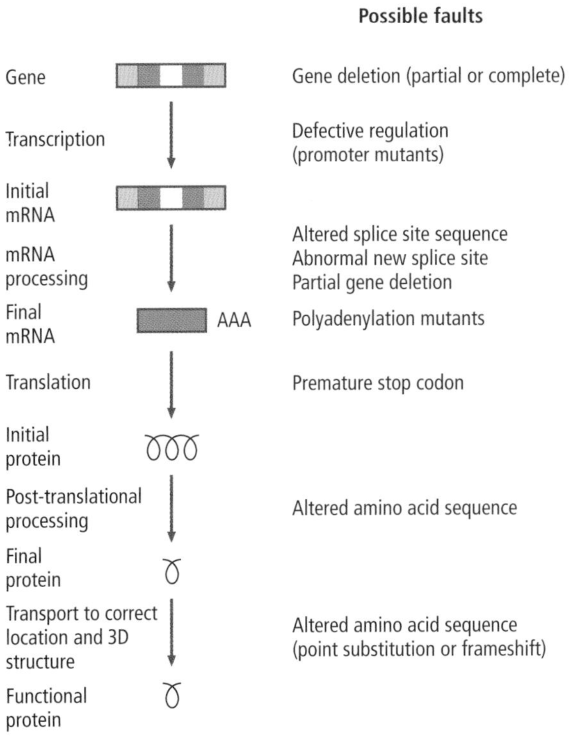

		Possible faults
Gene	▭	Gene deletion (partial or complete)
Transcription	↓	Defective regulation (promoter mutants)
Initial mRNA	▭	
mRNA processing	↓	Altered splice site sequence Abnormal new splice site Partial gene deletion
Final mRNA	▭ AAA	Polyadenylation mutants
Translation	↓	Premature stop codon
Initial protein	〇〇〇	
Post-translational processing	↓	Altered amino acid sequence
Final protein	〇	
Transport to correct location and 3D structure	↓	Altered amino acid sequence (point substitution or frameshift)
Functional protein	〇	

Fig. 3.17 Possible faults in protein biosynthesis.

cytosine residues are spared and hence CpG dinucleotides have a relatively high frequency in non-methylated CpG islands, which are associated with the 5′ ends of many genes. These C to T transitions most commonly occur in male germ cells (with a sevenfold higher frequency than in females) and this might reflect the heavy methylation of sperm DNA compared with oocyte DNA, which tends to be undermethylated.

Molecular pathology of single-gene disorders

For most single-gene disorders, a diversity of molecular lesions (occurring at any stage in the protein biosynthetic pathway) are found (Fig. 3.17). Generally, with length mutations (particularly those insertions and deletions that result in frameshifts), nonsense point mutations (chain terminators) and point mutations adjacent to the intron/exon boundaries, which interfere with splicing, the biological activity of the protein product is reduced in proportion to the reduction in amount of the protein. In this situation, commonly a truncated, absent or almost absent protein results and the mutation is termed null (or sometimes protein⁰ or cross-reacting material (CRM)-negative mutations). Interestingly, transcripts encoding trun-

cated proteins are often degraded by a process known as nonsense-mediated decay (see Glossary). In contrast, with missense mutations (amino acid substitutions), there is often a relatively normal amount of protein produced although its function may be impaired to some extent (sometimes referred to as leaky, protein⁺ or CRM-positive mutations). The level of protein that is expressed can be detected by laboratory techniques such as (i) immunohistochemistry, in which a protein-specific antibody is used to detect the protein, generally in a tissue section on a slide, or (ii) Western blotting, in which the proteins are extracted from fresh tissue (or cultured cells) and then separated by electrophoresis, prior to detection, again using a protein-specific antibody.

Most single-gene disorders can be caused by either length or point mutations, but for several, one particular type of pathology predominates. For example, length mutations due to trinucleotide repeat amplifications (see above) are the major pathology found in myotonic dystrophy, the fragile X syndrome (a cause of mental handicap) and Huntington disease (a cause of dementia). Rarely, all patients have the same point mutation; for example, in sickle-cell anaemia, all patients have a point mutation that results in substitution of valine in place of glutamic acid at amino acid position 7 in β-globin (counting from the initiator methionine, in accordance with the new nomenclature as described below). Where there is a range in the type of molecular pathology, geographical differences may be observed that reflect factors operating at a population genetic level. Thus, for example, two-thirds of Caucasian patients in the UK and USA with cystic fibrosis have a 3 bp deletion at amino acid position 508, whereas this mutation is found in less than one-third of Turkish or Arab patients with cystic fibrosis.

Classification of mutations by their effects on function

Mutations may usefully be classified by their effects on protein function into loss-of-function, gain-of-function and dominant-negative mutations.

Loss-of-function mutations cause a reduction in the activity or amount of the encoded protein and include most mutations (particularly the truncating mutations mentioned above, as well as most missense mutations). Loss-of-function mutations can underlie recessive inheritance, e.g. if the resulting 50% of protein activity in a carrier of such a mutation is sufficient for normal cellular function. If, instead, the 50% level of activity is insufficient, then the loss-of-function mutation is said to result in 'haploinsufficiency' and dominant inheritance results. This is the case, for instance, with mutations affecting the *SHOX* gene, with the resulting haploinsufficiency causing Léri–Weill dyschondrosteosis.

Gain-of-function mutations, in contrast, which are less common, result in a greater level of activity (e.g. as is the case

for those *RET* mutations that cause multiple endocrine neoplasia type 2), a greater amount of protein or, more rarely, acquisition of a new function (e.g. following a chromosomal translocation and generation of a new chimeric gene such as the *BCR–ABL* fusion).

Dominant-negative mutations are those that generally impair the function of the protein encoded by the mutant gene copy and also, as a result of protein–protein interactions (e.g. in a multi-subunit protein complex), reduce the function of the protein encoded by the normal copy of the gene. They include, for example, some mutations in *FBN1*, the gene that encodes fibrillin and is associated with Marfan syndrome. Both gain-of-function and dominant-negative types of mutations typically result in dominant inheritance.

Recommended nomenclature for sequence variants

The way in which mutations are described can occasionally give rise to confusion. According to recent guidelines drafted by the Human Genome Variation Society (http://www.HGVS.org/mutnomen/) designed to eliminate ambiguity, all sequence variants should, strictly, now be described at the DNA level (and preferably in relation to the coding DNA reference sequence) in a certain manner. For cDNA ('c.') sequences, the A of the ATG initiator methionine codon is denoted as nucleotide +1, with the nucleotide immediately 5′ to this being numbered −1. For genomic ('g.') reference sequences, the first nucleotide of the database reference sequence is generally denoted as 1. Substitutions are designated by a '>' symbol, e.g. c.90A>G for substitution of the A at coding sequence

Table 3.5 Examples of mutations causing cystic fibrosis

Mutation	Nomenclature	Consequence
3 bp deletion nt 1521–1523	p.F508del (ΔF508)	In-frame deletion of codon for phenylalanine at aa position 508 in exon 10
G → T at nt 1624	p.G542X (G542X)	Nonsense mutation with substitution of glycine by a stop codon at aa position 542
G → A at nt 1652	p.G551D (G551D)	Missense mutation with substitution of glycine by aspartic acid at aa position 551
Insertion of a T after nt 3773	c.3773_3774insT (3905insT)	Frameshift due to a 1 nt insertion
Deletion of 22 bp starting at nt 720	c.720_741del22 (852del22)	Frameshift due to a 22 bp deletion
G → A at nt 1 from 5′ junction of intron starting after nt 489	c.489+1G>T (621 + 1G → T)	Splice junction mutation
G → A at nt 1 from 3′ splice junction of intron ending before nt 1585	c.1585-1G>A (1717 − 1G → A)	Splice junction mutation
G or A at nt 1584	c.1584G>A (1716G/A)	Silent mutation that leaves the amino acid unaltered (Glu at aa position 528)

Nt: nucleotide; aa: amino acid.
Nomenclature is according to the new approved format (i.e. where the A of the initiator ATG is now numbered nucleotide 1) with the older nomenclature in parentheses.

nucleotide 90 by a G. Polymorphisms (i.e. genetic variants found at a frequency of 1% or greater in the population) should be similarly described. Deletions are indicated by 'del' with the range of affected nucleotides shown using the underscore ('_') symbol, e.g. c.85_87delCTA. Similarly, insertions should be described with the positions of the flanking nucleotides, e.g. c.70_71insA. Finally, intronic nucleotides located either within the first half of the intron (or at a central nucleotide) are described in relation to the number of the last nucleotide of the preceding exon (e.g. c.100+2G>A for a substitution of the second nucleotide of the intron that is located between nucleotides 100 and 101 of the coding sequence). Similarly, for intronic mutations located in the second half of the intron, the position is given relative to the first nucleotide of the next exon (e.g. c.101-3T>C for a substitution of the T located at the third last nucleotide of that intron).

Mutations can also be described at the protein level using the new standardised nomenclature, using the amino acid short code (Table 3.2) and the amino acid position within the protein (Table 3.5). They should be preceded by a 'p.' to designate a protein-level description (e.g. p.Trp26Cys or p. W26C). Strictly, when such protein-level descriptions are first given in a text, they should also include the DNA level description, e.g. 'c.1652G>A (p.G551D)' for a missense mutation or 'c. 1624G>T (p.G542X)' for a nonsense mutation. The initiator methionine is now designated codon 1.

■ The DNA molecule consists of two nucleotide chains, coiled clockwise forming a double helix with 10 nucleotides per turn. The two chains are held together by hydrogen bonds (in base pairing, A:T and G:C).

■ Nucleotides consist of a sugar (deoxyribose in DNA and ribose in RNA), a purine (adenine or guanine) or pyrimidine (thymine or cytosine) base and a phosphate group.

■ Most of the genome does not code for proteins and contains repeated sequences, which can be tandem (adjacent) satellite DNA repeats or interspersed (single) repeats.

■ For protein synthesis, a gene is first transcribed by an RNA polymerase into hnRNA, which is then spliced (removing the introns) to form mRNA. The mRNA diffuses to the cytoplasm where translation into polypeptides takes place at ribosomes and subsequent post-translational modifications can then take place.

■ Gene regulation at the transcriptional level depends on promoter and enhancer sequences, to which general and specific (tissue-restricted) transcription factors (proteins) may bind, respectively.

■ Mutations of DNA can be length mutations (deletions, duplications, insertions and trinucleotide repeat amplifications) or point mutations (single-nucleotide substitutions, which, in 70% of cases, lead to an amino acid change, i.e. a missense mutation).

SUMMARY

FURTHER READING

Albrecht A, Mundlos S (2005) The other trinucleotide repeat: polyalanine expansion disorders. *Curr Opin Genet Dev* **15**:285–93.

Antonorakis SE, Cooper DN (2006) Mutations in human genetic disease: nature and consequences. In *Emery and Rimoin's Principles and Practice of Medical Genetics*, 5th edn. Churchill Livingstone: Edinburgh.

Matera AG, Terns RM, Terns MP (2007) Non-coding RNAs: lessons from the small nuclear and small nucleolar RNAs. *Nat Rev Mol Cell Biol* **8**: 209–20.

Shaw CJ, Lupski JR (2004) Implications of human genome architecture for rearrangement-based disorders: the genomic basis of disease. *Hum Mol Genet* **1**:R57–64.

Strachan T, Read AP (2011) *Human Molecular Genetics*, 4th edn. Garland Science: London.

Walker FO (2007) Huntington's disease. *Lancet* **369**:218–28.

WEBSITE

Nomenclature for the description of sequence variations:
http://www.hgvs.org/mutnomen/

Self-assessment

1–4. Which of the following four statements are true?
1. The pyrimidine bases are cytosine and guanine
2. Base pairing is by hydrogen bonds
3. C pairs with T and A pairs with G
4. The sugar–phosphate backbone of the DNA molecule relies on covalent rather than hydrogen bonds

5. Which of the following does not play a role in the regulation of transcription?
A. Transcription factors
B. Enhancer sequences
C. Silencer sequences
D. The promoter
E. The spliceosome

6. Which of the following genetic alterations or repair defects is correctly paired with the associated disease?
A. Base excision repair defect and xeroderma pigmentosum
B. Nucleotide excision repair defect and *MutYH*-associated polyposis
C. Mismatch repair defect and Huntington disease
D. Trinucleotide repeat length mutation and colon cancer
E. Chromosomal microdeletion deletion and Williams syndrome

7. Which of the following would be least likely to result in a reduced amount or shortening of a protein encoded by a 20-exon gene?
A. A 2bp insertion in the second exon
B. A 1bp deletion in the third exon
C. A nonsense mutation in the sixth exon
D. A T to C nucleotide substitution in the middle of the fifth exon
E. Methylation of the cytosines surrounding the promoter

8. Which of the following is not a post-translational modification?
A. Phosphorylation
B. Polyadenylation
C. Glycosylation
D. Proline hydroxylation
E. Disulphide bond formation

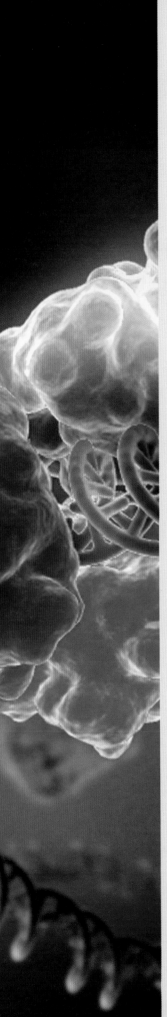

CHAPTER 4
DNA analysis

Key Topics

Introduction

Medical genetics utilises a wide range of DNA analysis techniques for both clinical practice and research. This chapter will mainly discuss the basic techniques and applications of most relevance to clinical practice, and suggestions for further reading are provided for those needing wider or more detailed coverage. These techniques generally start with DNA from an affected family member, which can be extracted from any nucleated cells. The lymphocytes from a 10 ml anticoagulated venous blood sample yield about 200–300 μg of DNA, which is sufficient for multiple DNA analyses.

The most widely used basic techniques for DNA analysis in the diagnostic laboratory include the polymerase chain reaction (PCR) and its adaptations, automated DNA sequencing and array comparative genomic hybridisation (aCGH). The range of techniques used is summarised in Table 4.1.

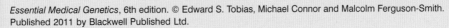

Essential Medical Genetics, 6th edition. © Edward S. Tobias, Michael Connor and Malcolm Ferguson-Smith.
Published 2011 by Blackwell Published Ltd.

Table 4.1 DNA-based detection methods used in diagnostic laboratories

Detection of point mutations

DNA sequencing

- Capillary-based automated fluorescent dideoxy (Sanger) cycle sequencing
- Massively parallel sequencing ('next-generation sequencing') (not yet in routine use in clinical laboratories)

Allele-specific PCR using allele-specific oligonucleotides (ASOs)

- For a known (e.g. recurring) single mutation
- Multiple as in an amplification refractory mutation system (ARMS) and oligonucleotide ligation assay (OLA)

Restriction digest and gel electrophoresis (e.g. if a restriction site is created or abolished by the mutation)

Detection of expanded trinucleotide repeats

Fluorescent PCR and product-length analysis on an automated DNA sequencer

Triplet repeat-primed PCR (TP-PCR)

Southern blotting (e.g. for fragile X syndrome) using radioactivity or chemiluminescence

Pre-sequencing mutation screening

Heteroduplex analysis by gel electrophoresis

Conformation-sensitive capillary electrophoresis (CSCE)

Denaturing high-performance liquid chromatography (dHPLC)

High-resolution melt curve analysis (HRM)

Detection of submicroscopic duplications and deletions

Multiplex ligation-dependent probe amplification (MLPA)

Multiplex (dosage) PCR (less commonly used than MLPA)

Array comparative genomic hybridisation (aCGH)

Rapid detection of aneuploidies

Quantitative fluorescent PCR (QF-PCR)

Basic methods

Polymerase chain reaction

PCR permits the production, within 3 h, of enormous numbers of copies of a specific DNA sequence (i.e. DNA amplification), starting with minute quantities (50 ng or less) of the initial target DNA.

The steps involved in PCR are illustrated in Fig. 4.1. Two oligonucleotide primers are required, which are designed to be complementary to the flanking sequences of the target segment of DNA that is to be amplified (which is commonly up to 1 kb in length, occasionally up to 10 kb). The primers direct repeated cycles or rounds of localised DNA replication to produce an exponential increase in the number of copies of the target sequence (Fig. 4.2). Each cycle consists of three steps: heat denaturation (i.e. rendering the DNA single stranded), primer annealing and strand elongation. A crucial component is a thermostable DNA polymerase, such as *Taq* polymerase, that can tolerate the high denaturation temperature of around 95 °C. After 25–35 cycles (which takes 2–3 h in an automated procedure), the target DNA will, in theory, have been amplified 2^{25} (or 3×10^7) to 2^{35} (or 3×10^{10}) fold and the corresponding product will constitute the bulk of all DNA present. The DNA amplification product can then be checked by direct visualisation under ultraviolet (UV) light following gel electrophoresis and staining with a DNA stain such as ethidium bromide (or a less mutagenic compound such as SYBR Safe). Commonly, to detect small changes such as nucleotide substitutions and small insertions or deletions, the DNA product will be sequenced by an automatic sequencing strategy (see below). Alternatively, in order to detect a specific sequence change, the DNA can be subjected to an appropriate restriction enzyme digest and the resulting fragments separated and visualised by gel electrophoresis and DNA staining.

The adaptations of PCR include quantitative fluorescent PCR (QF-PCR), allele-specific PCR such as in the amplification-refractory mutation system (ARMS), triplet repeat-primed PCR and multiplex ligation-dependent probe amplification (MLPA) (Table 4.1). These are discussed in more detail below.

Restriction digests

Restriction digests are reactions that use DNA cleavage enzymes, which will only cut at specific DNA sequences. These

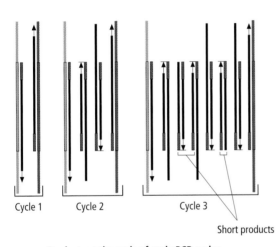

First round of the PCR

Products at the ends of early PCR cycles

Fig. 4.1 Steps involved in amplification of a DNA segment using PCR. After several cycles, the amplified target short products predominate. dNTP: deoxynucleotide triphosphate.

sequence-specific enzymes are called restriction enzymes and they are found naturally in bacteria where they function as a defence mechanism against the incorporation of foreign DNA. More than 400 different restriction enzymes have been described, which together possess over 100 different recognition sites for DNA cleavage. Each enzyme is named after the organism from which it was first isolated (e.g. *Eco*RI was found in *Escherichia coli*). The recognition site is commonly 4 or 6 bp in length and the cleavage may produce flush ('blunt') or staggered ('sticky') ends (Fig. 4.3). By convention, each recognition site is written 5′ to 3′ using the symbols A, T, C and G for specific bases, as well as N for any nucleotide, R for either purine (A or G) and Y for either pyrimidine (T or C). A single nucleotide substitution in a patient can eliminate a restriction

enzyme's target sequence and can therefore be detected by testing the ability of a restriction enzyme to cut the patient's DNA at that location (Fig. 4.4). However, with the increasing availability and efficiency of DNA sequencing technology and of allele-specific PCR (see below), the use of restriction digests in diagnostic laboratories has become much less common than previously.

Mutation detection

Pre-sequencing methods for mutation screening

Specific point mutations may be demonstrated by DNA sequencing (see below) in addition to a number of other methods that may be appropriate, depending on whether scanning for mutations or testing for a specific known mutation is being undertaken. Where mutation analysis is to be carried out to detect a possible base change of unknown location, a rapid screening strategy may be employed initially to identify a DNA segment (e.g. an exon) that may contain a mutation, prior to DNA sequencing of that region of the gene. Several such methods include heteroduplex analysis, which is designed to detect the abnormal properties (e.g. altered mobility upon electrophoresis through a non-denaturing polyacrylamide gel, or resistance to denaturation upon heating) of the heteroduplex molecules. These form (by base pairing between mutant and normal strands of DNA) in the presence of DNA containing heterozygous mutations. To perform these analyses, therefore, these heteroduplexes are allowed to form in the laboratory by heating the DNA to 95 °C and then cooling it to 25–40 °C. A more recent development, called conformation-sensitive capillary electrophoresis (CSCE), is similar to the gel electrophoresis heteroduplex analysis but instead involves fluorescent detection of the heteroduplexes, permitting automation and greater sensitivity.

A further related technique, known as denaturing high-performance liquid chromatography (dHPLC) detects the slightly reduced ability of such heteroduplexes to bind to a DNA-binding cartridge (Fig. 4.5). Although high sensitivity is possible, drawbacks of dHPLC include the necessity for the assays to be optimised for the specific DNA sequence being tested and the often subtle indications of the presence of a mutation. This method is usually reserved for the repeated analysis of multiple samples.

A more recently developed technique for pre-sequencing screening of DNA segments for the presence of heteroduplexes (indicating a likely heterozygous mutation), is high-resolution melt curve analysis (HRM). After allowing heteroduplexes to form (as above), the DNA molecules are heated very gradually from around 65 to 95 °C to cause the strands to slowly separate. When heteroduplexes are present, the strands will separate slightly earlier (detected as a reduction in the fluorescence emitted from double-stranded DNA-binding dye molecules), indicating the possible presence of a mutation. This would be followed by DNA sequencing of such regions of the gene.

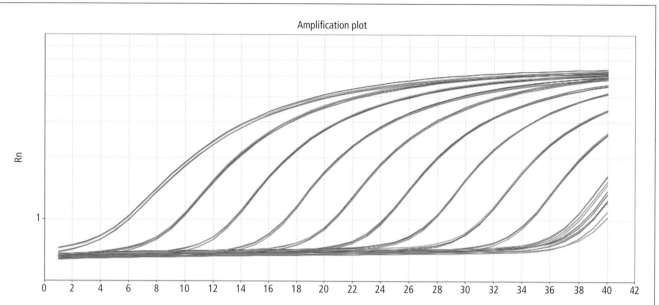

Fig. 4.2 Exponential increase in product formed by PCR with increasing number of cycles on real-time PCR analysis. Fluorescence intensity is represented on the *y*-axis (as normalised intensity of the reporter dye 'Rn') and PCR cycle number is represented on the *x*-axis. The different exponential curves, from left to right, indicate PCRs carried out using serial tenfold dilutions of the same template DNA. With a more dilute template, the number of cycles required to generate the same product level increases. All reactions eventually level off at a plateau level where no further product can be generated, probably due to the depletion of reagents and the accumulation of inhibitory products. Image kindly provided by Alexander Fletcher, University of Glasgow.

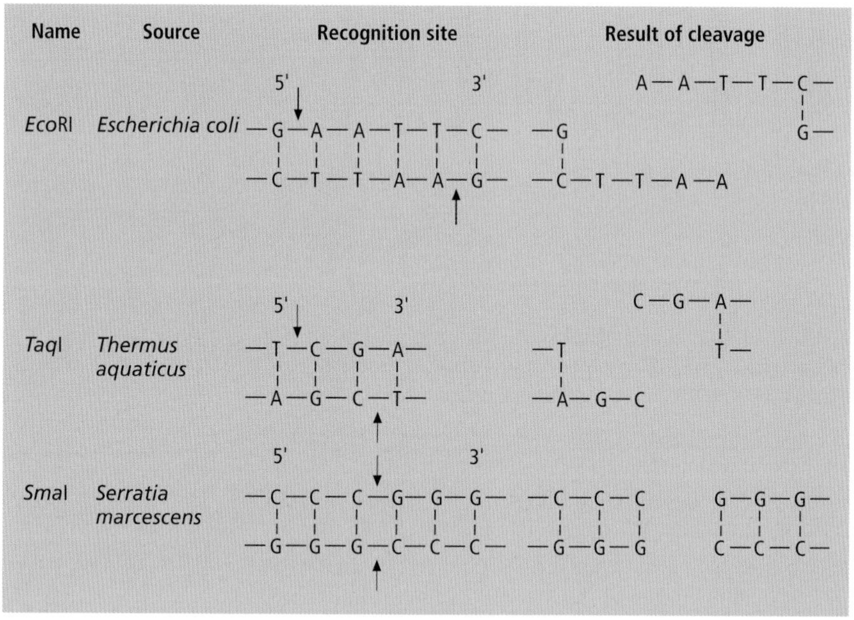

Fig. 4.3 Examples of restriction enzymes and their recognition sites.

Sanger (dideoxy) sequencing

DNA sequencing is the determination of the precise sequence of nucleotides in a section of DNA. In diagnostic laboratories, at present, the sequencing method most commonly used is fluorescent dideoxy chain termination (based on the method originally developed in 1975 by the double Nobel prize winner Frederick Sanger). This involves a PCR-like reaction (but with just a single forward or reverse oligonucleotide primer) and utilises a DNA template to generate a series of detectable single-stranded fragments of increasing length, each being 1 nucleotide longer than the last. In this method, a chemical reaction is first set up, which includes the DNA template (often, itself, a purified PCR product), a thermostable DNA polymerase, a single oligonucleotide primer and the four deoxynucleotide triphosphate (dNTP) substrates (dATP, dCTP,

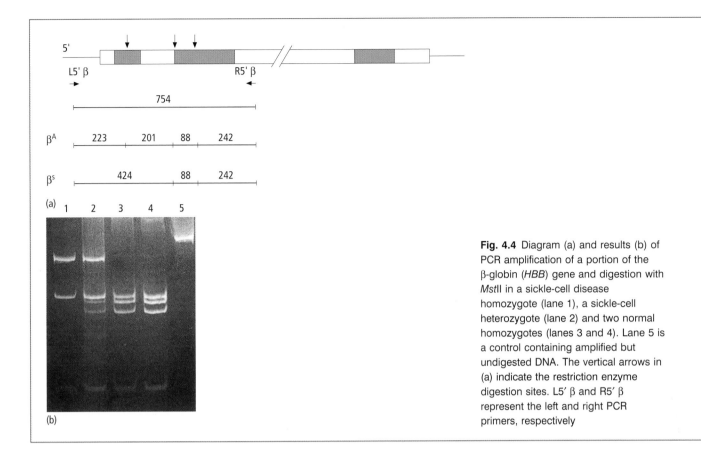

Fig. 4.4 Diagram (a) and results (b) of PCR amplification of a portion of the β-globin (*HBB*) gene and digestion with *Mst*II in a sickle-cell disease homozygote (lane 1), a sickle-cell heterozygote (lane 2) and two normal homozygotes (lanes 3 and 4). Lane 5 is a control containing amplified but undigested DNA. The vertical arrows in (a) indicate the restriction enzyme digestion sites. L5′ β and R5′ β represent the left and right PCR primers, respectively

dGTP and dTTP). In addition, a small quantity of dideoxy-nucleotide triphosphates (ddNTPs: ddATP, ddCTP, ddGTP and ddTTP) are included together in a single tube, each with a different attached fluorescent chemical label (each emitting a different wavelength or colour of light). DNA polymerisation takes place, incorporating dATP, dCTP, dGTP and dTTP, generating a new strand of DNA that is exactly complementary to the DNA template. Eventually, however, at some point, a ddNTP will be incorporated by chance instead of a dNTP substrate molecule. At this point, further elongation of that chain is halted, because a ddNTP lacks the 3′-OH group on the deoxyribose sugar that is necessary for the addition of the next nucleotide (Fig. 4.6).

The result is a series (all present together within a single tube) of partially completed product chains each with a particular fluorescent ddNTP at its 3′ end. Subsequently, in an automated sequencer machine, these product molecules can be separated on the basis of length by gel electrophoresis (in a very long capillary tube) and then electronically detected and identified (by the wavelength of the emitted fluorescence, upon excitation by a laser) as they migrate through the gel (Fig. 4.7). The order in which the four fluorescent labels are detected (corresponding to the sequence of the four different nucleotides in the DNA being analysed) can then be visualised and recorded using appropriate software (Figs 4.8 and 4.9). The two strands of the target region are synthesised separately, using either a forward or a reverse oligonucleotide primer. The two

resulting complementary sequences that are generated are then aligned by computer, allowing the user to check that any presumed mutation is detected in both directions (as occasional sequencing artefacts are generally manifest in just one of the two directions).

Massively parallel ('next-generation') sequencing

Although not yet in routine use in most clinical laboratories, new techniques for DNA sequencing, permitting very high throughput, have now become available. Several different methods have been developed, which are reviewed in detail by Tucker *et al.* (2009) (see Further reading).

An example is 'sequencing by synthesis' (on an Illumina Genome Analyzer). This technology involves the incorporation into a new strand, which forms along a genomic fragment template, of a single base (with a chemical block at its 3′-OH). This is sequentially followed by imaging of the fluorescence emitted by this newly added base, removal of the 3′-OH block and automated repetition of these three steps. This is carried out on millions of chains of nucleotides, elongating simultaneously upon a single surface (or 'chamber'), with high-resolution image capture and sophisticated processing.

Other technologies include 'pyrosequencing' of DNA attached to agarose beads within emulsion droplets (Roche GS-FLX 454). Several even newer sequencing technologies are now being developed. One of these essentially involves

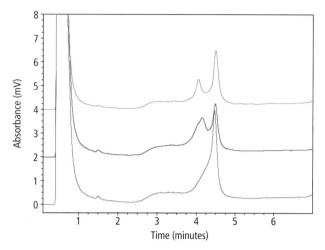

Fig. 4.5 Pre-sequencing analysis of a patient's DNA using dHPLC, following initial PCR and then heating and cooling to allow heteroduplex formation. In the lower fluorescence trace, the result (shown in red) can be seen for the PCR product for this region (exon 20 of the *BRCA2* gene) at a detection temperature of 55 °C. The middle trace (blue) represents the clearly abnormal result for that exon for a known mutation carrier (i.e. a positive control). The additional peak, to the left of the normal peak, is the result of the earlier release from a DNA-binding cartridge of the exon PCR product upon washing with a steadily increasing concentration of acetonitrile (with time shown on the *x*-axis). The additional peak represents the heteroduplex molecules, which elute (i.e. are released) earlier than the homoduplexes. In the upper trace (green), the additional peak is again clearly seen, indicating a possible sequence change in the sequence of this patient. This was an individual who was affected by familial breast cancer but for whom the *BRCA2* gene had not yet been sequenced. The result, therefore, suggested that DNA sequencing should be performed on exon 20 of *BRCA2* in that patient in order to determine whether or not a mutation was present. A single-nucleotide substitution was indeed subsequently found to be present. In practice, however, the changes in the output traces resulting from such mutations can be much less evident than that shown here.

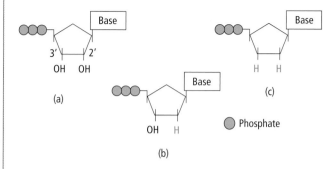

Fig. 4.6 Difference between (a) ribonucleotides, (b) deoxyribonucleotide triphosphates (dNTPs) and (c) dideoxyribonucleotide triphosphates (ddNTPs). Ribonucleotides, present in RNA, possess a hydroxyl (-OH) group at both the 2′ and 3′ positions of the ribose. The dNTPs, present in DNA, have a 3′-OH group (although not a 2′-OH group). The ddNTPs, however, cause DNA chain termination because they possess a hydrogen (-H) instead of the -OH group at the 3′ position and therefore cannot react further. Courtesy of Maria Jackson and Leah Marks, University of Glasgow.

patient's DNA fragments are all molecularly bar-coded or tagged with a short synthesised nucleotide sequence, allowing that patient's DNA sequence data to be extracted subsequently by the associated software.

At present, such machines are extremely expensive, although they are likely to become much cheaper. In addition, the lengths of DNA that such machines can 'read' are often much shorter than with current Sanger dideoxy sequencing. This necessitates sequence assembly, which can be difficult in repetitive or rearranged regions of the genome. There is also a higher error rate in the raw sequence data than with the Sanger method, although this is more than offset by the ability to sequence in great 'depth', i.e. to sequence the same region many times over (e.g. 40-fold). It should be noted, however, that, although such new technology can make the acquisition of DNA sequence data much more rapid, it will still be necessary for clinical laboratory scientists to prepare genomic template DNA that is appropriately enriched for the genes to be sequenced, by PCR or hybridisation methods. Moreover, the process of analysing the huge quantity of data generated, in order to detect pathogenic mutations (and to differentiate them from non-pathogenic sequence changes such as single-nucleotide polymorphisms or SNPs) will, of course, still be required, and is likely to be time-consuming, even with sophisticated software.

Screening for a set of recurrent mutations

If a mutation is one of a limited number of known recurrent specific base changes, its presence may be detected in several additional ways. For instance, allele-specific PCR may be carried out with primers known as allele-specific oligonucleotides (ASOs), which are specific at their extreme 3′ end for

electrophoretically pulling single DNA molecules through microscopic holes known as nanopores. If an electric charge is applied to the nanopore itself, then, as different nucleotides pass through, the DNA sequence can be determined from the distinguishable, although minute, sizes of the current that flows.

The result is the generation of an enormous quantity of sequence data (at least 2000 Mb, or 2 Gb, per day). This would potentially permit the analysis of the entire coding regions of multiple genes all at the same time. This would therefore be of particular value for conditions that exhibit marked locus heterogeneity, such as hypertrophic cardiomyopathy, deafness and retinitis pigmentosa. In addition, the DNA of several patients can be pooled and analysed simultaneously, provided that each

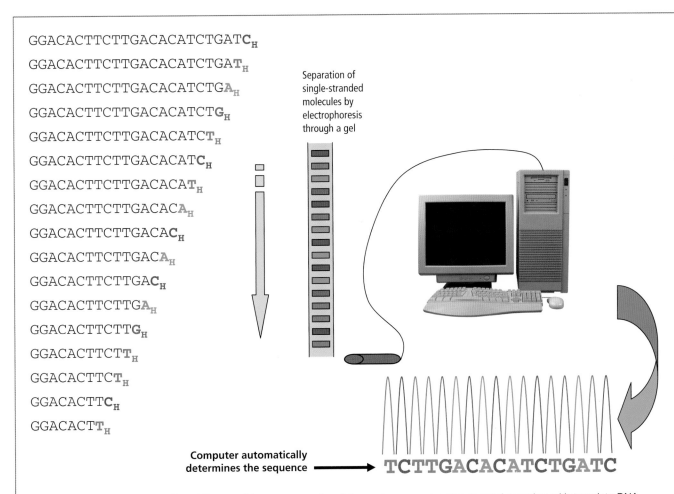

GGACACTTCTTGACACATCTGAT**C**_H

GGACACTTCTTGACACATCTGA**T**_H

GGACACTTCTTGACACATCTG**A**_H

GGACACTTCTTGACACATCT**G**_H

GGACACTTCTTGACACATC**T**_H

GGACACTTCTTGACACAT**C**_H

GGACACTTCTTGACACA**T**_H

GGACACTTCTTGACAC**A**_H

GGACACTTCTTGACA**C**_H

GGACACTTCTTGAC**A**_H

GGACACTTCTTGA**C**_H

GGACACTTCTTG**A**_H

GGACACTTCTT**G**_H

GGACACTTCT**T**_H

GGACACTTC**T**_H

GGACACTT**C**_H

GGACACT**T**_H

Separation of single-stranded molecules by electrophoresis through a gel

Computer automatically determines the sequence ⟶ **TCTTGACACATCTGATC**

Fig. 4.7 Diagrammatic illustration of Sanger dideoxy sequencing. A forward or reverse primer is used, together with template DNA consisting of a product from a previous standard PCR. Many single-stranded products will be generated, each prematurely terminated when, by chance, a ddNTP (shown in colour, with a subscript 'H' indicating the 3'-H instead of 3'-OH group) is incorporated into the new molecule instead of the more abundant dNTP. The ddNTPs lack the 3'-OH group on the deoxyribose sugar that is necessary for further extension of the chain. After generation of the mixture of many single-stranded products, terminated at different positions with ddNTPs, the products are separated by electrophoresis through a gel (generally within a long capillary tube). As each of the four different ddNTPs is fluorescently labelled with a different fluorophore, the identity of the base at each position can be determined by detecting the colour or wavelength of fluorescence of each ddNTP as it passes through a detector near the end of the capillary. A computer interprets the emitted fluorescence signals and thus automatically determines the sequence of the DNA. The computer-determined sequence indicated with an arrow at the foot of the diagram shows only the portion of the DNA sequence into which fluorescent ddNTPs were incorporated. It therefore does not show the nucleotide sequence for the DNA that immediately precedes this region (i.e. GGACACT). Courtesy of Maria Jackson and Leah Marks, University of Glasgow.

either the mutant or the normal sequence. The principle is that PCR amplification takes place only when the 3' nucleotide of the primer can correctly base-pair with the template DNA. This is the basis of the so-called amplification refractory mutation system or ARMS test. A related method for the detection of pre-defined mutations is the oligonucleotide ligation assay (OLA), in which the allele-specific primers for different mutations possess 5' tails of different lengths. In this OLA method, the 3' end of a correctly base-paired oligonucleotide is able to be ligated (i.e. joined via a 3'–5' phosphodiester covalent bond) to an adjacent common fluorescent primer and the ligated product can then be identified on a DNA sequencer. Several mutations can be tested simultaneously, the differing 5' tails permitting the products to be distinguished subsequently by their length. Methods based on ARMS and OLA have been used successfully in diagnostic laboratories for the detection of many common cystic fibrosis gene mutations (Fig. 4.10). Alternatively, in some cases it is possible to identify a mutation by the loss or gain of a specific restriction site, using PCR to amplify the region followed by an appropriate restriction digest and subsequent gel electrophoresis to check the products. Finally, DNA sequencing can, of course, be used to

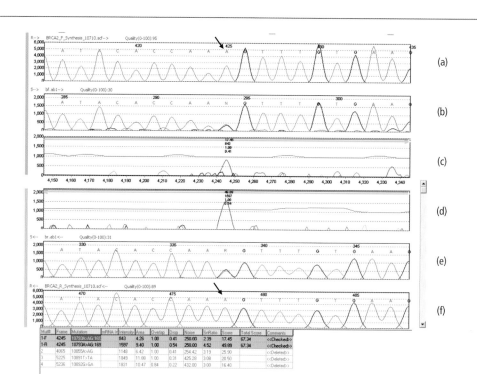

Fig. 4.8 Electropherogram showing the DNA sequencing results for a patient affected by familial breast cancer who possesses a *BRCA2* mutation. The result shows a single-nucleotide A to G substitution. This mutation (c.506A>G; p.Lys169Arg) can be seen to be heterozygous, as, at the substituted nucleotide (indicated by an arrow), there are two superimposed peaks, each resulting from the sequencing of one allele. The A is the nucleotide at that position in the wild-type or normal sequence, whereas the G represents the allele containing the mutation. The output shows the forward and reverse sequences, aligned so that the user can check that the sequence alteration has been detected by bidirectional sequencing to eliminate artefacts. A set of six traces is shown (a–f). The patient's DNA sequence is indicated in the electropherogram trace that is second from the top (for sequencing using the forward primer; trace b) and second from the bottom (e; reverse direction), with the Genbank reference normal sequences being represented in the top and bottom traces (a and f, respectively) and a computerised prediction of mutation likelihood visible in the middle two traces (c and d).

detect a pre-defined mutation although this may be less efficient when several samples are to be checked for the same set of specific base changes located in different exons.

Detection of deletions and duplications by DNA-based methods

Small length mutations may be identified by PCR followed by DNA sequencing. Larger changes in length can be detected by Southern blot analysis (see below) or by one of a range of more modern techniques. For instance, large expansions of trinucleotide repeats (e.g. of more than 100 triplets), particularly $(CTG)_n$ in myotonic dystrophy and $(GAA)_n$ in Friedreich's ataxia, can be detected by an alternative technique named triplet repeat-primed PCR (TP-PCR), which is described further in Chapter 16. The large $(CGG)_n$ repeat in fragile X syndrome, however, is more difficult to analyse by this method. This is perhaps due to the resulting very high CG content and consequent abnormally high levels of hydrogen bonding in this expansion, located in the promoter region of the associated

FMR1 gene. This is therefore one of the few conditions for which Southern blotting is currently still in use in diagnostic laboratories.

An increasingly used alternative method for the detection of large deletions and amplifications affecting specific genes is the technique known as multiplex ligation-dependent probe amplification (MLPA) in which PCR is used to simultaneously analyse the copy number at multiple points along a particular DNA sequence (Fig. 4.11). A range of commercially developed MLPA kits is now in routine use in diagnostic laboratories for the rapid detection of deletions affecting the genes responsible for various conditions including hereditary breast and colorectal cancer, neurofibromatosis type 1, Williams syndrome, velo-cardiofacial syndrome, Prader–Willi syndrome, Angelman syndrome and Smith–Magenis syndrome.

In general, deletions and duplications involving several exons (such as in many cases of Duchenne muscular dystrophy and often in several cancer genes such as *BRCA1* and *BRCA2*) are difficult to detect using DNA sequencing and are likely to be too small to detect by karyotyping or even fluorescence *in*

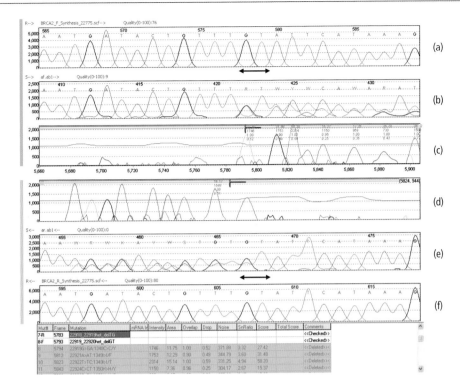

Fig. 4.9 Electropherogram similar to that shown in Fig. 4.8, but showing the DNA sequencing results for a different, unrelated, patient, similarly affected by familial breast cancer. This patient, in contrast, possesses a deletion of 2 bp (indicated by an arrow), again in *BRCA2*. This mutation (c.4043_4044delGT; p.Cys1348Tyr FsX 3) can again be seen to be heterozygous. In this output, from the position of the deletion onwards, the sequence is difficult to read. This is because the sequence trace from the mutant allele is advanced by 2 nucleotides relative to the normal sequence, onto which it is superimposed. In the forward sequencing of the patient's DNA (b), the traces appear to be disordered to the right of the start of the deletion, whereas in the reverse sequence (e), the disordered superimposed sequence is visible to the left of the deletion. The 'FsX 3' in the mutation nomenclature indicates that the frameshift in translation that results from the deletion of the 2 nucleotides causes protein truncation with a premature stop codon occurring just three codons downstream from the resulting amino acid substitution.

situ hybridisation (FISH). If available, a specific MLPA kit can be used to detect such abnormalities. An alternative, however, is to use PCR to amplify several regions of a gene simultaneously, by 'multiplex PCR', allowing a subsequent comparison to be made of the abundance of each of the resulting products, thus revealing regions of altered copy number (Fig. 4.12).

An increasingly used DNA-based method for the detection of relatively large (i.e. generally too large to be detected by DNA sequencing) submicroscopic genomic deletions or duplications is array comparative genomic hybridisation (aCGH), which is discussed in Chapter 7. This technique is particularly useful when the location of such an alteration is not already suspected and when the phenotype (e.g. significant dysmorphisms and learning difficulties) suggests that such a deletion may be present even though standard karyotyping has been apparently normal (see Chapter 18). Briefly, the technique involves comparing, at multiple defined positions across the genome, the abundance of an individual's test DNA relative to the abundance of a reference DNA. This is carried out by adding the fluorescently labelled subject's DNA and the reference DNA (e.g. labelled green and red, respectively) to microarrays that contain thousands of specific DNA sequences, then washing off the unbound DNA and laser scanning the microarrays (see Chapter 7 for further details).

Other uses of microarrays in DNA analysis

It should be noted that DNA hybridisation to microarrays can also be used to screen directly for the presence of point mutations in several genes simultaneously. For instance, microarrays can be used to check for a large number of possible mutations in the many genes that can cause childhood deafness (see Kothiyal *et al.*, 2010, in Further reading) or cardiomyopathy (see Zimmerman *et al.*, 2010, in Further reading). The arrays generally have to be custom-designed and they are not used widely in diagnostic laboratories in the UK at present for this purpose.

Alternatively, specific regions of genomic DNA can (after fragmentation of the genome) be 'captured' by hybridisation to custom-designed oligonucleotide arrays in order that these

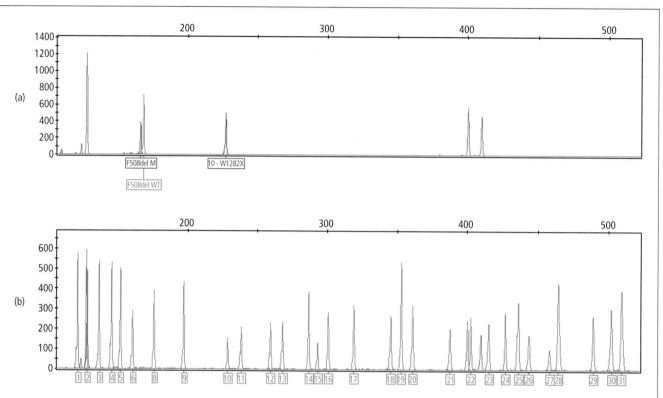

Fig. 4.10 Results of a fluorescent ARMS test for 31 cystic fibrosis gene (*CFTR*) mutations. A commercial kit was used to analyse the commoner *CFTR* mutations in an affected patient. Two sets of fluorescent allele-specific primers were used. These were specific for individual mutants (the products being represented as blue peaks in a) or for individual normal sequences at those sites (shown in green, predominantly in b). The red traces represent PCR products from control primers included in both sets, designed to check that the test has worked. This patient is a compound heterozygote, with two different *CFTR* mutant alleles: ΔF508 (labelled as F508del) and W1282X.

selected DNA regions can subsequently undergo next-generation sequencing as above. This hybridisation-mediated method of DNA enrichment can even be used to select for all protein-encoding exons (i.e. the human 'exome') prior to massively parallel sequencing.

Southern blotting

An additional technique, which is now used less frequently than previously, is Southern blotting. This method can be used to detect large changes in the length of a region of DNA, for instance those resulting from a large deletion or duplication. Deletions may be evident as absent bands or bands of reduced molecular weight. In diagnostic laboratories, one of its few remaining uses is to detect a major expansion of a trinucleotide repeat, in particular that associated with fragile X syndrome. Figure 4.13 illustrates the steps involved in Southern blot analysis (named after its inventor, Professor Sir Edwin Southern). The DNA is cleaved into fragments using a specific restriction enzyme and the fragments are then separated according to size by gel electrophoresis (with the smallest fragments migrating furthest in the gel). At this stage, the multi-

tude of fragments can be visualised as a continuous smear (Fig. 4.13a). These fragments are then transferred to a DNA-binding filter and the fragments of interest are identified using a specific DNA probe (Fig. 4.13b). These probes are sections of DNA, ranging from tens of base pairs to several kilobases (kb) in size, which are used to identify complementary base sequences. Prior to their hybridisation to the filters that contain the patient's DNA, the probes are labelled to permit subsequent detection.

Probe labelling is achieved by the incorporation of modified nucleotides that are either radioactive or, alternatively, have an attached molecule (e.g. digoxigenin) that can subsequently be used to trigger an enzymatic reaction that emits light (a 'chemiluminescent' reaction). The probe and its (filter-bound) target sequences are firstly denatured to render them single-stranded and then incubated together. Upon recognition of their complementary sequence(s), the single-stranded probe and target DNA molecule hybridise (i.e. bind together in a sequence-specific manner) to form a labelled double-stranded molecule that can then be visualised following exposure of the filter to sensitive X-ray film (Fig. 4.13c). This type of analysis, however, relies on starting with sufficient numbers of copies of

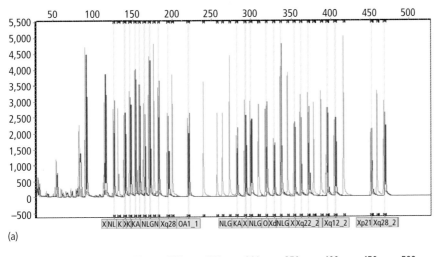

(a)

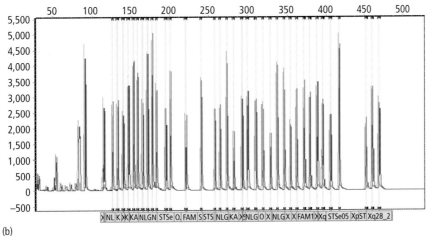

(b)

Fig. 4.11 Results of MLPA for (a) the DNA of a male patient with an *STS* gene (X chromosome) deletion, revealed by the virtually absent blue (patient DNA) peaks for many PCR products relative to the red peaks (control DNA) and (b) a control patient. Fluorescence units are shown on the *y*-axis. Product lengths (in bp) are shown above the top *x*-axis and gene probe names are shown, compressed, below the bottom *x*-axis.

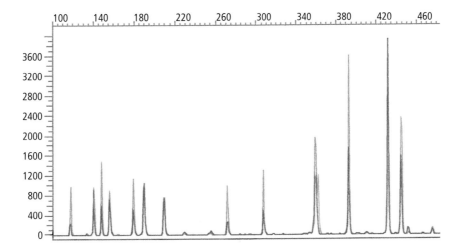

Fig. 4.12 Results from a multiplex 'dosage' PCR test for deletions/duplications in the Duchenne muscular dystrophy (*DMD*) gene. In this analysis, DNA from a female DMD obligate carrier was analysed using multiple sets of fluorescently labelled PCR primers that were designed to be individually specific for many different *DMD* exons. The results are shown in blue, with arbitrary units of fluorescence intensity shown on the *y*-axis and product length in base pairs on the *x*-axis. The red peaks represent the control PCR products (using DNA from a normal control individual) shown together with the blue peaks to allow the user to compare the relative heights of the patient and control peaks (reflecting the abundance of the corresponding PCR products). This permits the user to determine which exons, if any, appear to be present as just one copy in the case of a deletion (or three, in the case of a duplication) rather than two copies. In this case, the blue peaks for several exons (actually *DMD* exons 45–52) are reduced to approximately half the intensity of the red control peaks for those exons, indicating a probable intragenic deletion affecting these exons.

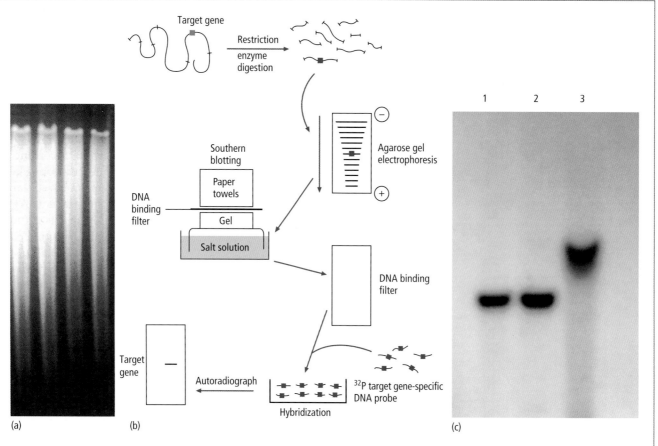

Fig. 4.13 (a) Smear of DNA fragments of various sizes after digestion of four DNA samples and gel electrophoresis (visualised under UV light after staining with ethidium bromide). (b) Diagram of the steps involved in involved in Southern blot analysis. (c) A Southern blot showing the results from two normal males (with *Eco*R1 restriction digest products of 5.2 kb in size in lanes 1 and 2) and an affected male (in lane 3). The DNA product from the affected male, of approximately 6.7 kb, is 1.5 kb larger than that from the unaffected males, as a result of an expansion of approximately 500 trinucleotide repeats.

the DNA target, usually requiring much more DNA than PCR-based techniques (e.g. 5–10 µg) and takes days to produce a result. In the future, Southern blotting is likely to gradually be replaced in diagnostic laboratories by more rapid methods.

Indirect mutant gene tracking

Gene tracking utilises DNA sequence variations to follow the inheritance of mutant (and normal) genes within a family, for instance when no specific pathogenic mutation has been identified. The use of this technique has become much less frequent as the identification of pathogenic mutations has become easier with improvements in DNA sequencing methods. In order to be useful for distinguishing the mutant gene from its partner, the sequence variations at a site are ideally multiple and frequent. By definition, frequent (involving 1% or more of the population) discontinuous genetic variations are called polymorphisms and hence these markers are usually referred to as DNA polymorphisms (Table 4.2). For this purpose,

Table 4.2 DNA polymorphisms useful for indirect mutant gene tracking

Length polymorphisms (variable number of tandem repeats, VNTRs)
Microsatellites, such as the frequently used (CA)$_n$ repeats
Minisatellites (rarely used)
Site polymorphisms
DNA point variations or single nucleotide polypmorphisms (SNPs) (by analysis of restriction fragment length polymorphisms (RFLPs), by sequence-specific fluorescent probes or the use of allele-specific oligonucleotides (ASOs))

microsatellite markers, e.g. (CA)$_n$, are frequently used, on account of their high degree of polymorphism, ease of analysis and large numbers in the genome (see below). Previously, individual restriction fragment length polymorphisms (RFLPs) were used. These are essentially particular SNPs (see below) that alter a restriction enzyme's target sequence and result in a detectable altered DNA product length following PCR of the surrounding region, specific restriction digestion and gel electrophoresis. About one in six SNPs may be identified by using a specific restriction enzyme as described above.

Indirect mutant gene tracking, using adjacent (or internal) polymorphic markers, however, needs DNA samples from multiple family members and relies on an accurate clinical diagnosis and the absence of locus heterogeneity to permit the selection of the appropriate markers. It also has an error rate due to recombination if markers are located at some distance from the mutant gene, and non-paternity can interfere with the analysis. Direct mutant gene analysis, in contrast, needs fewer samples and the demonstration of a mutation often confirms the clinical diagnosis. It is not susceptible to errors due to recombination or non-paternity, and hence it has become the procedure of first choice for DNA analysis for genetic counselling applications. Its drawbacks are that, although the DNA sequence of the human genome is now known, it is not yet known for all diseases which genes are responsible. In addition, the underlying specific genetic alterations need to be defined for each family as a result of the diversity of causative genetic alterations, which is evident for most single-gene disorders. This is complicated by the technical challenge of finding point mutations and small length mutations in genes that are often very large, containing many exons.

Analysis of DNA length polymorphisms

SNPs due to DNA point variations show only two forms (presence or absence of the base change) and hence, at most, only one-half of the population will be heterozygous at a site. In practice, this is an important limitation because, if key individuals in a family are homozygous for the marker, it can no longer be used for genetic prediction. This limitation can be avoided by the use of DNA length polymorphisms, which often have multiple alleles and correspondingly high heterozygosity frequencies.

Length polymorphisms due to variable numbers of tandem repeats are subdivided according to length into microsatellite repeats and minisatellite repeats (see Chapter 3). Microsatellite repeats are under 1 kb in length and the most common repeat motifs are A, CA, AAN (where N is any nucleotide) and GA. CA repeats commonly have 10–60 repeats (with corresponding lengths of 20–120 bp) and are found every 30 kb. In about 70% of individuals, the number of repeats differs between the two homologous chromosomes and thus the length of a DNA fragment (generated by PCR or restriction enzyme digestion) that carries the repeat will vary in length. Moreover, accurate determination of the PCR product length is possible on an automated DNA sequencer if one of the PCR primers is fluorescently labelled (Fig. 4.14). These polymorphic microsatellite DNA markers can therefore be used, as mentioned above, to track neighbouring mutant genes within families (when the pathogenic point mutation itself has not been detected).

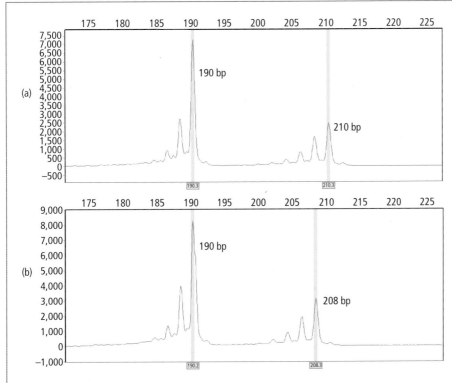

Fig. 4.14 A (CA)$_n$ microsatellite length analysis (performed on an automated sequencer) following fluorescent PCR across an intragenic polymorphic marker. The traces for two siblings, affected by the same autosomal dominant condition known to be caused by this gene, are shown (a and b). Of the three main products (190, 208 and 210 bp, respectively), which result from different repeat lengths, the one that has been inherited by both affected siblings and therefore is most likely to represent the pathogenic allele of the gene, is the 190 bp product.

DNA fingerprinting

Historically, a subsequent development of minisatellite polymorphism analysis was to carry out Southern blotting using probes that simultaneously detected multiple minisatellite loci. Minisatellite repeats are usually 1–3 kb in length and have longer repeat motifs than microsatellite repeats. They again show marked variation in repeat number so that about 70% of individuals are heterozygous for each polymorphism. The result, known as a DNA fingerprint, consists of multiple bands of different sizes that are specific to an individual. Half of the bands are inherited from each parent and thus DNA fingerprinting has been widely used for disputed paternity cases, for resolving family relationships in immigration disputes and for forensic identification of tissue samples at crime scenes (Fig. 4.15).

On account of technological improvements, the preferred method for forensic genetic fingerprinting is now the analysis of multiple (at least ten) highly polymorphic, single-locus, tetranucleotide repeat microsatellites, which, on account of their smaller size compared with minisatellites, can be analysed by PCR rather than by Southern blotting. Owing to the much greater sensitivity of PCR, this permits the successful use of much smaller quantities of DNA. In fact, the use of fluorescent PCR primers and the consequent automated recovery of the resulting marker profiles has led to the rapid entry of such data into DNA databases. The National DNA Database (NDNAD) in the UK now contains well over 5,000,000 DNA profiles and has permitted the identification in the past year alone, of over 11,000 suspects by the identification of matches between these profiles and crime scene DNA samples (see Jeffreys, 2005, in Further reading for an excellent review of the technology, its uses and the surrounding ethical issues). It should be noted that DNA fingerprinting analysis is usually carried out in forensic, rather than in diagnostic, DNA laboratories.

Quantitative fluorescent PCR

A different technique that, unlike DNA fingerprinting, is carried out in diagnostic laboratories but that again involves the analysis of tetranucleotide repeats is quantitative fluorescent PCR (QF-PCR). It is used as a rapid means of prenatally detecting a trisomy of chromosome 21, 18 or 13. In this technique, selected tetranucleotide repeats are amplified by PCR using fluorescent primers and the products analysed on an automated DNA sequencer. Several markers are used for each chromosome, as some markers will be uninformative if the maternal and paternal alleles contain the same number of tetranucleotide repeats at that locus. The user can then compare the signal intensities of the chromosome-specific marker PCR products. Trisomies are detected by the presence of three peaks, representing three alleles instead of two, for individual markers or by a trisomic diallelic pattern, i.e. two peaks with a 2:1 size ratio (see Chapter 7 for further details). The technique is less reliable for the detection of deletions.

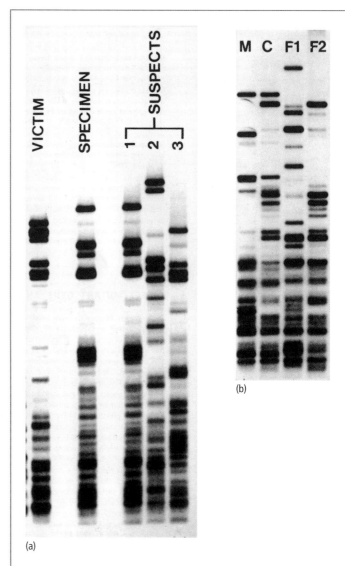

(a)

(b)

Fig. 4.15 DNA fingerprints. (a) From a rape victim, the semen specimen and three suspects. Which suspect which matches the specimen? (b) From a family where paternity was disputed: M, mother; C, child; F1 and F2 are the potential fathers. See questions 6 and 7 in Self-assessment. As mentioned in the text, DNA fingerprinting is now more commonly performed using microsatellite analysis by fluorescent PCR.

Analysis of single-nucleotide polymorphisms

As discussed in Chapter 3, SNPs occur every 200–500 bp in the genome and the majority are thought to be of no clinical significance as they occur in non-coding DNA and do not result in amino acid substitutions within coding DNA (silent mutations). In research laboratories, SNP detection can be carried out by PCR and sequencing of the region that contains it or, more efficiently, by the use of a mixture of two slightly different DNA probes (each with a different attached fluorescent label) that are designed to bind either the normal or the variant sequence, respectively. Such techniques allow the rapid analysis of many different SNPs in hundreds or even thousands of individuals. More modern methods have also now been developed for high-throughput genotyping involving the simultaneous detection of thousands of SNPs across the entire genome using microarray technology. As discussed in Chapter 14, an increasing number of SNPs, have, using such methods, been found to be associated with modest (usually less than twofold) increases in an individual's risk of developing common medical conditions such as type 2 diabetes (see Wellcome Trust Case Control Consortium, 2007, in Further reading). In addition, the presence or absence of various SNPs can be associated with altered pharmacokinetics and drug responses. The analysis of SNPs for either the determination of disease risk or the prediction of drug kinetics or response has not yet been widely adopted in clinical diagnostic laboratories. This may change in the future, however, particularly with the continued expansion of such testing in commercial laboratories.

SUMMARY

- The technique of PCR, in 2–3 h, permits the generation of many millions of copies from a segment of DNA of up to approximately 10 kb in length. PCR requires template DNA, two oligonucleotide primers that are complementary to sequences flanking the target DNA segment, deoxyribose nucleotides and a thermostable DNA polymerase. The PCR product can subsequently be analysed by DNA sequencing or by restriction enzyme digestion and gel electrophoresis. PCR can thus be used to detect small sequence alterations such as substitutions.

- Several methods have been developed to permit the screening of multiple DNA samples for the presence of mutations prior to full DNA sequencing. These methods include heteroduplex analysis on non-denaturing gel electrophoresis, CSCE, dHPLC and HRM analysis.

- Automated DNA sequencing currently uses the fluorescent dideoxy chain termination (Sanger) method. Newer 'next-generation' or 'massively parallel' sequencing methods are currently being developed and tested. These will permit much greater numbers of DNA molecules to be sequenced simultaneously.

- Detection of a set of several recurrent mutations in a specific gene (e.g. the cystic fibrosis *CFTR* gene) can be achieved using ASOs in the PCR-based methods ARMS and OLA.

- Methods for the detection of large duplications/insertions or deletions include Southern blotting, multiplex ('dosage') PCR and more modern methods such as MLPA and aCGH (particularly useful when the chromosomal location of the suspected abnormality is unknown).

- Triplet repeat-primed PCR is helpful for the detection of certain triplet repeat expansions, e.g. in myotonic dystrophy and Friedreich's ataxia.

- When the precise identity of the gene responsible for a family's condition is known but the specific mutation has not been identified, indirect mutant gene tracking can be undertaken. This requires intragenic or adjacent polymorphic DNA markers e.g. $(CA)_n$ repeat microsatellite markers, plus DNA samples from relatives

- QF-PCR is a rapid method used to detect trisomies of chromosome 21, 18 or 13 in prenatal diagnosis. It involves PCR analysis of several tetranucleotide repeats using fluorescent primers.

FURTHER READING

Jeffreys AJ (2005) Genetic fingerprinting. *Nat Med* **11**: 1035–9.

Kothiyal P, Cox S, Ebert J, Husami A, Kenna MA, Greinwald JH, Aronow BJ, Rehm HL (2010) High-throughput detection of mutations responsible for childhood hearing loss using resequencing microarrays. *BMC Biotechnol* **10**:10.

Strachan T, Read AP (2011). *Human Molecular Genetics*, 4th edition. Garland Science: London.

Tucker T, Marra M, Friedman JM (2009) Massively parallel sequencing: the next big thing in genetic medicine. *Am J Hum Genet* **85**:142–54.

Wellcome Trust Case Control Consortium (2007) Genome-wide association study of 14,000 cases of seven common diseases and 3000 shared controls. *Nature* **447**:661–78.

Zimmerman RS, Cox S, Lakdawala NK, Cirino A, Mancini-DiNardo D, Clark E, Leon A, Duffy E, White E, *et al* (2010) A novel custom resequencing array for dilated cardiomyopathy. *Genet Med* **12**:268–78.

Self-assessment

1. Which of the following are required in order to carry out a polymerase chain reaction (PCR)?
A. Single-stranded oligonucleotides
B. Heat-stable RNA polymerase
C. DNA template
D. Deoxynucleotide triphosphates (dNTPs)
E. Approximately 2–3 days

2. Standard PCR and DNA sequencing are useful for the detection of which of the following?
A. A 2 bp deletion
B. A 100 kb duplication
C. A 3 bp deletion
D. An A to G substitution
E. A centric fusion translocation

3. Methods for screening DNA to detect possible mutations prior to DNA sequencing, include which of the following?
A. Conformation-sensitive capillary electrophoresis (CSCE)
B. High-resolution melt curve analysis (HRM)
C. Triplet repeat-primed PCR (TP-PCR)
D. Multiple ligation-depended probe amplification (MLPA)
E. Denaturing high-performance liquid chromatography (dHPLC)

4. Which factors are helpful for indirect mutant gene tracking?
A. The presence of an intragenic microsatellite repeat
B. A microsatellite repeat located very close to the gene
C. The existence of several different causative genes for the condition
D. The existence of a pseudogene
E. DNA sample availability from several affected and unaffected relatives

5. Which of the following are helpful in order to perform quantitative fluorescent PCR (QF-PCR) for the detection of trisomy 18?
A. Fluorescent primers
B. DNA-binding filter or membrane
C. The presence of tetranucleotide repeat markers on chromosome 18
D. DNA polymerase
E. An automated DNA sequencer

6. In Fig. 4.15a showing DNA fingerprints, which of the three suspects matches the specimen?

7. In Fig. 4.15b, which of the two potential fathers (F1 and F2) is the father of the child?

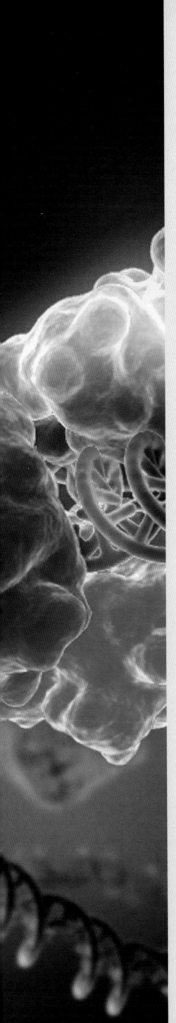

CHAPTER 5
Chromosomes

Key Topics

Introduction

Despite the rapid development and refinement of DNA-based laboratory techniques for the investigation of genetic disorders, the analysis of chromosomes by microscopy currently remains a widely-used and important technique. This chapter discusses the structure of chromosomes, as well as karyotyping and fluorescence *in situ* hybridisation. In addition, the features of mitochondrial chromosomes and the process of mitosis are described.

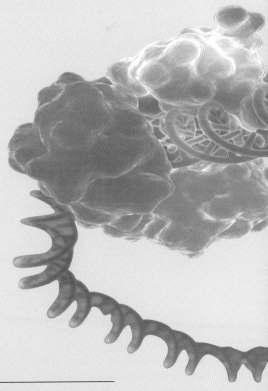

Essential Medical Genetics, 6th edition. © Edward S. Tobias, Michael Connor and Malcolm Ferguson-Smith.
Published 2011 by Blackwell Published Ltd.

Chromosome structure

Chromosomes are named for their ability to take up certain stains (Greek: *chromos* = coloured; *soma* = body). They are present in all nucleated cells and contain DNA with associated acidic and basic proteins in an imperfectly understood arrangement. The basic structure is the elementary fibre, which is 10 nm in diameter. This is composed of repeating units called nucleosomes, each consisting of eight histone molecules, around which 146 bp of the DNA molecule is coiled 1.75 times (Fig. 5.1). The elementary fibre of linked nucleosomes (which appears under the electron microscope as a string of 10 nm 'beads') is, in turn, coiled into a chromatin fibre of 30 nm diameter.

The metaphase chromosome has a central scaffold formed of acidic protein to which the chromatin fibre is attached at scaffold attachment regions (SARs) containing AT-rich repeated sequences. This results in loops of fibre ('Laemli loops' each containing 30–150 kb of DNA) radiating out from the scaffold to form the body of the chromatid, some 0.6 μm in diameter. The loops are attached to the central scaffold by proteins such as scaffold attachment factor-A (SAF-A) multimers. While the details are unclear, this method of compaction allows approxi-mately 2 m of double-stranded DNA to be packaged for cell division into metaphase chromosomes, which range in size from 10 μm (chromosome 1, containing 249 Mb of DNA) to 2 μm (chromosome 21, containing 48 Mb of DNA). It is likely that topoisomerase II, an enzyme that is a major component of the chromosomal scaffold, plays an important role in regulating the chromatin compaction necessary for mitosis (see Hizume *et al.*, 2007, in Further reading). Topoisomerase II achieves this by making a double-stranded cut in the DNA and passing an unbroken double strand through the gap before repairing it.

In addition to facilitating chromatin compaction, individual Laemli loops appear to be fundamental functional units, as each appears to contain only active euchromatin or inactive heterochromatin. Histones, around which DNA is coiled as described above, undergo at least eight different modifications. These can determine the 'chromatin environment' (i.e. euchromatin or heterochromatin, where DNA is kept either accessible or inaccessible for transcription, respectively; see Kouzarides, 2007, in Further reading). The methylation of lysine 9 of histone H3, for instance, is associated with heterochromatin (see Grewal and Jia, 2007, in Further reading). The subsequent transcriptional activation within the euchromatin region is

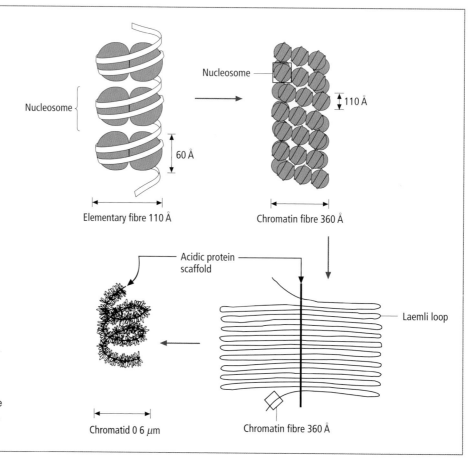

Fig. 5.1 A possible arrangement of DNA and its associated protein in the nucleosome, a chromatin fibre and a chromatid.

dependent in part on various other modifications to histones and in part on the local absence of 5-methylcytosine methylation of DNA. For instance, the access of transcriptional machinery to euchromatin is facilitated by histone modifications that include acetylation of various histone tail amino acids and methylation of lysines 4, 36 and 79 of histone H3. Methylation of lysines 9 and 27 of histone 3 or of lysine 20 of histone H4, are, however, associated with the transcriptional repression of genes. In contrast to areas of euchromatin, areas of heterochromatin contain few active genes and replicate late during S phase. Heterochromatic areas are commonly located close to the telomeres (tips) and centromeres (central chromosomal constrictions; see below) and often contain macrosatellite DNA repeats (see Chapter 3).

Chromosome analysis

Chromosomes are most conveniently studied in peripheral blood lymphocytes, but almost any growing tissue including bone marrow, cultivated skin fibroblasts or cells from amniotic fluid or chorionic villi can also be used. A sample containing 5–10 ml of heparinised venous blood is ideal. The heparin prevents coagulation that would otherwise interfere with the later separation of the lymphocytes. Samples need to be delivered without delay, but a karyotype can still usually be obtained on a blood sample delivered by first-class post.

In the cytogenetics laboratory, phytohaemagglutinin is added to cultures set up from each blood sample and this stimulates the T lymphocytes to transform and divide. After a 48–72 h incubation, cell division is arrested at metaphase by the addition of colchicine (which interferes with the production of spindle microtubules), and a hypotonic solution is added to cause the cells to swell and to separate the individual chromosomes before fixation. The fixed cell suspension is dropped onto microscope slides and air dried to spread the chromosomes out in one optical plane.

The chromosomes may be stained with numerous stains, but for routine karyotyping, G-banding (Giemsa banding) is usually preferred. This produces 550–600 alternating light and dark bands, which are characteristic for each chromosome pair (Figs 5.2 and 5.3) and which reflect different degrees of chromosomal condensation. With G-banding, the dark bands appear to contain relatively few active genes, to be AT-rich and to replicate late in S phase. Light bands contain about 80% of the active genes, including all housekeeping genes (see Chapter 3), are relatively GC-rich and replicate early in S phase. Alternatively, a similar banding pattern can be produced by staining in quinacrine and examining under ultraviolet light (Q-banding). Modern banding allows precise identification of each chromosome and missing or additional material of 4000 kb (4 Mb) or more can be visualised on routine chromosome analysis. Improved resolution of smaller defects is possible by earlier arrest of the dividing cell (promet-

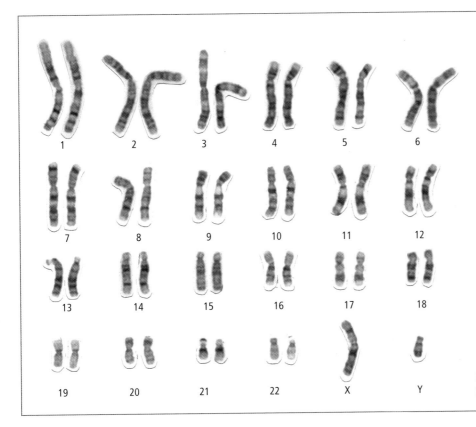

Fig. 5.2 Normal human male karyotype (G-banding, 300 bands).

Fig. 5.3 Normal human female karyotype (G-banding, 800–1000 bands).

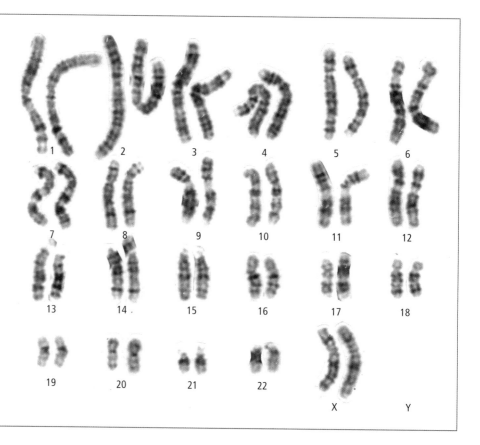

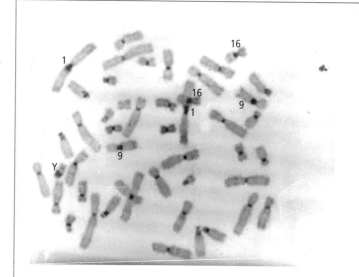

Fig. 5.4 Normal male karyotype (C-banding).

aphase banding, Fig. 5.3), fluorescence *in situ* hybridisation, flow cytometry (see Fig. 5.7) or analysis of the DNA using, for instance, array comparative genomic hybridisation (aCGH; see below and Chapter 7).

The chromosomes can also be treated in a number of different ways to show features such as: highly repetitive macrosatellite repeat DNA in heterochromatin at the centromeres, especially in chromosomes 1, 9 and 16, and the long arm of Y (C-banding, Fig. 5.4); active nucleolus organiser regions (NORs), which contain the ribosomal RNA genes in the satellite stalks (see below) of the acrocentrics (silver NOR stain, Fig. 5.5); the late-replicating X chromosome (5-bromodeoxyuridine (BrdU) staining with incorporation towards the end of DNA synthesis); or the centromeric heterochromatin of 1, 9 and 16 together with distal Yq and proximal 15p (DAPI/distamycin A staining). Some laboratories routinely use R-banding (reverse banding), in which the bands stain in the opposite fashion from that seen with G-banding; this is achieved by heating the chromosomes in a saline buffer before staining with Giemsa and may be useful if the telomeres are involved in aberrations.

Computerised systems for image capture and automated karyotyping are being introduced into an increasing number of diagnostic cytogenetic laboratories. Such systems have the ability to identify cells possessing metaphases of a suitable quality and to perform karyotyping automatically. A trained cytogeneticist is, however, required subsequently to verify the karyotype and to identify any cytogenetic abnormalities. Such systems can greatly reduce the time required for the preparation of a karyotype, permit the electronic storage of images, perform image enhancement when required and permit the

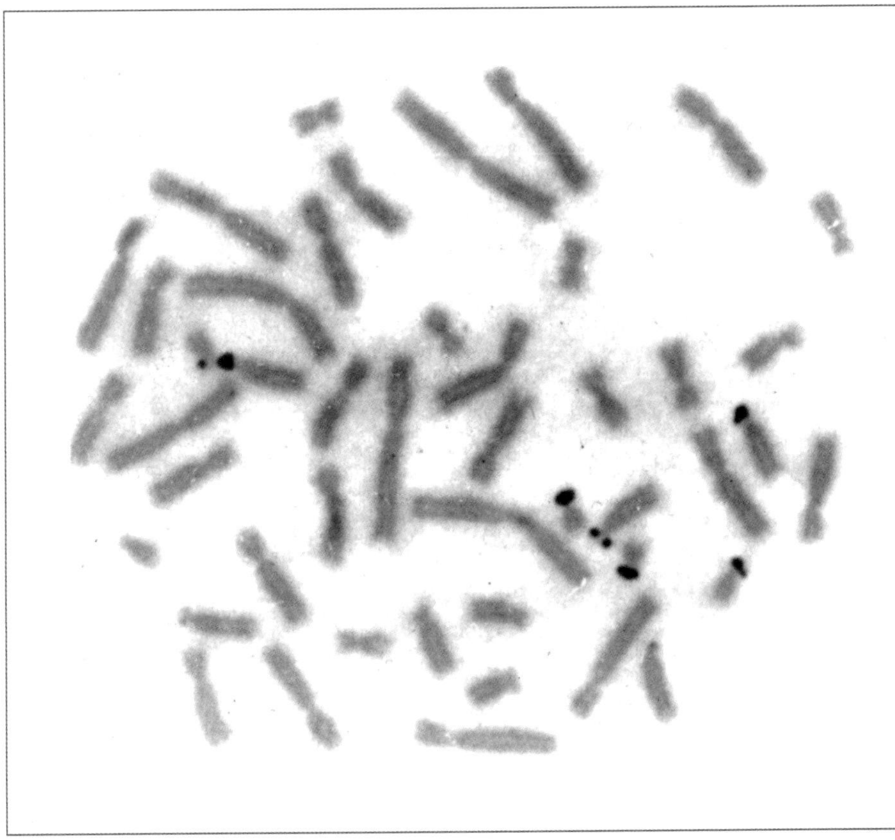

Fig. 5.5 Normal male karyotype (silver NOR stain). Note that not all acrocentrics are stained – this reflects NOR activity.

user to examine specific chromosomes quickly in a series of cells.

The normal human karyotype

Figure 5.3 shows a normal human female karyotype. In total, there are 46 chromosomes, which are arranged in order of decreasing size as 23 matching or homologous pairs. They are divided into the autosomes (numbers 1–22 inclusive) and the sex chromosomes, which consist of two X chromosomes in a normal female. Thus, in such an individual, one of each pair of the autosomes and one X is of maternal origin and the other 23 chromosomes are of paternal origin. In a normal male, there are again 46 chromosomes with 22 pairs of autosomes but a different pattern of sex chromosomes, namely one X chromosome together with a smaller Y chromosome (Fig. 5.2). One of each pair of autosomes and the X are of maternal origin, while the father contributes the Y and the remaining autosomes.

Each chromosome has a narrow waist called the centromere, which is the site of attachment of the spindle fibres by which the two chromatids are drawn to opposite poles of the spindle during cell division. The position of the centromere is constant for a given chromosome, and three subgroups are identified on the basis of the position of the centromere: metacentric – centromere in the middle of the chromosome; acrocentric – centromere close to one end; and submetacentric – intermediate position of centromere. Each chromosome has

a long and a short arm. The short arm is labelled p (from French: *petit*) and the long arm q. The tip of each arm is called the telomere.

Chromosomes 1, 3, 16, 19 and 20 are metacentric or nearly so. Chromosomes 13, 14, 15, 21, 22 and Y are acrocentric, and the remainder are submetacentric. As mentioned above, metaphase chromosomes often show a lack of condensation in the NOR of the short arms of chromosomes 13–15, 21 and 22 due to activity of their clustered ribosomal genes (Chapters 2 and 3) in the formation of the nucleoli. Thus, the ends of the short arms appear as 'satellites', separated from the rest of the chromosome arm by narrow stalks, also known as secondary constrictions (Fig. 5.5).

Karyotypes may be described using a shorthand system of symbols (Paris nomenclature). In general, this has the order: total number of chromosomes, sex chromosome constitution and a description of any abnormality.

Thus, a normal female karyotype is 46,XX whereas that of a normal male is 46,XY. Table 5.1 lists the other commonly used symbols. A standardised numbering system is used for the bands seen with G-banding and this is shown diagrammatically in the human idiogram (Fig. 5.6). This permits the accurate description of breakpoints in chromosome rearrangements and is useful for describing the location of genes in the chromosomal map. Each chromosome in this idiogram is divided into a number of chromosome regions using the ends, centromere and most prominent G-bands as landmarks. The centromere

Table 5.1 Symbols used for karyotype description

p	Short arm
q	Long arm
pter	Tip of short arm
qter	Tip of long arm
cen	Centromere
h	Heterochromatin
del	Deletion
der	Derivative of a chromosome rearrangement
dic	Dicentric
dup	Duplication
i	Isochromosome
ins	Insertion
inv	Inversion
mat	Maternal origin
pat	Paternal origin
r	Ring chromosome
t	Translocation
::	Breakage with reunion
/	Mosaicism
+/−	Before a chromosome number indicates gain or loss of that whole chromosome
+/−	After a chromosome number indicates gain or loss of part of that chromosome
upd	Uniparental disomy

divides the chromosome into short (p) and long (q) arms. Most arms are divided into two or more regions by prominent bands, and each region is further subdivided according to the number of visible bands. Thus, band Xp21.2 is to be found in the short arm (p) of the X chromosome, in region 2, band 1, sub-band 2.

Flow karyotyping

It is possible to harness the technique of flow cytometry to measure the DNA content of individual chromosomes as they pass in a fluid stream through the laser beam of a fluorescence-activated cell sorting (FACS) machine at a speed of 2000 chromosomes per second. The suspension of chromosomes is first stained by a fluorescent dye (usually ethidium bromide), and the fluorescence generated by the laser beam in each chromosome is collected in a photomultiplier and stored in a computer. After several minutes, sufficient individual measurements have been collected to generate a histogram or flow karyotype (Fig. 5.7), which groups the chromosome measurements according to increasing DNA content. Many chromosomes form separate peaks, and the median of each peak

provides an accurate and reproducible measure of the relative DNA content of a particular pair of chromosomes. The area under each peak represents the relative number of chromosomes in each group. As shown in Fig. 5.7, male and female flow karyotypes are clearly distinguished by the size of the X chromosome peak, females having twice the size of the male peak. The technique can be used for assessing variation in individual chromosomes (see Fig. 5.12) and for identifying chromosome aberrations, in particular microdeletions, as its lower limit of resolution is 1–2 Mb compared with 4 Mb for the light microscope. As FACS can also sort chromosomes according to their DNA content, sufficient individual chromosomes or groups of chromosomes can be collected for the preparation of chromosome-specific DNA libraries.

The technique of dual laser flow cytometry allows chromosomes to be resolved not only by their DNA content but also by their AT:GC ratio. The chromosomes are stained by a mixture of two dyes (Hoechst 33258, which has an affinity for AT-rich DNA, and chromomycin A3, which has an affinity for GC-rich DNA) and pass sequentially through the laser beams, which allows the fluorescence generated by each dye to be analysed separately. Figure 5.8 shows bivariate flow karyotypes which not only resolve each chromosome more efficiently than the univariate karyotype but also demonstrate separation of individual homologues.

In situ hybridisation

Sensitive molecular methods can help to characterise individual chromosomes under the microscope by their DNA content. The principle is based on the property of double-stranded DNA to denature on heating to form single-stranded DNA. On cooling, the single-stranded DNA reanneals with its complementary sequence to re-form double-stranded DNA. If an appropriately labelled segment of DNA (a probe) is added to denatured chromosomes on a microscope slide during the process of reannealing, some of the labelled DNA will hybridise to its complementary sequence in the chromosome. Detection of the labelled DNA under the microscope identifies the chromosomal site of its complementary sequence. Initially, radioactive isotopes were used to label DNA probes, but these have been superseded by non-isotopic labels such as biotin; this label can be detected by a fluorochrome coupled to streptavidin. Alternatively, the fluorochrome can be coupled to a nucleotide (e.g. FITC-11-dUTP) used in the preparation of the DNA probe. Fluorescence in situ hybridisation (FISH) is widely used in the diagnosis of chromosome defects (see Chapter 7). It is, for instance, now a useful method of detecting deletions of individual disease-associated chromosomal regions (such as the velocardiofacial syndrome locus at 22q11). The multiple ligation-dependent probe amplification (MLPA) DNA analysis technique (see Chapter 7) now provides an additional method by which specific deletions can be identified but utilises extracted DNA rather than metaphase chromosome preparations.

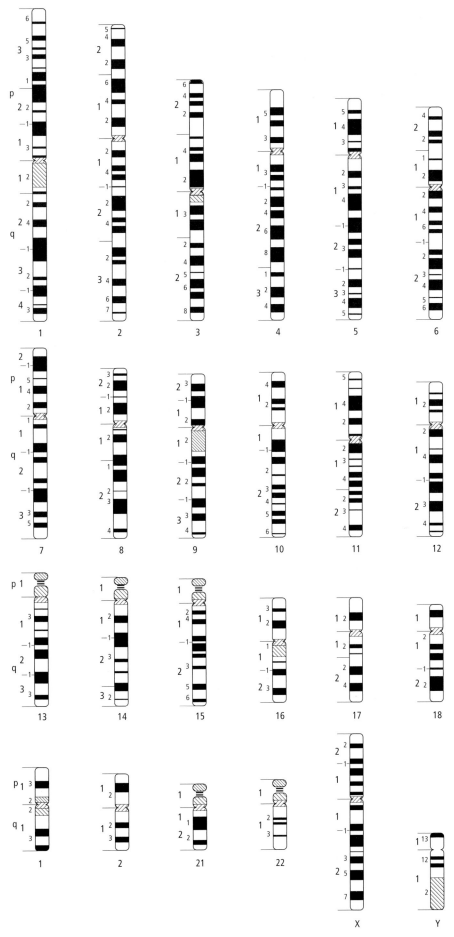

Fig. 5.6 Human idiogram (only the more prominent bands are numbered).

Fig. 5.7 Flow karyotypes of a normal male and a normal female. The peaks correspond to individual chromosome pairs or groups of chromosomes as indicated.

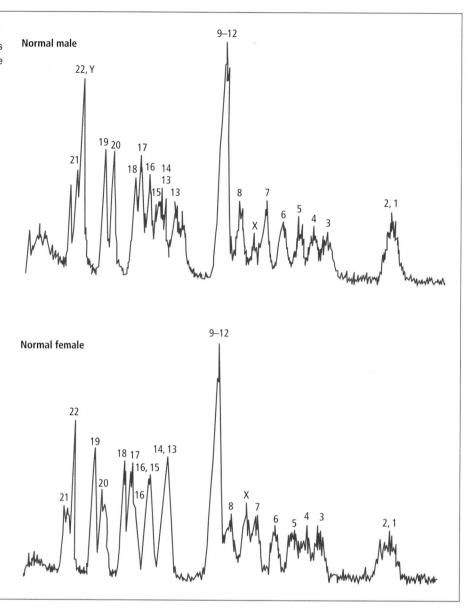

FISH is currently being increasingly used clinically in pre-implantation genetic diagnosis (PGD) in order to determine the fetal sex and to detect unbalanced translocation products in situations where there is a family history of an X-linked recessive genetic condition or a known apparently balanced parental chromosome translocation, respectively (see Chapters 1 and 12).

A useful clinical research technique is to use bacterial artificial chromosome (BAC) probes to carry out FISH in order to locate a specific breakpoint in individuals who have a clinical phenotype and an apparently balanced chromosomal translocation. Once a breakpoint-spanning BAC is identified, it is possible, using online database information, to identify candidates for the likely disrupted causative gene. This research technique was employed (see Johnson *et al.*, 2006, in Further reading) to confirm the *CHD7* gene on chromosome 8 as an important cause of CHARGE association, a syndrome com-prising colobomata, choanal atresia, developmental delay and malformations of the heart and ear.

Complex DNA probes made from multiple fragments of chromosome-specific DNA from flow-sorted or microdissected chromosomes are available that 'paint' the whole chromosome. Multicolour FISH (M-FISH) is a modification of this procedure in which combinations of several different fluorochromes are used to paint all chromosomes simultaneously in different colours allowing analysis of the whole karyotype in one hybridisation (see Chapter 7).

DNA fibre FISH

Microscopic chromosome analysis at the highest resolution is achieved by techniques that release the elementary chromosome fibre from its associated proteins within the chromosome

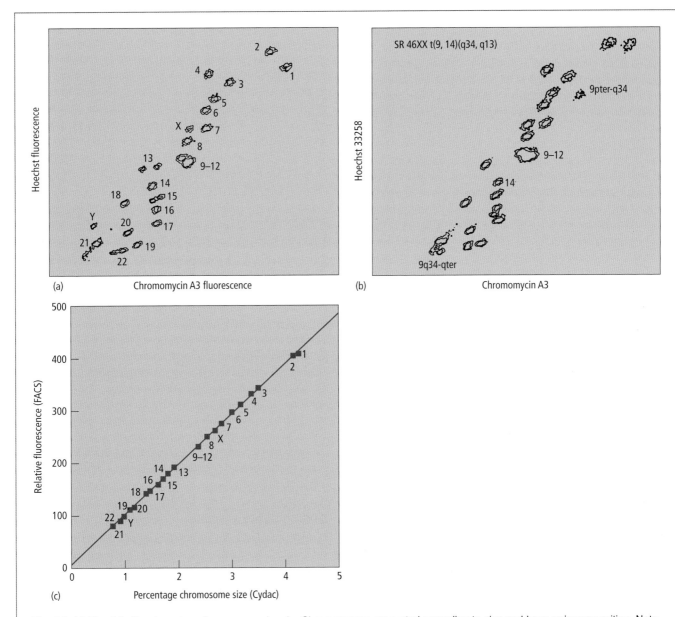

Fig. 5.8 (a) Bivariate flow karyotype from a normal male. Chromosomes are sorted according to size and base-pair composition. Note that chromosomes 13, 15 and 22 resolve into their separate homologues. (b) Bivariate flow karyotype from a female patient (SR) with a 9 : 14 translocation with break points in 9q34 and 14q13. The derivative chromosomes sort near chromosome 3 and 21, respectively. (c) Comparison of the DNA content of chromosomes as measured by microdensitometry and flow cytometry reveals an excellent correlation ($r^2 = 0.999$; $y = 8.4822 + 94.781x$). Note particularly that by both techniques chromosome 19 is smaller than 20 and chromosome 21 smaller than 22. The identity of these chromosomes was defined before DNA measurement was refined.

scaffold. Greatly extended fibres of several megabases in length may be obtained by decondensation of chromatin using detergents and enzymes. When DNA probes are hybridised by FISH to these fibres fixed onto microscope slides, sequences less than 5 kb apart may be separated readily, and distances down to 1 kb have been claimed. Fibre preparations have been particularly useful in determining the order and arrangement of components of centromeric and other types of heterochromatin, and in high-resolution gene mapping.

Chromosome heteromorphisms

Detailed DNA measurements by flow cytometry or microdensitometry reveal that all chromosomes show interindividual variation in DNA content, which is heritable. The Y chromosome shows most variation, while the X chromosome is least variable. The most obvious differences in the appearance of the chromosomes can be seen under an oil-immersion lens in at least 30% of the population. Such differences are called heteromorphisms and are examples of genetic polymorphisms (discontinuous genetic variants present in 1% or more of the population). Size polymorphisms usually involve repetitive DNA, and the degree of variation shows a normal distribution. Four main groups of chromosome heteromorphisms are known: size of Yq, size of centromeric heterochromatin, satellite polymorphisms and fragile sites.

Size of Yq

The commonest chromosomal polymorphism relates to the length of the long arm of the Y chromosome. About 10% of clinically normal males have a Y that is obviously longer or shorter than usual (Fig. 5.9). The long arm of the Y contains non-transcribed repetitive DNA and fluoresces intensely under ultraviolet light with dyes such as quinacrine (Q-banding). This fluorescent region may be visible in an interphase nucleus and is referred to as Y-chromatin (Fig. 5.10).

Size of centromeric heterochromatin

Variations in the size of the centromeric heterochromatin are relatively frequent for chromosomes 1, 9 and 16. Figure 5.11 shows a large chromosome 16 due to excess centromeric heterochromatin, which was present in several healthy family members. Figure 5.12 shows the flow karyotype of an individual with this heteromorphism.

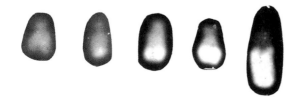

Fig. 5.9 Yq polymorphisms.

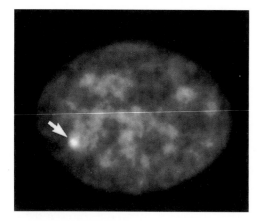

Fig. 5.10 Fluorescent Y-chromatin.

Satellite polymorphisms

Variation in size of the satellites and in the degree of intensity with which they stain by Q-banding may be seen for the acrocentric chromosomes 13, 14, 15, 21 and 22. Much of the variation is due to repetitive DNA, but variation in the number of ribosomal genes also occurs. Size variation, due to differences in DNA content, may occur as a result of mispairing during meiosis at sites of repetitive DNA. This is often termed unequal crossing-over (see Fig. 3.12), and an example of tandem duplication involving a NOR on chromosome 15 is shown in Fig. 5.13.

Fragile sites

Constrictions at sites other than the centromere may be seen and these secondary constrictions may be particularly liable to chromatid breaks. There are at least 89 common fragile sites, which can be induced at low levels in all individuals by aphidicolin and which usually involve both homologues. In addition, 30 rare fragile sites have been described, which collectively occur in about 5% of the population. Most of these are induced by antifolate agents in culture and almost all are autosomal (e.g. at 2q13, Fig. 5.14). These rare autosomal fragile sites, which usually involve only one homologue, show Mendelian inheritance. Most are not associated with any clinical abnormality (except for the X chromosomal fragile site at Xq27.3, which is associated with mental handicap; see Chapter 16). The molecular basis of these fragile sites appears to involve tracts of trinucleotide repeats that have been amplified beyond a critical threshold.

Copy number variation

While the heteromorphisms described above are visible under the microscope, lesser degrees of the same chromosomal variations are detectable using molecular cytogenetic techniques. These variations can also involve repetitive DNA and include transposable elements and gene families. They vary from large segmental duplications up to several Mb in size, to smaller copy number variants. Most appear to have no phenotypic effect, despite being important in initiating chromosome rearrangements through non-allelic homologous recombination (Fig 7.13). These submicroscopic deletions and duplications can be identified by high-resolution aCGH (see Chapter 7).

Chromosomes in other species

With light microscopy, the chromosomes appear essentially similar in all races of man. Among primates, the X chromosome is remarkably constant in size and banding pattern. Other chromosomes are more variable and the variation in chromosome number and appearance is in proportion to the timing of evolutionary separation of the species (Table 5.2). The gorilla, chimpanzee and orang-utan have 48 chromosomes, and the autosomes are similar to those in humans, with the

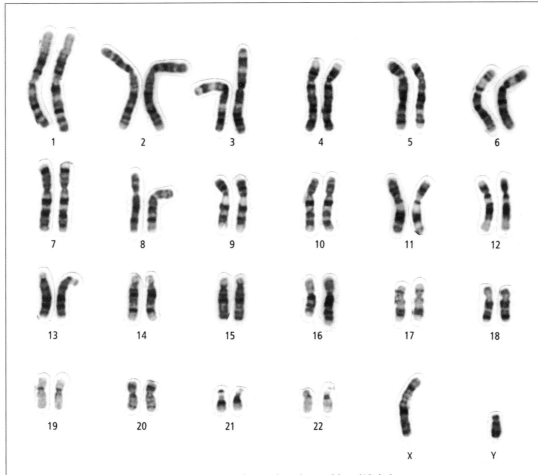

Fig. 5.11 Chromosome 16 centromeric heterochromatin polymorphism (16qh+).

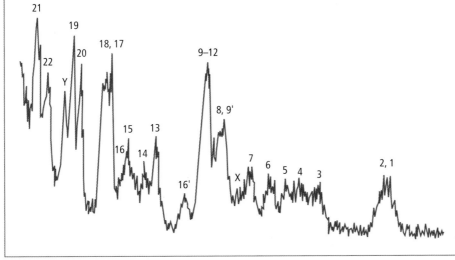

Fig. 5.12 Flow karyotype of 16qh+.

exception of human chromosome 2, which appears to have been derived from two ape acrocentrics after separation of the species (Fig. 5.15). Interestingly, the fragile site on human chromosome 2 seems to mark the site of this ancient fusion (see Fig. 5.14). Large chromosomal segments are conserved even between non-primate mammals and humans. Cross-species chromosome painting studies using chromosome-specific fluorescent DNA probes have been particularly useful in analysing patterns of chromosome homology. Interestingly, analyses of homologous 'synteny' blocks between mammalian species

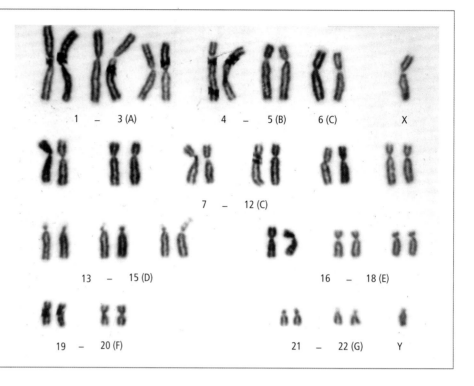

Fig. 5.13 Tandem duplication involving a NOR on chromosome 15 (aceto-orcein staining).

1 – 3 (A)   4 – 5 (B)   6 (C)   X

7 – 12 (C)

13 – 15 (D)   16 – 18 (E)

19 – 20 (F)   21 – 22 (G)   Y

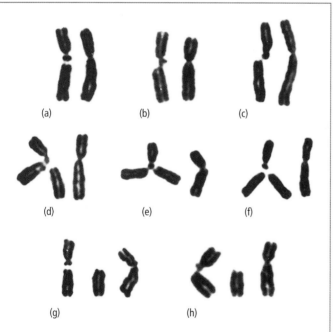

(a)   (b)   (c)

(d)   (e)   (f)

(g)   (h)

Fig. 5.14 Fragile site on chromosome 2 (at 2q13). (a) Site shown as a gap. (b, c) Site shown as chromatid break at gap. (d–f) Triradial chromosomes produced by chromatid breaks in previous division followed by non-disjunction of distal fragment. (g, h) Acentric fragments generated by chromatid breaks.

Table 5.2 Numbers of chromosomes and protein-encoding genes in different species

Species	Chromosome number	Approximate number of protein-encoding genes
Man	46	21,600
Gorilla	48	21,000
Mouse	40	22,700
Dog	78	19,300
Japanese pufferfish (*Takifugu rubripes*)	94	18,500
Drosophila	8	13,800
Escherichia coli	1	4,400
Epstein–Barr virus	1	85
Human immunodeficiency virus type 1	1	10

Mitochondrial chromosomes

Human mitochondria are cytoplasmic organelles that have their own chromosomes in the form of about ten single circular double helices of DNA. These are self-replicating and contain, in their 16,569 bp, 37 genes. These encode 22 mitochondrial transfer RNAs, the two types of mitochrondrial ribosomal RNA and 13 polypeptides, which are synthesised on the mitochondrial ribosomes and are subunits involved in the various steps of cellular oxidative phosphorylation. Human

indicate that, in independent mammalian evolutionary lineages, inter-chromosomal rearrangements have often occurred at apparently identical chromosomal breakpoints. Moreover, these regions tend to be gene-rich. For further details, see Ferguson-Smith and Trifonov (2007) in Further reading.

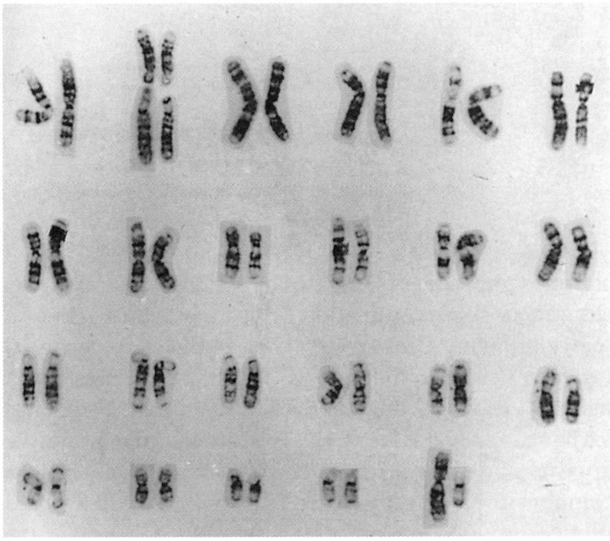

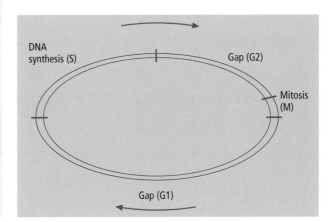

Fig. 5.15 Normal gorilla karyotype.

Fig. 5.16 Diagram of the cell cycle.

mitochondrial DNA differs from nuclear DNA with respect to the codon recognition pattern for several amino acids (e.g. UGA codes for tryptophan rather than chain termination). Furthermore, it has no introns and both strands are transcribed and translated, with around 66% of the mitochondrial genome being protein-coding sequence, in comparison with approximately 1.1% of the nuclear genome. Each cell contains hundreds of mitochondria and, as they are found in the cytoplasm, they are transmitted in the egg from a mother to all of her children (i.e. maternal inheritance). For further details of the composition of mitochondrial chromosomes and the importance of mitochondrial DNA mutations in human disease, see the review by Tuppen *et al.* (2010) in Further reading.

Mitosis

Mitosis is the type of division in somatic cells whereby one cell produces two identical daughter cells. Mitotic cell division occurs in all embryonic tissues and continues at a lower rate in most adult tissues other than end cells, e.g. neurones. Thus, mitosis is vital for both tissue formation and maintenance. In cultured mammalian cells, the duration of the cell cycle varies but is usually about 24 h. Mitosis itself occupies only 20 min to 1 h of the total, whereas DNA synthesis for replication takes 6–8 h (Fig. 5.16).

Five arbitrary stages are apparent in mitosis (Fig. 5.17): interphase, prophase, metaphase, anaphase and telophase. A cell that is not actively dividing is in interphase. This phase thus includes G_1 (gap 1), S (DNA synthesis) and G_2 (gap 2) periods of the cell cycle and during this phase the nuclear material appears relatively homogeneous. Replication of DNA occurs during the S phase, so that the nucleus in G_2 contains twice the diploid amount of DNA present in G_1. Each chromosome

has its own pattern of DNA synthesis, and some segments replicate early (e.g. housekeeping genes and expressed tissue-specific genes) and some late (e.g. centromeric heterochromatin and non-expressed tissue-specific genes). The inactive X is always the last chromosome to complete replication. As the cell prepares to divide, the chromosomes condense and become visible. At this stage, it can be seen that each chromosome consists of a pair of long thin parallel strands, or sister chromatids, which are held together at the centromere. Cross-overs, with exchange of material between sister chromatids, may occur at this stage. BrdU staining may be used to demonstrate these sister chromatid exchanges (Fig. 5.18). The nuclear membrane disappears and the nucleolus becomes undetectable as its component particles disperse. The centriole divides and its two products migrate towards opposite poles of the cell.

Metaphase begins when the chromosomes have reached their maximal contraction. They move to the equatorial plate of the cell and the spindle forms. The acrocentrics are often clustered at this stage (satellite association). Anaphase begins when the centromeres divide and the paired chromatids separate, each to become a daughter chromosome. The spindle fibres contract and draw the daughter chromosomes, centromere first, to the poles of the cell. Anaphase is triggered when a large protease named separase becomes activated following the destruction of its inhibitory regulator, securin. In fact, a surveillance mechanism known as the 'spindle assembly checkpoint' operates in which centromeres that are not properly attached to spindle microtubules (i.e. in chromosomes that are not yet fully aligned on the spindle) prevent securin degradation and thus prevent the onset of anaphase (see Nasmyth, 2005, in Further reading). Separase, once activated, cleaves a component of a complex called cohesin. As it is this complex that holds the sister chromatids together at the centromeres and the chromosome arms, separase activity allows anaphase

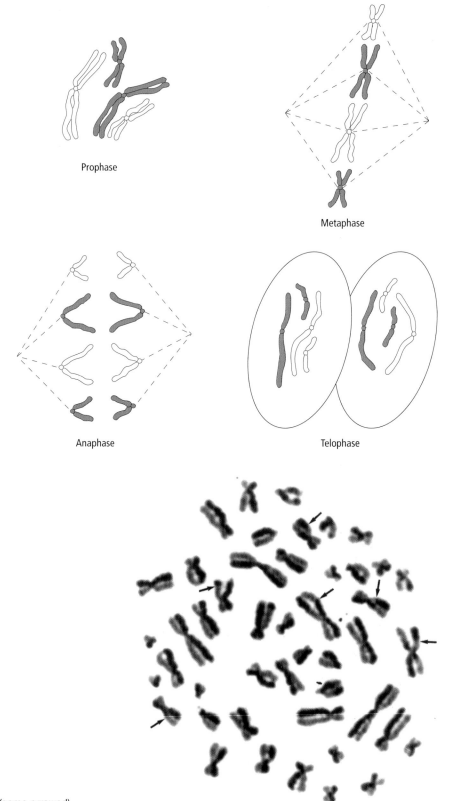

Fig. 5.17 Mitosis. Only two chromosome pairs are shown; the chromosomes from one parent are in outline, while those from the other are coloured.

Prophase

Metaphase

Anaphase

Telophase

Fig. 5.18 Sister chromatid exchanges (some arrowed).

to then proceed. When the daughter chromosomes reach each pole of the cell and following the degradation of the cell separation regulator, cyclin B (with the consequent inactivation of its cyclin-dependent kinase, CDK1), telophase can begin (see Pines, 2006, in Further reading). The cytoplasm divides, the cell plate forms and the chromosomes start to unwind. The nuclear membrane reforms at this stage.

Thus, mitosis results in two daughter cells, each with an identical genetic constitution. Rarely, somatic recombination may occur during mitosis with transfer of segments between homologous chromosomes, at a site known as a chiasma, resulting in homozygosity at gene loci for which the rest of the body cells are heterozygous (Fig. 5.19). This can be an important step in the genesis of some cancers (see Fig. 13.3).

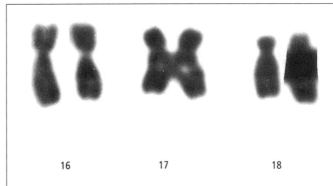

16   17   18

Fig. 5.19 Chiasma formation in a somatic cell.

SUMMARY

- The DNA molecule is packaged into chromosomes by successive layers of compaction that include the formation of nucleosomes, chromatin fibres and Laemli loops.
- Chromosomes can be analysed by staining and light microscopy, with a resolution of approximately 4 Mb.
- Greater resolution can be achieved using FISH, aCGH or flow karyotyping, when available.
- Well-recognised genetic polymorphisms in chromosome content, termed heteromorphisms, include Yq size, centromeric heterochromatin size, satellite polymorphisms and fragile sites.

- In addition, submicroscopic polymorphic chromosome region copy number variants are increasingly being detected by high-resolution techniques such as aCGH (see Chapter 7).
- Mitochondrial chromosomes are circular, possess a distinct genetic code, are maternally inherited and replicate independently of the nuclear chromosomes. They encode 37 genes and possess no introns with 66% of the mitochondrial genome representing protein-coding DNA.

FURTHER READING

Ferguson-Smith MA, Trifonov V (2007) Mammalian karyotype evolution. *Nature Rev Genet* **8**:950–62.

Grewal SI, Jia S (2007) Heterochromatin revisited. *Nat Rev Genet* **8**:35–46.

Hizume K, Araki S, Yoshikawa K, Takeyasu K (2007) Topoisomerase II, scaffold component, promotes chromatin compaction in vitro in a linker-histone H1-dependent manner. *Nucleic Acids Res* **35**:2787–99.

Johnson D, Morrison N, Grant L, Turner T, Fantes J, Connor JM, Murday V (2006) Confirmation of CHD7 as a cause of CHARGE association identified by mapping a balanced chromosome translocation in affected monozygotic twins. *J Med Genet* **43**:280–4.

Kouzarides T (2007) Chromatin modifications and their function. *Cell* **128**:693–705.

Nasmyth K (2005) How do so few control so many? *Cell* **120**:739–46.

Pines J (2006) Mitosis: a matter of getting rid of the right protein at the right time. *Trends Cell Biol* **16**: 55–63.

Tuppen HA, Blakely EL, Turnbull DM, Taylor RW (2010) Mitochondrial DNA mutations and human disease. *Biochim Biophys Acta* **1797**:113–28.

WEBSITES

DECIPHER database:
https://decipher.sanger.ac.uk/application/

Wellcome Trust Sanger Institute: Copy Number Variation Project:
http://www.sanger.ac.uk/humgen/cnv/

Self-assessment

1. Factors that are associated with reduced gene transcription include:
A. 5-Methylcytosine methylation of DNA
B. Acetylation of histone tail amino acids
C. Heterochromatin formation
D. Early replication in S phase
E. Chromosomal regions containing macrosatellite DNA repeats

2. Which of the following most closely approximates the resolution that is achieved by chromosomal staining and light microscopy?
A. 40 Mb
B. 4 Mb
C. 400 kb
D. 40 kb
E. 4 kb

3. Well-recognised genetic polymorphisms with regard to chromosomes include:
A. Yq size
B. Centromeric heterochromatin size
C. Variation in the number of ribosomal genes
D. Submicroscopic duplications of more than 1 Mb in size
E. Constrictions at sites other than the centromere

4. Features of mitochondrial chromosomes include:
A. Double-stranded linear structure
B. Distinct genetic code
C. More than 20 introns
D. The presence of only 37 genes
E. Maternal inheritance

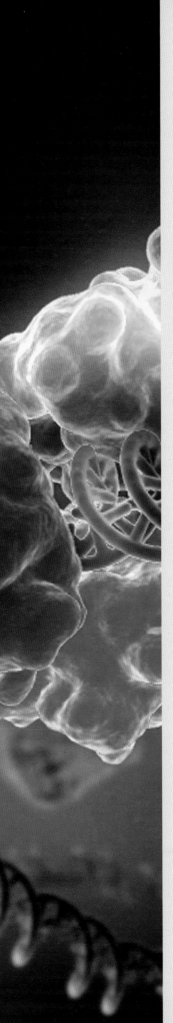

CHAPTER 6
Gametogenesis

Key Topics

Introduction

Gametogenesis (the production of gametes) occurs in the gonads. The somatic diploid chromosomal complement is halved to the haploid number of a mature gamete in such a way as to ensure that each gamete contains one member of each pair of chromosomes. This reduction is achieved by meiotic cell division. Fusion of the sperm and egg restores the diploid number in the fertilised egg. The uniqueness of each gamete is assured by random segregation of maternal and paternal homologues and by recombination during the prophase of the first meiotic (reduction) division. The latter involves the exchange of DNA between maternal and paternal chromosomes. Meiotic cell division is found only in the gonads and is thus less readily studied than mitosis, and as the testis is more accessible than the ovary for biopsy most human information relates to male meiosis. Furthermore, much of the prophase of female meiosis is completed during embryonic development and thus can only be studied in the fetus.

Essential Medical Genetics, 6th edition. © Edward S. Tobias, Michael Connor and Malcolm Ferguson-Smith.
Published 2011 by Blackwell Published Ltd.

Meiosis

Meiosis consists of two successive divisions, the first and the second meiotic divisions (Fig. 6.1), in which the DNA replicates only once before the first division.

First meiotic division (reduction division)

Prophase of the first meiotic division is complex, and five stages can be recognised by microscopy: leptotene (threadlike), zygotene (pairing), pachytene (thickening), diplotene (appearing double) and diakinesis (further condensation).

Leptotene starts with the first appearance of the chromosomes (Fig. 6.2). At this stage, each chromosome consists of a pair of sister chromatids (replication having occurred during the S phase of premeiotic interphase). Homologous chromosomes pair (starting at the telomeres and proceeding towards the centromere) during zygotene to form bivalents, which are

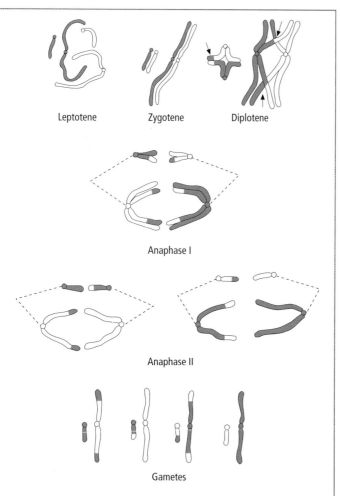

Fig. 6.1 Diagram of meiosis. Only two pairs of chromosomes are shown; chromosomes from one parent are in outline, while those from the other are coloured (cross-overs are indicated by arrows).

bound closely together by the synaptonemal complex (Fig. 6.3). The precise mechanism by which homologous chromosomes pair in humans is unclear, but dispersed blocks of repetitive DNA are suspected to be involved in the initial alignment and protein complexes ('synaptonemal complexes') are involved. The X and Y chromosomes undergo synapsis (pairing) only at the distal end of both short arms (the pairing or pseudoautosomal regions). They form a sex bivalent, which is out of phase with the others and is condensed early in pachytene as the sex body. The non-pairing, or differential, parts of the X and Y are transcriptionally silenced (meiotic sex chromosome inactivation) by phosphorylation of the nucleosomal histone, and their early condensation is important in preventing crossing-over between the non-pairing regions. Pachytene is the main stage of chromosomal thickening, and the pattern of chromosome condensation appears to correspond to the banding pattern seen at mitosis (Figs 6.4 and 6.5). Each chromosome is now seen to consist of two chromatids; hence, each bivalent is a tetrad of four strands (Figs 6.1 and 6.5). Satellite association of the acrocentrics also occurs at pachytene, due to the synapsis of homologous repetitive sequences on non-homologous chromosomes. Diplotene, which follows, is very short and difficult to study in humans. During diplotene, the bivalents start to separate. Although the two chromosomes of each bivalent separate, the centromere of each remains intact, so the two chromatids of each chromosome remain together. During longitudinal separation, the two members of each bivalent are seen to be in contact at several places, called chiasmata (Fig. 6.6). These mark the location of cross-overs, where the chromatids of homologous chromosomes have exchanged material in late pachytene (Fig. 6.7). On average, there are about 52 chiasmata per human male cell with at least one chiasma per chromosome arm (with the exception of the short arms of the acrocentrics and chromosome 18). Short chromosomes with a single chiasma appear as a rod or cross, longer chromosomes with two chiasmata appear as a ring and those with three have a figure-of-eight appearance. At diplotene, the sex bivalent opens out and the X and Y chromosomes can be seen attached to one another by the tiny pairing segments at the ends of their short arms indicating homology of these regions. This pairing region at the tip of the short arms is called the pseudoautosomal region 1 (PAR1) as, in contrast to the remainder of the X and Y in the male, crossing-over is usual in this area during male meiosis, and sequences mapping to this region appear to show autosomal rather than sex-linked inheritance. The PAR1 pairing region is particularly well demonstrated in electron microscopy (EM) preparations of the synaptonemal complex stained by silver nitrate (Fig. 6.8). The much smaller PAR2, present at the tip of Xq, in contrast, possesses a much lower rate of recombination and is not usually apparent at diakinesis. Diakinesis is the final stage of prophase, during which the chromosomes coil more tightly and so stain more deeply.

Metaphase begins when the nuclear membrane disappears and the chromosomes move to the equatorial plane. At anaphase, the two members of each bivalent separate, one going

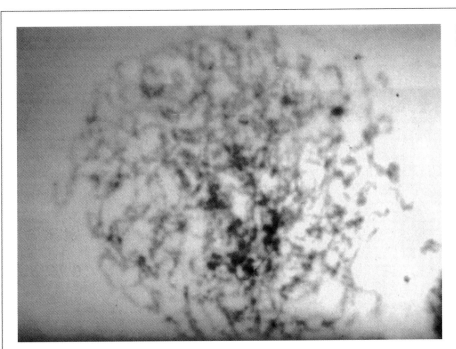

Fig. 6.2 Human primary spermatocyte in leptotene.

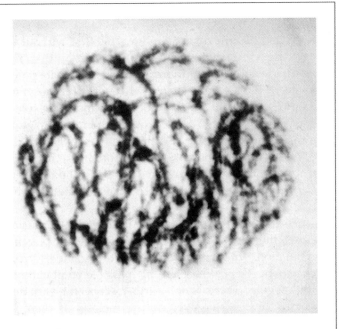

Fig. 6.3 Zygotene.

to each pole. These bivalents are assorted independently to each pole. The cytoplasm divides, and each cell now has 23 chromosomes, each of which is a pair of chromatids, differing from one another only as a result of crossing-over.

Second meiotic division

The second meiotic division follows the first without an interphase. It resembles mitosis, in that the centromeres now divide

Table 6.1 Comparison of mitosis and meiosis

	Mitosis	**Meiosis**
Site	All tissues	Gonads
Timing	All of life	Post-puberty in males, suspended until puberty in females
Result	Diploid daughter cells	Haploid gametes

and sister chromatids pass to opposite poles. However, the second meiotic division chromosomes are rather more coiled than mitotic ones and show splaying of the chromatids. The X and Y chromosomes in the male are exceptions, and this may be related to the fact that, except for the tips of their short arms, they are not involved in recombination (Fig. 6.9). Thus, meiosis differs from mitosis in several respects as outlined in Table 6.1.

As the chromosomes assort (i.e. move to the gametes) independently during meiosis, this results in 2^{23} or 8,388,608 different possible combinations of chromosomes in the gametes from each parent. Hence, there are 2^{46} possible combinations in the zygote. There is still further scope for variation provided by crossing-over during meiosis. If there is, on average, only one cross-over per chromosome and a 10% paternal/maternal allele difference, then the number of possible zygotes exceeds 6×10^{43}. This number is greater than the number of human beings who have so far existed and so emphasises our genetic uniqueness.

Meiosis thus has three important consequences:

1. Gametes contain only one representative of each homologous pair of chromosomes.

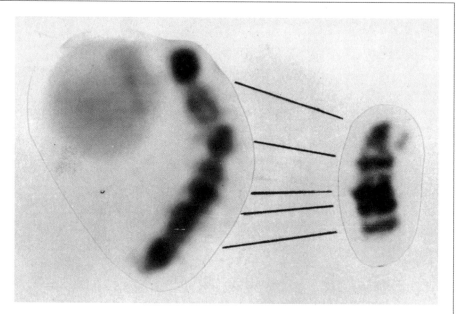

Fig. 6.4 Homology of the banding pattern from meiotic (left) and mitotic chromosomes (chromosome 13 shown). Note the nucleolus arising from the short arm (top) of the bivalent.

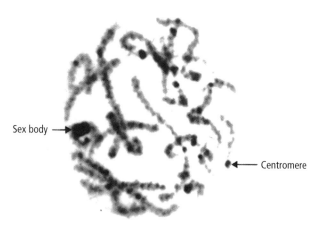

Fig. 6.5 Pachytene.

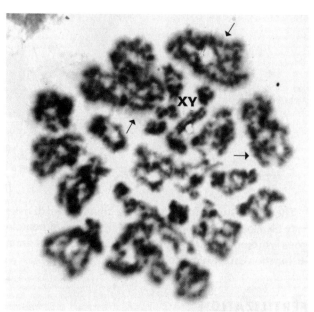

Fig. 6.6 Early diakinesis. Note the multiple chiasmata (some indicated by arrows).

2. There is random assortment of paternal and maternal homologues.
3. Crossing-over ensures uniqueness by further increasing genetic variation.

Spermatogenesis

Spermatogenesis occurs in the seminiferous tubules of the male from the time of sexual maturity onward (Fig. 6.10). At the periphery of the tubule are spermatogonia, of which some are self-renewing stem cells and others are already committed to sperm formation. The primary spermatocyte is derived from a committed spermatogonium. The primary spermatocyte undergoes the first meiotic division to produce two secondary spermatocytes, each with 23 chromosomes. These cells rapidly undergo the second meiotic division, each forming two spermatids, which mature without further division into sperm. This process of production of a mature sperm from a committed spermatogonium takes about 61 days.

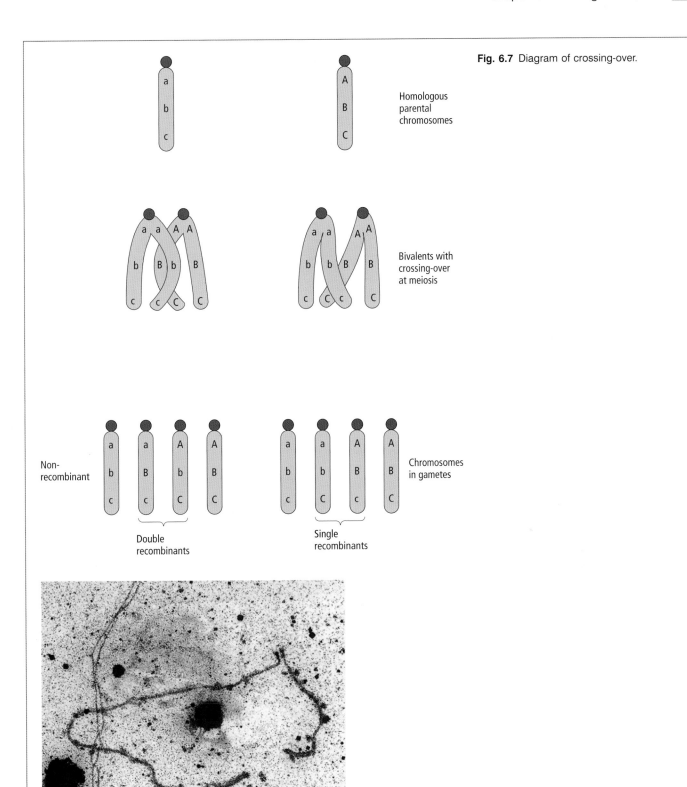

Fig. 6.7 Diagram of crossing-over.

Homologous parental chromosomes

Bivalents with crossing-over at meiosis

Non-recombinant

Chromosomes in gametes

Double recombinants

Single recombinants

Fig. 6.8 EM photomicrograph of the sex bivalent at pachytene showing the X chromosome (left) and the Y chromosome (right) attached by their pairing segments (top).

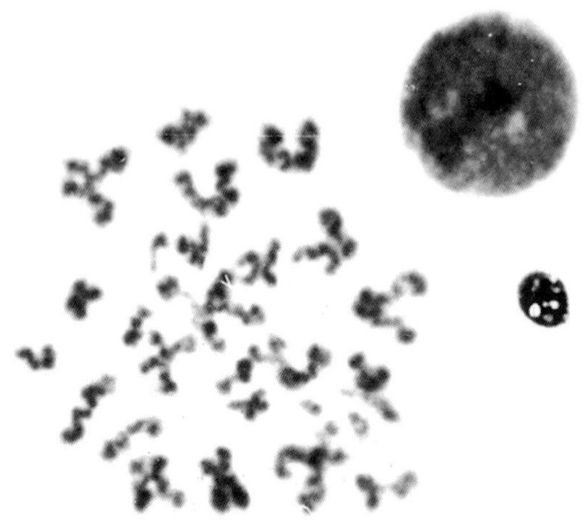

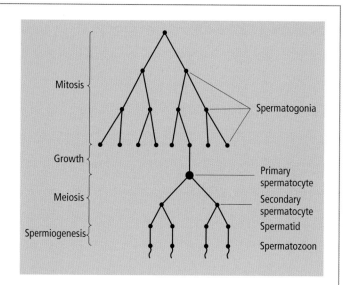

Fig. 6.9 Second meiotic metaphase showing a single condensed X chromosome.

Fig. 6.10 Spermatogenesis.

Normally semen contains 50–100 × 10⁶ sperms per ml. Sperm production continues, albeit at a reduced rate, into old age, and the total lifetime sperm production of a male exceeds 10^{12}. The numerous replications increase the chance for mutation, and the risk for several single-gene mutations has already been shown to be increased in the offspring of older men.

Oogenesis

In contrast to spermatogenesis, the process of oogenesis is largely complete at birth. Oogonia are derived from the primordial germ cells, and each oogonium is the central cell in a developing follicle. By about the third month of fetal life, the oogonia have become primary oocytes, and some of these have already entered the prophase of first meiosis. The primary oocytes remain in suspended prophase (dictyotene) until sexual maturity. Then, as each individual follicle matures and releases its oocyte into the Fallopian tube, the first meiotic division is completed. Hence, completion of the first meiotic division in the female may take over 40 years.

The first meiotic division results in an unequal division of the cytoplasm, with the secondary oocyte receiving the great majority in contrast to the first polar body (Fig. 6.11). The second meiotic division is not completed until after fertilisation in the Fallopian tube and results in the mature ovum and a second polar body. The first polar body may also divide at this stage. Thus, whereas spermatogenesis produces four viable sperm per meiotic division, oogenesis produces only one ovum.

The maximum number of germ cells in the female fetus is 6.8×10^6 at 5 months. By birth, the number is 2×10^6 and by puberty it is less than 200,000. Of this number, only about 400 will ovulate.

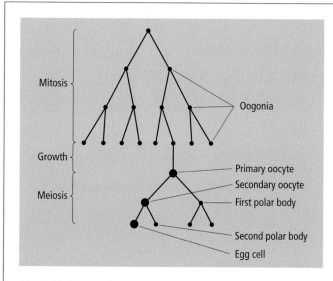

Fig. 6.11 Oogenesis.

The long resting phase during the first meiotic division may be a factor in the increased risk of failure of homologous chromosomes to separate during meiosis (non-disjunction) in the older mother.

Fertilisation

Fertilisation usually occurs in the Fallopian tube. As the sperm penetrates the ovum, a chemical change occurs that normally prevents the entry of other sperm. After entry, the sperm rounds up as a male pronucleus. The ovum now completes the second

Table 6.2 Embryonic and fetal milestones

Stage	Gestation from last menstrual period	Crown–rump length	Comment
Embryo	Conception (2 weeks)		
	4 weeks	1 mm	X-inactivation, first missed period, implantation complete, chorionic villi develop, primitive streak appears
	5 weeks	2 mm	Neural tube starts to fuse, organ primordia form, pregnancy test positive
	6 weeks	4 mm	Neural tube closed, limb buds appear, heart starts to contract, membranes apparent on ultrasound
	8 weeks	3 cm	Major organogenesis completed, fetal movements seen on ultrasound
Fetus	12 weeks	8 cm	External genitalia recognisable, chorionic villus sampling possible
	16 weeks	14 cm	Usual time for amniocentesis
	18 weeks	16 cm	Usual time for fetal blood sampling and detailed ultrasound scanning
	40 weeks	36 cm	Term pregnancy

meiotic division and produces the female pronucleus. These fuse to form the zygote, and embryogenesis commences.

By a series of mitotic divisions, the zygote produces the estimated 2×10^{12} cells found in the neonate and subsequently the 5×10^{12} cells found in the adult. Table 6.2 summarises the major milestones in embryonic and fetal life of medical genetic importance.

X-inactivation and dosage compensation

Inactivation of one of the two X chromosomes in female somatic cells is the process by which the dosage of X-linked genes is balanced between two Xs in females and one X in males. It is common to all placental mammals and, in humans, as evidenced by the appearance of the *XIST* (X-inactivation-specific transcript) RNA (see below), begins as early as the eight-cell stage. Inactivation only occurs in somatic cells, as in the germ line both X chromosomes need to remain active. For each somatic cell, it is random whether the paternal X or maternal X is inactivated, but the choice is fixed for all subsequent descendants of that cell (Fig. 6.12). As only one X is active in the female the product levels for most genes on the X chromosome are similar in females and males where the single X always remains active, except in primary spermatocytes where it becomes part of the condensed sex body.

X-inactivation affects most genes carried on the human X chromosome, but there are interesting exceptions, including the genes located within the blocks of sequence identity between the X and Y chromosomes, PAR1 and PAR2, located at the tips of Xp and Xq, respectively. There are at least 25 genes within PAR1 and four within PAR2, all of which escape X-inactivation with the exception of the two most proximal genes within PAR2. Only one of these 29 PAR genes, however, is known to be associated with human disorders. Deficiency of this short stature homeobox gene (*SHOX*), which encodes a

transcription factor important for chondrocyte function, can cause isolated short stature. Deficiency of *SHOX*, however, can result in skeletal malformations in addition to short stature, causing Léri–Weill dyschondrosteosis (with the so-called Madelung deformity of the forearm) and its more severe homozygous (or compound heterozygous) form, Langer mesomelic dysplasia. Loss of one copy (causing haploinsufficiency, i.e. inadequate protein product) of the *SHOX* gene is also thought to be responsible for some of the features of Turner syndrome (see below). Many non-PAR X chromosome genes (e.g. *ZFX*, a zinc finger protein gene) also appear to escape inactivation, totalling around 20% of all X chromosome genes. The majority of these have functional homologues on the Y chromosome.

In contrast, the locus *XIST*, which maps to Xq, is only active on the inactive X and this locus plays an important role in regulating the inactivation process itself. It encodes long non-coding *XIST* RNA molecules, which coat the chromosome and initiate transcriptional silencing. The mechanism by which *XIST* spreads along the X chromosome is unclear but may involve repeated sequences on the X chromosome, such as the many long interspersed elements (LINEs) acting as 'boosters'. The silencing by *XIST* appears to depend on repeated sequences in its 5′ end that each fold into two 'stem–loop' RNA structures. These may permit direct or indirect binding of repressor proteins such as those of the polycomb group. Following initiation of silencing by *XIST* and binding of repressor proteins, maintenance of X chromosome inactivation throughout subsequent cell divisions involves other factors including hypoacetylation of histone H4 and also DNA methylation. For instance, the CpG islands (see Chapter 3) of housekeeping genes on the inactive X are hypermethylated, while the reverse is true of the active X. In addition, the inactive X completes its replication later in mitosis than any of the other chromosomes, and thus is out of phase with the

Fig. 6.12 Diagram of X-inactivation. Xm: maternal X chromosome; Xp: paternal X chromosome. Inactive X chromosomes are shaded.

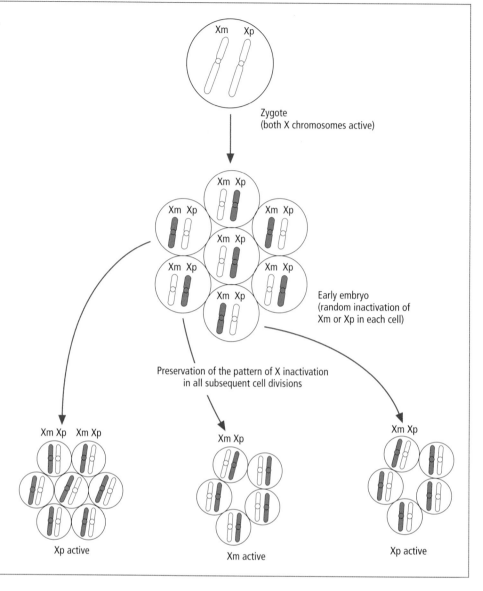

active X. For further details regarding *XIST*, and in particular how its own transcription is regulated, see Senner and Brockdorff (2009) in Further reading.

In females with loss of material from one X chromosome, the structurally abnormal X is preferentially inactivated. In contrast, females with an X–autosome translocation preferentially inactivate the normal X. If this were not the case, the inactivation could spread from the inactivation centre in Xq13 into the autosomal genes, leading to autosomal monosomy.

The inactive X remains condensed during most of interphase and is visible in a variable proportion of the nuclei in most tissues as a densely stained mass of chromatin known as the Barr body or X chromatin (Fig. 6.13). Only about 30% of cells from a buccal smear of a normal female show X chromatin, as this depends upon the stage each cell is at in the cell cycle. If a cell has more than two X chromosomes, then the extra ones are also inactivated and more than one Barr body will be seen in some cells. Thus, the maximum number of Barr bodies per cell will be one less than the total number of X chromosomes in the karyotype. The sex chromatin may also be seen in 1–10% of female neutrophils as a small drumstick (Fig. 6.14).

Thus, a female has a mixture of cells, some of which have an active paternal X chromosome and some of which have an active maternal X chromosome. The relative proportions vary from female to female (even in identical twins) due to the randomness of the inactivation process. This accounts for the patchy expression of mutant X-linked genes in carrier females.

Sex chromosome aberrations

45,X (Turner syndrome)

The overall incidence of Turner syndrome is between 1 in 2000 and 1 in 5000 female births. The frequency at conception is

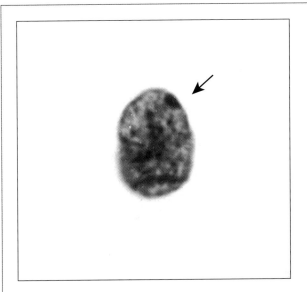

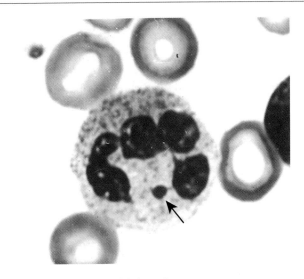

Fig. 6.14 Neutrophil drumstick (arrow).

Fig. 6.13 Barr body (arrow).

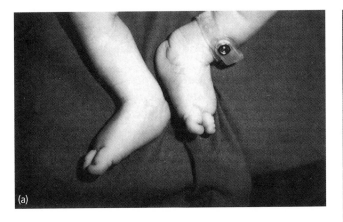

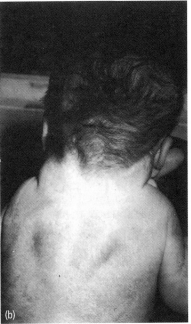

Fig. 6.15 (a) Neonatal lymphoedema in Turner syndrome. (b) Redundant neck skin in Turner syndrome.

much higher but over 99% of affected fetuses spontaneously abort.

Clinical features

The diagnosis may be suggested in the newborn by redundant neck skin and peripheral lymphoedema (Fig. 6.15). However, not infrequently, the diagnosis is only made later, during the investigation of short stature or primary amenorrhoea.

Proportionate short stature is apparent from early childhood. No adolescent growth spurt occurs, and the mean adult height, if untreated, is 145 cm with a correlation to midparental height. The chest tends to be broad, with the impression of widely spaced nipples, the hair line is low and the neck may be webbed. The elbow carrying angle may be increased and the fourth metacarpals short. Hypoplasia of the nails and multiple pigmented naevi are common. Peripheral lymphoedema occurs at some stage in 40% of patients. The ovaries develop normally until the 15th week of gestation, but then ova begin to degenerate and disappear, so that at birth the ovaries are represented by streaks, and this results in failure of secondary sexual development. Occasionally, ovarian degeneration is incomplete, menses may occur (10–15%) and, rarely, a pregnancy may be possible.

Cardiac abnormalities, including, most commonly, a bicuspid aortic valve, but also coarctation of the aorta, atrial septal defect and aortic stenosis, are present in up to 50% of patients. There is also an increased risk of unexplained systemic hypertension (27%), renal malformations, Hashimoto thyroiditis, Crohn disease and gastrointestinal bleeding. Intelligence and lifespan are normal. Sex hormone replacement will allow the development of secondary sexual characteristics, and treatment with growth hormone in childhood has been shown to increase the final height by at least 5 cm (see Donaldson *et al.*, 2006, in Further reading). Normal childbirth has been achieved by *in vitro* fertilisation using donor oocytes.

Genetic aspects

Monosomy X may arise from non-disjunction in either parent. In 80% of patients with monosomy X, only the maternal X chromosome is present, and thus the error occurred in spermatogenesis or post-fertilisation. This accounts for the lack of a maternal age effect. In monosomy X, the sex chromatin body is absent from nuclei. Overall, 50% of patients have 45,X, 17% have an isochromosome of the long arm of X, 24% are mosaics, 7% have a ring X and 2% have a short arm deletion of one X. In general, deletion of the short arm of the X is associated with the Turner phenotype, while long-arm deletions alone produce streak ovaries without the associated dysmorphic features. In 4% of patients, mosaicism with a second cell line containing a Y chromosome is found. In these patients, there is a risk of up to 20% that the streak gonad will develop a gonadoblastoma (which can progress to a dysgerminoma), and gonadal removal is generally recommended. The genotype/phenotype correlation is otherwise rather poor, possibly as a result of varying extents of mosaicism for a normal cell line (45,X/46,XX) in different tissues. It is likely that the short stature, which is present in around 95% of cases, is caused at least in part by haploinsufficiency (reduced dosage) of the *SHOX* gene located on Xp, which encodes a transcription factor that is especially important during limb development (see above).

Recurrence risk

The recurrence risk does not appear to be increased above the general population risk.

47,XYY

The incidence of 47,XYY is 1 in 1000 male births, but it accounts for approximately 20 per 1000 adult males who are in institutions on account of significant learning difficulties or criminal behaviour. There is no apparent parental age effect.

Clinical features

This chromosome disorder is often asymptomatic and most 47,XYY men do not have learning difficulties or criminal behaviour. Intelligence (overall IQ score) tends to be 10–15 points less than their normal siblings, and behaviour problems with easy frustration and aggression may occur. Patients tend to be tall, but have normal body proportions and no other clinical signs.

Genetic aspects

47,XYY arises from the production, by non-disjunction, of a YY sperm at the second paternal meiotic division, or from post-fertilisation non-disjunction of the Y chromosome. The recurrence risk is probably not increased for the parents of an affected child. For a person with 47,XYY, the expected ratio of offspring would be 2 XXY to 2 XY to 1 XX to 1 XYY. In practice, fertility appears unimpaired in most cases, and only XX and XY offspring have been observed.

47,XXY (Klinefelter syndrome)

Overall, the birth incidence of 47,XXY is 1 in 1000 males, with an increased risk at increased maternal age. The frequency is increased amongst azoospermic infertile males (1 in 10) and in males with significant learning difficulties (1 in 100).

Clinical features

The diagnosis is generally made during adult life at the investigation of infertility, as this is the single commonest cause of hypogonadism and infertility in men. The testes are small (less than 2 cm long in the adult) and fail to produce adult levels of testosterone. This leads to poorly developed secondary sexual characteristics and gynaecomastia (in 40% of patients). The limbs are elongated from early childhood and the upper to lower segment ratio is abnormally low with a mean adult height close to the 75th centile. Scoliosis, emphysema, diabetes mellitus (8%) and osteoporosis may occur, and the frequency of carcinoma of the breast (7%) is similar to that for normal females.

Testosterone replacement therapy from early adolescence will improve secondary sexual characteristics and help to prevent osteoporosis, but infertility is the rule, except in mosaic patients. In some males, fertility has been achieved using testicular sperm aspiration and intracytoplasmic sperm injection (ICSI). There is a 10–20-point reduction in verbal skills, but performance scores are usually normal and severe learning difficulties are uncommon. Behavioural problems are common in childhood.

Genetic aspects

The extra X chromosome is of maternal origin in 56% and paternal in 44% of patients. It usually arises by non-disjunction at the first (or occasionally the second) maternal meiotic division and rarely as a mitotic error after fertilisation. In the male, it arises when the first meiotic division produces an XY sperm and this is favoured if the normal single XY cross-over is lost or fails to occur during male meiosis. About 15% of patients are mosaic 46,XY/47,XXY. The recurrence risk does not appear to be increased above the general population risk. Patients with 48,XXXY and 49,XXXXY have severe learning difficulties and proximal radioulnar synostosis is a common skeletal defect.

47,XXX

The birth frequency is 1 in 1000 females with a maternal age effect.

Clinical features

Individuals appear clinically normal, but 15–25% have mild learning difficulties.

Genetic aspects

47,XXX may arise from non-disjunction at either the first (65%) or second (24%) maternal meiotic divisions, as a post-zygotic mitotic error (3%) or from non-disjunction at the male second meiotic division (8%). The recurrence risk does not appear to be increased above the general population incidence. About three-quarters of affected females are fertile. One-half of their offspring would be expected to be affected, but in practice they are usually normal.

Women who have more than three X chromosomes (as is the case for men who have more than two) often have significant learning difficulties, with the severity increasing according to the number of extra X chromosomes.

Sex determination and differentiation

Studies of structural aberrations of the human Y chromosome reveal that maleness is determined by a testis-determining factor (TDF) located on the short arm of the Y chromosome. If this region is absent, the undifferentiated gonad becomes an ovary and sex differentiation occurs along female lines. If the TDF region is present, a testis forms, which produces two hormones that act locally. The Sertoli cells of the seminiferous tubules secrete a Mullerian duct inhibitor, anti-Mullerian hormone (AMH), which causes regression of the primitive uterus and Fallopian tubes, and the interstitial cells of the testis secrete testosterone, which both stimulates the Wolffian ducts to differentiate into the epididymis, vas deferens and seminal vesicles, and also masculinises the external genitalia. The gene *SRY* (sex-determining region of the Y) has been confirmed as the master-switch TDF in humans and mice by mutation analysis in cases of sex reversal. In addition, the gene maps within the sex-determining region, is expressed in the undifferentiated gonad at an appropriate time in development and, in the mouse, causes sex reversal when introduced into female pre-embryos (see Wilhelm and Koopman, 2006, in Further reading for a review of the role of the *SRY* gene in male development). The SRY protein binds to DNA at a specific 6-nucleotide target sequence and is believed to act as a transcription factor by causing the DNA to bend through a specific angle. An important downstream effector of SRY is thought to be the *SOX9* gene on human chromosome 17. In turn, the SOX9 protein appears to regulate the expression of AMH. Interestingly, the *SOX9* gene is highly dosage-sensitive, as duplication of the gene has been reported to induce male development in the absence of *SRY* (i.e. causing XX sex reversal), while *SOX9* haploinsufficiency can prevent male development in the presence of *SRY* (i.e. causing XY sex reversal).

The normal pairing of the X and Y chromosomes in first meiosis and their regular segregation into different secondary spermatocytes achieves approximately equal numbers of male and female conceptions. The location of *SRY* outside the pairing segment on the short arm of the Y normally ensures that recombination does not transfer the TDF to the X chromosome (which would thus separate it from other determinants carried on the long arm of the Y that are necessary for spermatogenesis).

Rare exceptions to the rule that sex determination depends on the presence or absence of the Y chromosome occur in XY females, some of which may have deletions or mutations affecting *SRY*, and XX males, in whom *SRY* has been transferred from the Y to the X by accidental recombination.

Genomic imprinting (parental imprinting)

At most autosomal loci, both alleles are, together, either active or inactive, but at approximately 100 loci, only one allele is active. At these loci, the allele chosen for inactivation depends upon its parental origin. Thus, for example, only the paternally inherited allele of the insulin growth factor 2 (*IGF2*) gene on 11p is active. This imprint is established during gametogenesis and, as with other imprinted genes, involves methylation differences at specific sites adjacent to the gene. Methylation at these sites in the germ line may be determined by specific secondary DNA structures resulting from the short direct repeat sequences that are found close to both maternally and paternally methylated imprinting control regions (ICRs) or imprinting control centres. At different loci, the mechanisms by which differential ICR methylation results in monoallelic gene expression are different and often complex, frequently involving clusters of coregulated imprinted genes. For example, *IGF2* expression is prevented on the maternal allele because a nearby ICR is able, in its unmethylated state, to bind a so-called boundary factor, CTCF. When the CTCF protein is bound to the ICR, it prevents the interaction of the *IGF2* promoter from interacting with its enhancers, which are located on the other side of the ICR. On the paternal allele, in contrast, methylation acquired during spermatogenesis prevents CTCF binding, subsequently permitting the *IGF2* promoter to interact with its enhancers and thus leading to efficient *IGF2* expression. Adding to this complexity is the finding that the expression of another gene at the same locus, *H19*, is reciprocally regulated, as the *H19* promoter competes with that of *IGF2* for the same enhancers.

The reason for such imprinting is unknown, but one consequence is the difference in the clinical appearance for particular chromosomal disorders depending upon the parent of origin. Thus, for example, a deletion of the proximal long arm of chromosome 15 on a maternal chromosome results in mental handicap and clinical features of Angelman syndrome (see below), whereas a similar deletion on a paternal chromosome results in a clinically distinct condition called Prader–Willi syndrome (see below). This is because at this locus it is only the paternally inherited copies of the *SNRPN*, *MKRN3*, *NDN* and *MAGEL2* genes that are normally expressed in the tissues involved (e.g. in the brain) whereas *UBE3A*, a different gene at the same locus, is normally transcriptionally active only on the maternally inherited allele.

The most extreme imbalance of maternal and paternal contributions, however, occurs in hydatidiform moles, which have a double paternal contribution and no maternal contribution. The chromosomes look normal but no fetus develops and the placenta is grossly abnormal.

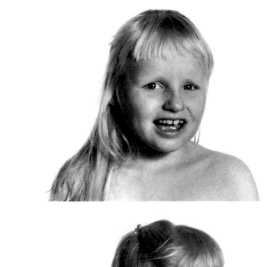

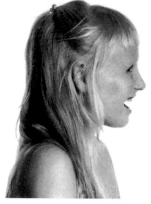

Fig. 6.16 Facial appearance in Angelman syndrome. Image kindly provided by Dr John Tolmie, Clinical Genetics Department, Yorkhill Hospitals, Glasgow, UK.

Angelman syndrome

Clinical features

The clinical features of Angelman syndrome include developmental delay, very poor speech, jerky movements, paroxysms of inappropriate laughter, reduced hair and skin pigmentation, facial dysmorphisms (Fig. 6.16) and microcephaly. An electroencephalogram is always abnormal with posterior high-voltage sharp waves and a posterior spike and wave on eye closure.

Genetic aspects

The frequency is 1 in 20,000 and about 50% of patients show a visible cytogenetic microdeletion at 15q12. A deletion can be identified in a further 25% using fluorescence *in situ* hybridisation (FISH) or DNA analysis with probes from the deleted region. Other recognised causes include paternal uniparental disomy (UPD) in which both copies of chromosome 15 are contributed by the father (approximately 5%), a mutation in the *UBE3A* gene (10-20%) and an imprinting defect (3%). In contrast to Prader–Willi syndrome, which shows a similar cytogenetic microdeletion, the deleted chromosome 15 is always maternal in origin in Angelman syndrome. The recurrence risk in families with a *de novo* deletion is low, with

familial recurrences being more likely if, for example, a parent possesses a chromosomal translocation or if the proband possesses an inherited *UBE3A* mutation or an inherited imprinting control centre (IC) deletion (see Chapter 16 for additional information). The *UBE3A* gene encodes a ubiquitin protein ligase enzyme that normally catalyses the marking of specific proteins (with ubiquitin tags) for subsequent degradation. Thus, the neurological abnormalities in Angelman syndrome may result from the absence of UBE3A and the consequent abnormal accumulation of these target proteins.

Prader–Willi syndrome

Clinical features

In the newborn with Prader–Willi syndrome, hypotonia and poor swallowing may be marked. The face is flat with a tented upper lip, and the external genitalia are hypoplastic. In later childhood, the hypotonia improves and overeating with obesity occurs. The forehead tends to be prominent with bitemporal narrowing. The palpebral fissures are almond-shaped and the hands and feet are small (Fig. 6.17). Mental handicap is usual, with an IQ range of 20–80 and a mean of 50.

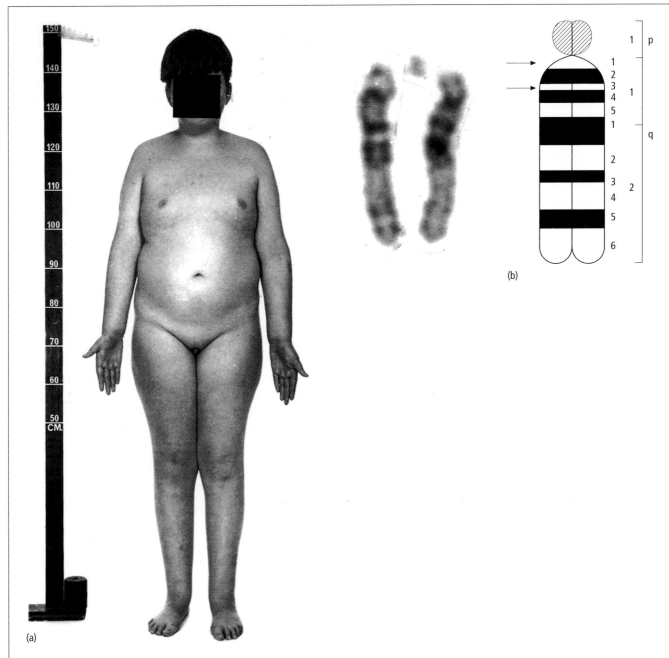

Fig. 6.17 (a) Prader–Willi phenotype. (b) Interstitial deletion of chromosome 15 (q11–q13).

Genetic aspects

The frequency is 1 in 10,000 and in 50% a cytogenetic micro-deletion is apparent at 15q11–13. In a further 25%, a deletion of chromosome 15q of variable size can be detected by FISH or DNA analysis with probes from the deleted region (Fig. 6.18). In contrast to Angelman syndrome, the deleted chromosome in Prader–Willi syndrome is invariably paternal in origin. Recurrence is very unlikely where the child has a *de novo* deletion, but 2% arise from a parental structural rearrangement and here prenatal diagnosis needs to be considered. In the remaining 25% of Prader–Willi patients, there is no 15q deletion, but DNA analysis reveals maternal uniparental disomy or, alternatively, in 1% of cases, an IC mutation or IC micro-deletion (either of which can be inherited from a parent). The consequent lack of paternally expressed genes such as *SNRPN* (a small nuclear ribonucleoprotein gene involved in alternative mRNA splicing) from the critical region results in the phenotype.

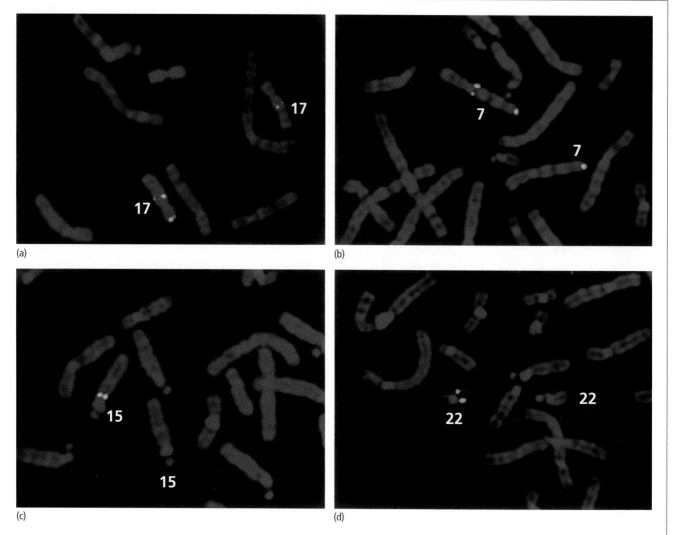

Fig. 6.18 Microdeletion detection using specific FISH probes, with the deletions being identified by the absence of the locus-specific signal on one of the two chromosomes analysed in each case: (a) Hybridisation to a Miller-Dieker syndrome probe (PAFAH1B1, at 17p13.3) with a 17q-specific control probe reveals a deletion at the Miller-Dieker syndrome locus on one chromosome 17. (b) Hybridisation to a Williams syndrome probe (ELN, at 7q11.2) with a 7q-specific control probe shows a deletion at the Williams syndrome locus on one chromosome 7. (c) Hybridisation to a Prader-Willi/Angelman syndrome probe (SNRPN, at 15q11-q13) shows a deletion at the Prader-Willi/Angelman syndrome region on one chromosome 15. (d) Hybridisation to a DiGeorge/velocardiofacial syndrome probe (22q11.2) reveals a deletion at the 22q11.2 microdeletion syndrome region on one chromosome 22.

SUMMARY

- Meiosis comprises two successive cell divisions but DNA replication occurs only prior to the first meiotic division. This division results in two cells, each containing 23 chromosomes, with each chromosome consisting of two chromatids that differ only due to prior crossing-over.
- The second meiotic division resembles mitosis in that the centromeres divide, with sister chromatids passing to opposite poles.
- Enormous genetic variation results from the crossing-over that occurs between chromatids belonging to homologous chromosomes, in addition to the random assortment of paternal and maternal homologues.
- In oogenesis, but not spermatogenesis, there is a long resting phase during the first meiotic division.
- X-chromosome inactivation occurs early in female embryonic development. It involves coating of the X chromosome by *XIST* non-coding RNA molecules that are expressed from the *XIST* locus on Xq. The X chromosome genes that possess functional

homologues on the Y chromosome, however, such as *SHOX*, which is located in the pseudo-autosomal region at the tip of Xp, escape X inactivation.

■ Male sex determination involves the *SRY* gene on the Y chromosome, probably acting via the autosomal *SOX9* gene and the subsequent production of anti-Mullerian hormone.

■ At a few autosomal loci, gene expression is limited to just one allele and is determined by its parental origin. This genomic imprinting can result in different clinical phenotypes depending on whether, for example, a deletion at that locus affects the chromosome that is inherited from the mother or the one from the father.

FURTHER READING

Blaschke RJ, Rappold G (2006) The pseudoautosomal regions, SHOX and disease. *Curr Opin Genet Dev* **16**:233–9.

Donaldson MDC, Gault EJ, Tan KW and Dunger DB (2006) Optimising management in Turner syndrome: from infancy to adult transfer. *Arch Dis Child* **91**:513–20.

Lalande M, Calciano MA (2007) Molecular epigenetics of Angelman syndrome. *Cell Mol Life Sci* **64**:947–60.

Senner CE, Brockdorff N (2009) *Xist* gene regulation at the onset of X inactivation. *Curr Opin Genet Dev* **19**:122–6.

Wallis M, Waters P, Graves JAM (2008) Sex determination in mammals – before and after the evolution of SRY. *Cell Mol Life Sci* **65**:3182–95.

Wilhelm D, Koopman P (2006) The makings of maleness: towards an integrated view of male sexual development. *Nat Rev Genet* **7**, 620–31.

Wood AJ, Oakey RJ (2006) Genomic imprinting in mammals: emerging treatments and established theories. *PLoS Genet* **2**:e147.

Self-assessment

1. Which of the following are true of meiosis?
A. It consists of two cell divisions
B. DNA replication occurs twice
C. It results in chromosomes that each consist of a pair of identical chromatids
D. In a male, pairing occurs between the X and Y chromosome along their length
E. The first meiotic division in an oocyte is not completed until after the onset of puberty

2. With regard to X-inactivation, which of the following are correct?
A. It normally occurs in every female somatic cell and results in inactivation of one of the two X chromosomes
B. It is regulated by an active *XIST* locus on the long arm of the X chromosome that is inactivated
C. It occurs by a process that involves non-coding RNA molecules as well as DNA methylation
D. It may account for phenotypic variability between female carriers of an X-linked recessive disorder within a family
E. Many genes on the X chromosome are not inactivated by this process

3. Which of the following is not associated with Turner syndrome?
A. Peripheral lymphoedema
B. Short fourth metacarpals
C. Low hair line
D. Bicuspid aortic valve
E. Chance of recurrence of approximately 3–5%

4. Which of the following are true of sex determination and differentiation in humans?
A. Male sex determination requires the testis-determining factor (TDF) located on the Y chromosome
B. The key TDF is the *SRY* gene
C. The *SRY* gene encodes a structural tail protein of spermatozoa
D. Male sex determination involves activation of the *SOX9* gene on the Y chromosome
E. XX males may result if the *SRY* gene has previously been transferred from a Y chromosome to an X chromosome by recombination

5. In relation to genomic imprinting, which of the following are correct statements?
A. For those genes affected, it results in just one allele being active, with the selection being dependent upon the parental origin of the allele
B. The imprint is established during gametogenesis
C. It is regulated by the *XIST* gene
D. Angelman syndrome often results from a deletion located on the long arm of the maternal chromosome 15
E. A well-recognised cause of Prader–Willi syndrome is paternal uniparental disomy

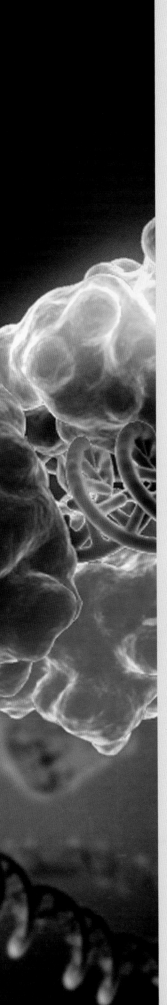

CHAPTER 7
Chromosome aberrations

Key Topics

Introduction

Mutations sometimes involve very large parts of the chromosome, and when these are large enough to be visible under the light microscope they are termed chromosome aberrations. With routine light microscopy, the smallest visible addition or deletion from a chromosome is about 4 Mb. Using the distance from London to New York as the length of the haploid DNA, this would be equivalent to a distance of about 8 km, and on this scale the average gene would be about 30 m in length. Thus, any visible abnormality usually involves many contiguous genes.

Abnormalities of the chromosomes are usually classified into numerical abnormalities, where the somatic cells contain an abnormal number of normal chromosomes, and structural aberrations, where the somatic cells contain one or more abnormal chromosomes. They may involve either the sex chromosomes or the autosomes and may occur either as a result of a germ cell mutation in the parent or a more remote ancestor, or as a result of somatic mutation, in which case only a proportion of cells will be affected.

Numerical aberrations

Normally, human somatic cells contain 46 chromosomes and are termed diploid (as the number is twice the haploid number of 23 as found in gametes). A chromosome number that is an exact multiple of the haploid number and exceeds the diploid number is called polyploidy, and one that is not an exact multiple is called aneuploidy (Table 7.1).

Aneuploidy

Aneuploidy usually arises from the failure of paired chromosomes or sister chromatids to disjoin at anaphase (non-disjunction). Alternatively, aneuploidy may be due to delayed movement of a chromosome at anaphase (anaphase lag). Thus, by either of these mechanisms two cells are produced, one with an extra copy of a chromosome (trisomy) and one with a missing copy of that chromosome (monosomy) (Fig. 7.1). The cause of meiotic non-disjunction is not known, but it occurs at increased frequency with increasing maternal age, with maternal hypothyroidism, and possibly after irradiation or viral

Table 7.1 Examples of numerical chromosomal aberrations

Karyotype	Description
92,XXYY	Tetraploidy
69,XXY	Triploidy
47,XX,+21	Trisomy 21
47,XY,+18	Trisomy 18
47,XX,+13	Trisomy 13
47,XX,+16	Trisomy 16
47,XXY	Klinefelter syndrome
47,XXX	Trisomy X
45,X	Turner syndrome
49,XXXXY	Variant of Klinefelter syndrome

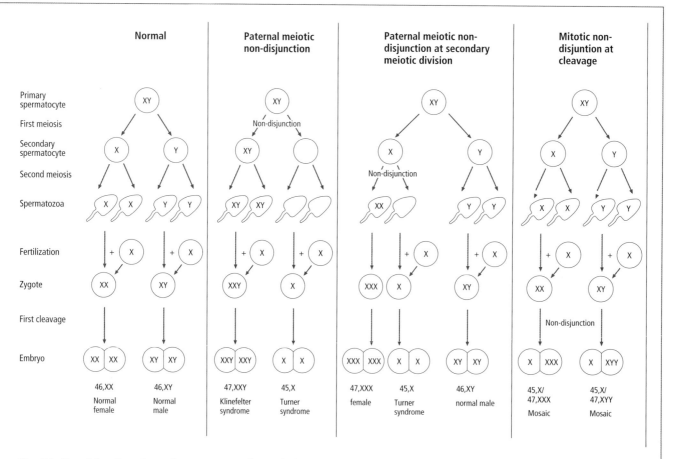

Fig. 7.1 Non-disjunction of sex chromosomes at first meiosis, at second meiosis and at early cleavage.

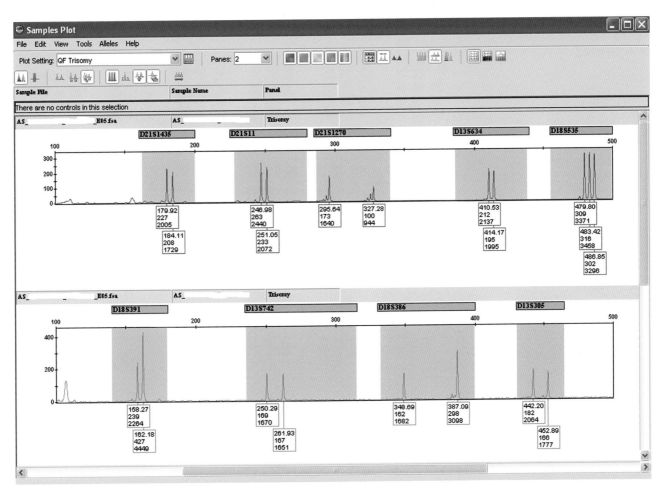

Fig. 7.2 Detection of trisomy 18 using QF-PCR. Diagnosis of trisomy requires a clear trisomic pattern on a chromosome indicated by at least two informative markers. The chromosome number is indicated after the prefix 'D' in the marker label above each set of peaks (e.g. D21S11). The product length (in bp) is represented on the *x*-axis and by the first of three measurements given in each small box. The other two measurements represent the peak height and area, respectively. Two signals of approximately equal amplitude are detected for the markers on chromosomes 21 and 13 (which are disomic). For the polymorphic markers tested on chromosome 18, however, there are three signals (trisomic triallelic as for the marker D18S535) or, alternatively, two peaks with one peak being of approximately twice the size of the other (trisomic diallelic, as for the marker D18S391).

infection or as a familial tendency. It is probably associated with a reduced frequency of recombination, but it is unknown whether or not this is causal (see Bugge *et al.*, 2007, in Further reading). The cause of mitotic non-disjunction is also unknown, although it has been suggested that it results from the altered expression of proteins involved either in kinetochore microtubule attachment or in the spindle assembly checkpoint described in Chapter 5 (see Cimini and Degrassi, 2005, and King, 2008, in Further reading).

Trisomy of chromosome 13, 18 or 21 (in addition to sex chromosome aneuploidy, if required) can be detected prenatally, without the need for prior cell culture, by fluorescence *in situ* hybridisation (FISH) (see Chapter 5) carried out in interphase or by quantitative fluorescent polymerase chain reaction (QF-PCR). In this increasingly used technique (see below), which can be completed in a few hours, the signal intensity of several chromosome-specific marker PCR products are

compared with each other (Fig. 7.2). This is achieved using multiplex PCR reactions with fluorescent oligonucleotide primers and subsequent detection using an automated DNA sequencer with dedicated software.

Aneuploidy can arise during either meiosis or mitosis, as mentioned above, and meiotic non-disjunction may occur at either the first or the second meiotic divisions (Fig. 7.1). If non-disjunction occurs at the first meiotic division, then the gamete with the extra chromosome will contain both (non-identical) homologues of that chromosome, whereas if it occurs at the second division then the normal and the extra copy of that chromosome will be identical. Sometimes the origin of the non-disjunctional event can be determined from the knowledge that two alleles at one locus are contributed by one parent, or by analysing the inheritance of chromosomal or DNA polymorphisms. Complete failure of synapsis of a pair of parental homologues at first meiosis (non-conjunction) may

Fig. 7.3 Triploidy detected at amniocentesis.

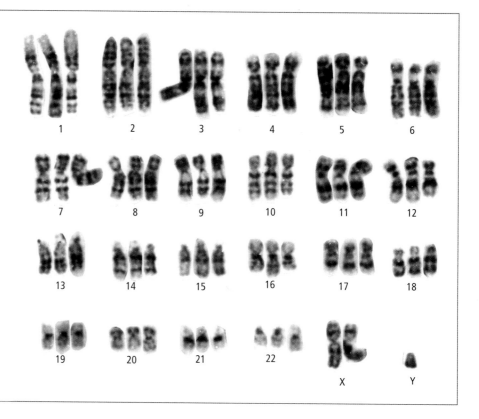

also lead to aneuploidy, and this is revealed by a total lack of recombination between parental loci.

Aneuploidy arising at a mitotic cell division may result in a mosaic, i.e. an individual with cell lines of two or more different chromosomal complements derived from a single zygote (Fig. 7.1).

Polyploidy

A complete extra set of chromosomes will raise the total number to 69, and this is called triploidy (Fig. 7.3). This usually arises from fertilisation by two sperms (dispermy), or from failure of one of the maturation divisions of either the egg or the sperm, so that a diploid gamete is produced. Thus, the chromosomal formula for a triploid fetus (which will usually miscarry) would be 69,XXY (most common), 69,XXX or 69,XYY, depending upon the origin of the extra chromosomal set.

Tetraploidy, or four times the haploid number, is usually due to failure to complete the first zygotic division. A proportion of polyploid cells occurs normally in human bone marrow, as megakaryocytes usually have 8–16 times the haploid number. Tetraploid cells are also a normal feature of regenerating liver and other tissues.

Structural aberrations

Structural aberrations result from chromosomal breakage and abnormal reunion. They can be induced experimentally by ionising radiation and mutagenic agents. When a chromosome breaks, two unstable sticky ends without telomeres are produced. Generally, repair mechanisms rejoin these two ends without delay. However, if more than one break has occurred, or if the double-strand break DNA repair system is defective following the inactivation of the breast cancer-related BRCA1 protein (see Chapter 13), then, as the repair mechanisms cannot distinguish one sticky end from another, there is the possibility of rejoining the wrong ends. The spontaneous rate of chromosomal breakage is markedly increased by exposure to ionising radiation, either environmental or therapeutic, and is also increased in some rare inherited conditions such as Fanconi anaemia. X-rays produce double-stranded breaks at any stage of the cell cycle in a dose-dependent linear fashion, but without any increase in the number of sister chromatid exchanges. In contrast, chemical mutagens, which are S phase-dependent, induce sister chromatid exchanges rather than chromatid break and exchange abnormalities. Chromosomal breakage is not randomly distributed, and for all translocations the spontaneous mutation rate is 1 in 1000 gametes.

Most structural chromosome aberrations in both somatic and germ cells arise from errors of recombination. Recombination is preceded by synapsis of homologous chromosomes, which involves the recognition by one homologue of complementary sequences in the other homologue. Mismatching can occur, particularly in regions of repetitive DNA, followed by unequal crossing-over (see Fig. 7.13), leading to duplication or deletion. Similarly, synapsis between homologous regions on non-homologous chromosomes can lead to accidental recom-

Table 7.2 Examples of structural chromosomal aberrations

Karyotype	Description
46,XY,t(5;10)(p13;q25)	Balanced reciprocal translocation involving chromosomes 5 and 10 (breakpoints indicated)
45,XX,der(13;14)(q10;q10)	Robertsonian (centric fusion) translocation of chromosomes 13 and 14
46,XY,del(5)(p15.2)	Short-arm deletion of chromosome 5, cri du chat syndrome
46,X,i(X)(q10)	Isochromosome of Xq
46,XX,dup(2)(p13p22)	Partial duplication of the short arm of chromosome 2 (p13 → p22)
46,XY,r(3)(p26q29)	Ring chromosome 3 (p26 → q29)
46,XY,inv(11)(p15q14)	Pericentric inversion of chromosome 11

bination between non-homologous chromosomes, resulting in chromosome rearrangements. Sites of non-allelic homologous recombination (NAHR) are characterised by low copy number region-specific repeats. Thus, rearrangement breakpoints tend to occur within segmental duplications, retrotransposons, copy number variants and other duplications with up to 97% homology. They tend to be located at pericentromeric and subtelomeric chromosomal regions and may be in direct or inverted orientation with respect to one another. Thus, the most frequent constitutional chromosome aberrations can be traced to NAHR. Other, less frequent mechanisms include non-homologous end joining and centromere repositioning.

Recombination can also occur between homologous chromosomes in somatic cells, and examples of chromosome pairing and chromatid exchange are occasionally seen during routine chromosome analysis (see Fig. 5.19). It is likely that most of the complex chromosome rearrangements in cancer cells arise by NAHR.

Variation between the karyotypes of different species has a similar origin, often using the same breakpoint sites, although the number of rearrangements that become fixed in evolution is comparatively small due to the high level of genome conservation revealed by chromosome painting (see Ferguson-Smith and Trifonov, 2007, in Further reading). However, there is evidence that breakpoint sites of evolutionary rearrangements may be re-used during the divergence of species.

Structural aberrations are subdivided into translocations, deletion and ring chromosomes, duplications, inversions, isochromosomes and marker chromosomes (Table 7.2).

Translocations

A translocation is the transfer of chromosomal material between chromosomes. The process requires breakage of both chromosomes with repair in an abnormal arrangement, or accidental recombination between non-homologous chromosomes during meiosis. This exchange usually results in no significant loss of DNA and no gene disruption. The individual is usually clinically normal and is said to have a balanced translocation. The medical significance is for future generations, because a bal-

anced translocation carrier is at risk of producing chromosomally unbalanced offspring.

Three types of translocation are recognised: reciprocal, Robertsonian (centric fusion) and insertional.

Reciprocal translocations

In a reciprocal translocation, chromosomal material distal to breaks in two chromosomes is exchanged. Either the long or the short arm may break and any pair of chromosomes may be involved (either homologous or non-homologous). Thus, in Fig. 7.4a, breaks have occurred in the long arm of chromosome 10 and the long arm of chromosome 11 with reciprocal exchange, while Fig. 7.5a shows a balanced 5;10 reciprocal translocation. The carrier of either of these balanced translocations is healthy, but during gametogenesis unbalanced gametes may be produced. When these chromosomes pair during meiosis, a cross-shaped quadrivalent is formed, which allows homologous segments to be in contact (Fig. 7.4b–d). This later opens into a ring or chain held together by chiasmata (Fig. 7.5b,c). At anaphase, these four chromosomes must segregate to the two daughter cells. Fourteen possible different gametes may be seen in each case. Figure 7.5d shows the six of these that result from a two-to-two segregation (i.e. two chromosomes passing to each daughter cell). Of these six possibilities, only one gamete is normal and one is a balanced translocation. The other four result in various imbalances of the amounts of chromosomes 5 and 10. Such visible imbalance involves large numbers of genes, and affected conceptions may miscarry, or, if liveborn, learning disability and multiple congenital malformations would be found. Three-to-one segregation results in a further eight (of the 14) gametes, but the chromosomal imbalance in each of these is so gross that early spontaneous miscarriage would be expected. Thus, in the liveborn offspring of the carrier of either of these translocations, one would expect a ratio of 1 normal : 1 balanced : 4 unbalanced. In practice, some of the unbalanced fetuses miscarry, and there may also be selection against the unbalanced gametes, so the actual risk of unbalanced offspring is always lower than expected (also see Chapter 16).

Fig. 7.4 (a) Reciprocal translocation between chromosomes 10 and 11. The normal chromosome is shown on the left for each pair. (b) Meiotic quadrivalent configuration in a 10;11 translocation. Chromosome 10 is shown at the top and chromosome 11 at the bottom. Normal chromosomes 10 and 11 are shown on the top right and lower left, respectively. (c) Meiotic quadrivalent at pachytene in a 10;11 translocation carrier (arrow). For simplicity, in the diagrammatic representation of the quadrivalent, whole chromosomes, rather than their individual chromatid components, are shown. (d) Electron micrograph of the synaptonemal complex of a 9;20 translocation observed at pachytene in a translocation carrier (stained with silver nitrate).

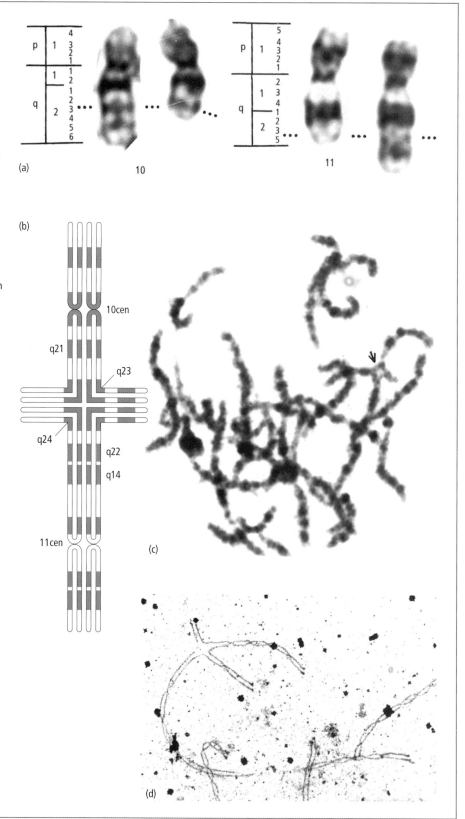

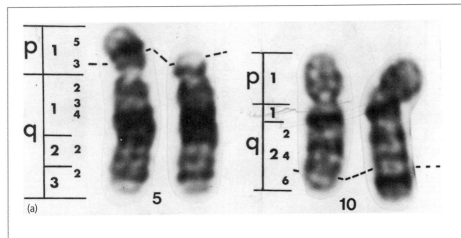

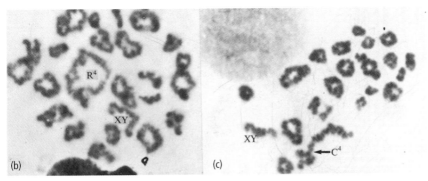

Fig. 7.5 (a) Reciprocal translocation between chromosomes 5 and 10. The normal chromosome is shown on the left for each pair. (b) Meiotic ring quadrivalent (R⁴) for a balanced 5;10 reciprocal translocation at first meiosis. (c) Meiotic chain quadrivalent (C⁴, arrow) at diakinesis. (d) Three types of 2:2 segregation for a balanced 5;10 reciprocal translocation at first meiosis. Note that the four types of 3:1 segregation are not shown. Except in specific translocations, such as an 11;22 translocation, the unbalanced offspring resulting from a 3:1 segregation would not be viable and a miscarriage would result from the gross chromosomal imbalance. For simplicity, the two individual chromatids that would be present are not shown in the first and final stages of this figure and are represented instead by a single chromosome.

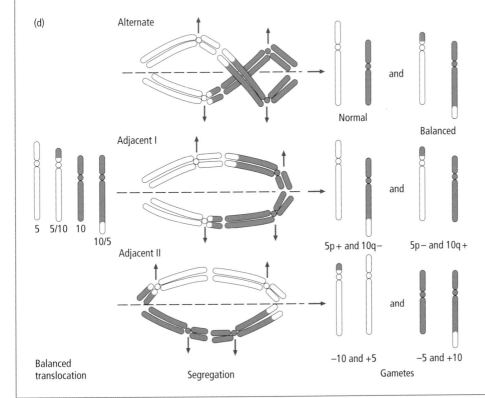

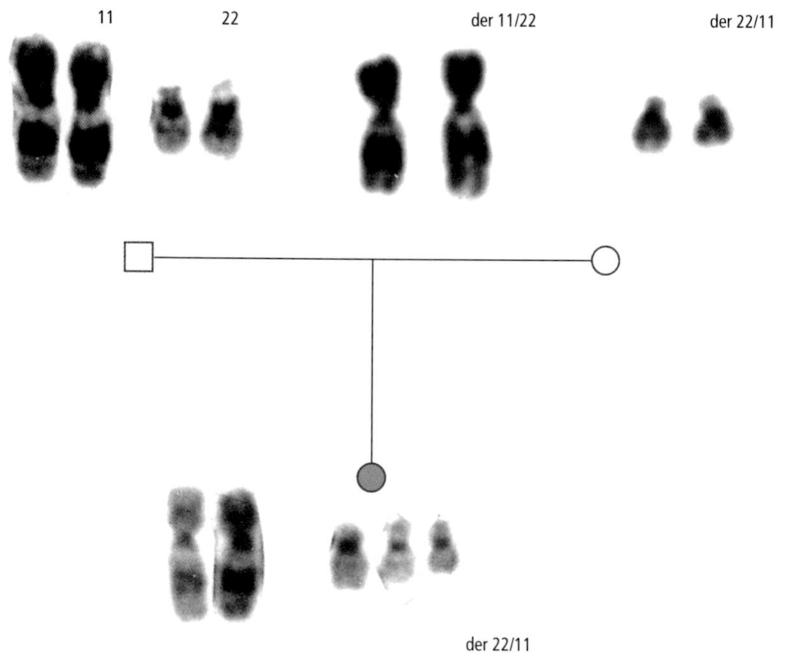

Fig. 7.6 Maternal reciprocal translocation between chromosomes 11 and 22 with 3 : 1 segregation to produce partial duplication of chromosomes 11 and 22 in a daughter with significant learning disability. In the 3 : 1 segregation, the daughter inherited the mother's der(22;11) in addition to the mother's normal chromosome 11 and normal chromosome 22.

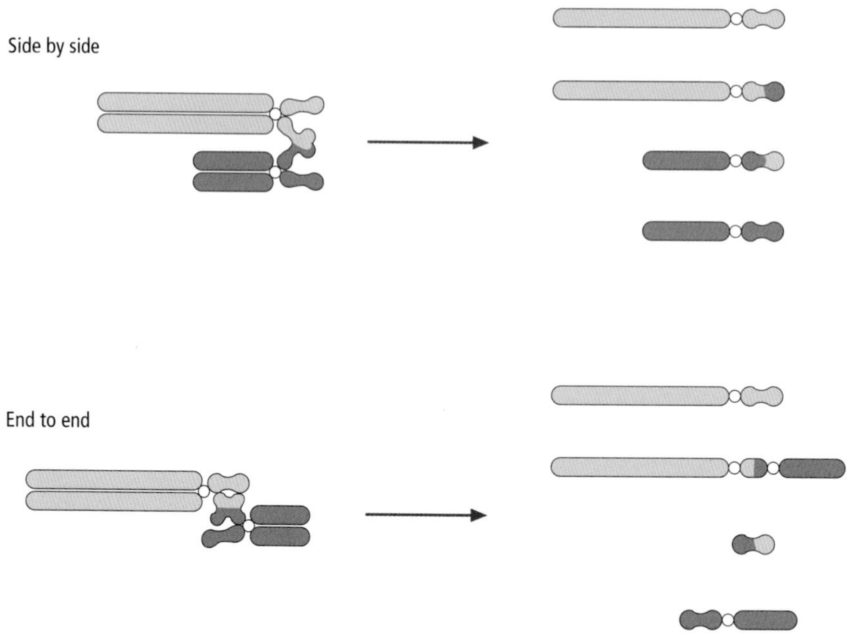

Fig. 7.7 Accidental recombination between homologous regions of non-homologous chromosomes during meiosis as a cause of dicentric centric fusion chromosomes.

For particular translocations, unbalanced offspring produced by a three-to-one segregation may be viable, e.g. with partial triplication of chromosome 22 (Fig. 7.6).

Robertsonian (centric fusion) translocations

Robertsonian translocations arise from breaks at or near the centromere in two acrocentric chromosomes with cross-fusion of the products. In most cases, the breaks are just above the centromere and so the products are a single chromosome with two centromeres (dicentric) and a fragment with no centromere (acentric) bearing both satellites. An acentric fragment cannot undergo mitosis and will usually be lost at a subsequent cell division. The most likely cause is NAHR occurring at homologous sequences within the acrocentric short arms during first meiosis (Fig. 7.7).

Centric fusion of chromosomes 13 and 14 is the single most frequent type of translocation in humans, and this is followed in frequency by centric fusion of 14 and 21. Figure 7.8 shows the partial karyotype of a balanced 14;21

Robertsonian translocation. This combined chromosome is dicentric, and the acentric fragment has been lost, so leaving only 45 chromosomes in total. Again, such an individual is healthy, but problems may arise at gametogenesis. When the chromosomes pair during meiosis a trivalent is formed, which allows homologous segments to be in contact (Fig. 7.9). At anaphase, these three chromosomes must segregate to the gametes, and Fig. 7.10 shows the six possible gametes. Only one is normal; one is balanced and four are unbalanced. Again, in practice, spontaneous abortion and gametic selection result in a lower observed frequency of unbalanced offspring than predicted (also see Chapter 16).

Insertional translocations

For an insertional translocation, three breaks are required in one or two chromosomes. If between two chromosomes, this results in an interstitial deletion of a segment of one, which is inserted into the gap in the other (Fig. 7.11). Again, the balanced carrier is healthy but may produce unbalanced offspring with *either* a duplication *or* a deletion, but not both.

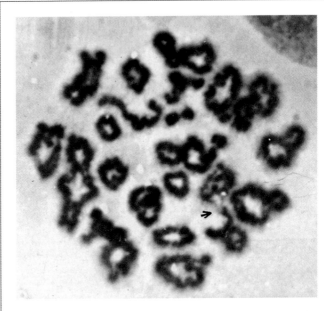

Fig. 7.9 Meiotic trivalent for a t(13;14) Robertsonian translocation (arrow).

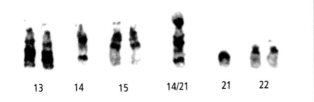

13	14	15	14/21	21	22

Fig. 7.8 Robertsonian translocation of chromosomes 14 and 21.

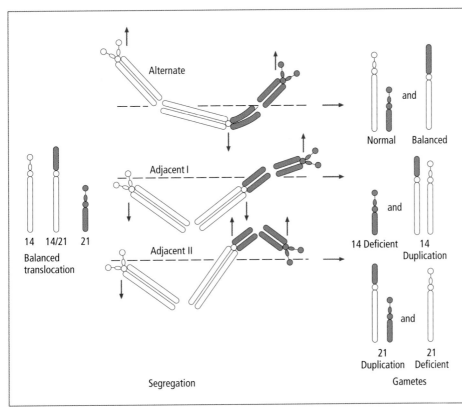

Fig. 7.10 Segregation of a Robertsonian translocation at first meiosis. For simplicity, as in Figs 7.4 and 7.5, whole chromosomes rather than their individual component chromatids are shown.

Alternate

Adjacent I

Adjacent II

14   14/21   21
Balanced
translocation

Segregation

Normal   Balanced

and

14 Deficient   14
Duplication

and

21   21
Duplication   Deficient

and

Gametes

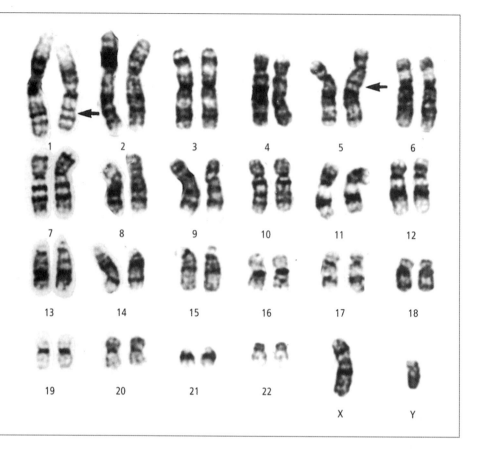

Fig. 7.11 Insertional translocation showing interstitial deletion of band 1q31 and insertion into band 5q13 (arrows).

Deletions and ring chromosomes

A loss of any part of a chromosome is a deletion. Deletions arise from loss of a portion of the chromosome between two breakpoints (interstitial deletions), as a result of unequal crossing-over, as a result of a parental translocation or as a terminal deletion. In the latter instance, the deletion continues proximally until a DNA region homologous to telomere sequences is reached. Here, the enzyme telomerase is able to synthesise a new telomere and so arrest the deletion. The deleted portion lacks a centromere (an acentric fragment) and will be lost at a subsequent cell division. A ring chromosome arises from breaks in both arms of a chromosome: the terminal ends are lost and the two proximal sticky ends unite to form a ring. If the ring has a centromere, then it may be able to pass through cell division. A sister chromatid exchange within a ring results in a dicentric ring of twice the size in subsequent divisions (Fig. 7.12).

As the smallest visible loss from a chromosome is about 4 Mb, individuals with visible deletions are rendered monosomic for large numbers of contiguous genes, and with autosomal deletions learning disability and multiple congenital malformations are usual. Deletions of a size close to the limit of resolution with the light microscope are termed microdeletions (see Fig. 6.18) and molecular techniques have been developed to aid their detection (see Chapter 5).

Duplications

In a duplication, an additional copy of a segment of a chromosome is present. It may originate by unequal crossing-over during meiosis, and the reciprocal product is a deletion (Fig. 7.13). A duplication can also result from meiotic events in a parent with a translocation, inversion or isochromosome.

Duplications are more common than deletions and are generally less harmful. Indeed, tiny duplications at the molecular level (repeats) may play an important role in permitting gene diversification during evolution.

Inversions

Inversions arise from two chromosomal breaks with inversion through 180° of the segment between the breaks. If both breaks are in a single arm, then the centromere is not included (paracentric inversion) (Fig. 7.14a), whereas if the breaks are on either side of the centromere it is included (pericentric inversion) (Fig. 7.14b). Generally, this change in gene order does not produce clinical abnormality. The medical significance lies with the increased risk of generating unbalanced gametes.

Inversions interfere with the pairing of homologous chromosomes during meiosis, and crossing-over tends to be suppressed within the inverted segment. For homologous

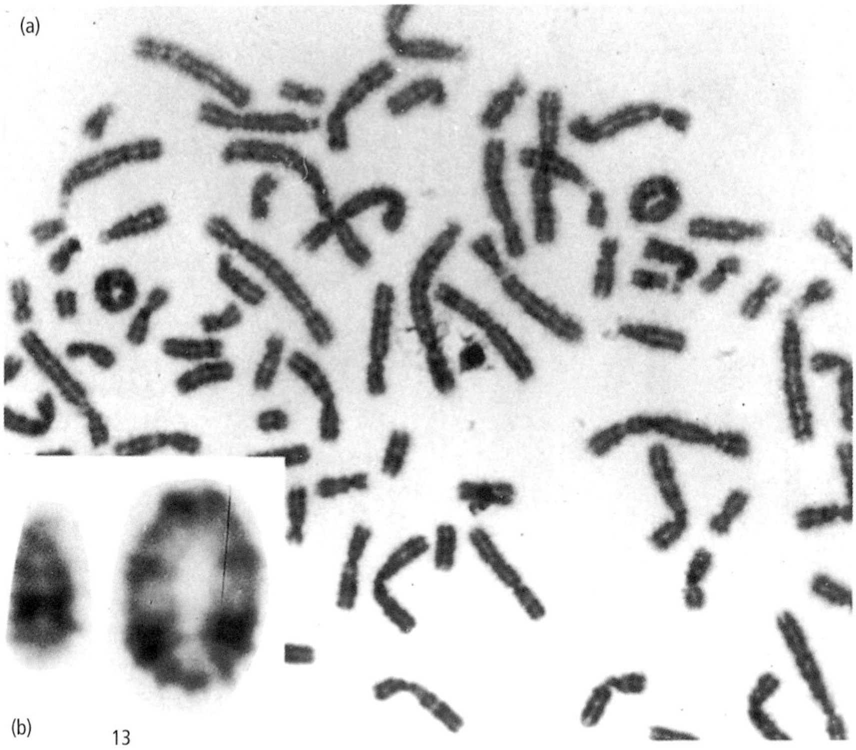

(a)

(b)   13

Fig. 7.12 (a) Ring chromosomes, dicentrics and acentric fragments following exposure to irradiation. (b) Double-ring chromosome 13.

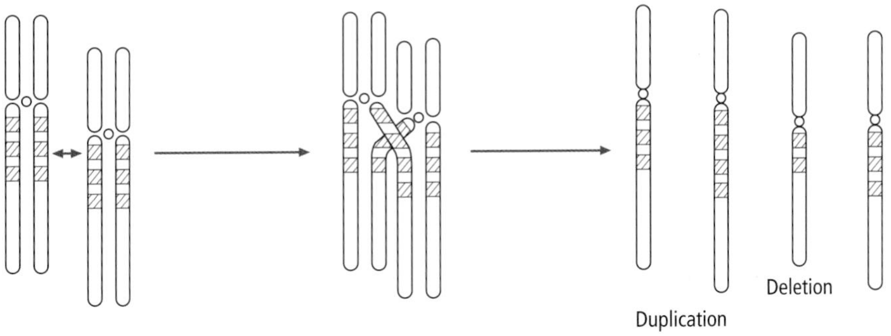

Duplication   Deletion

Fig. 7.13 Results of unequal crossing-over.

chromosomes to pair, one member must form a loop in the region of the inversion (Fig. 7.15) or the chromosome arms distal to the inversion fail to pair. For a paracentric inversion, if a cross-over does occur within the loop, then this will result in a dicentric chromatid and an acentric fragment. Both of these are unstable and rarely result in abnormal offspring. In contrast, for a pericentric inversion, if an uneven number of cross-overs occurs within the loop, then each of the two chromatids produced will have both a deletion and a duplication, and abnormal offspring may be produced (Figs 7.16 and 7.17). These unbalanced products always show a deletion of the segment distal to one of the breakpoints and duplication of the segment distal to the other. The closer both breakpoints are to the telomeres, the smaller the duplication and deletion and thus the higher the likelihood of survival of the fetus until birth.

It is important to distinguish inversions from centromere repositioning in which there is no change in gene order and little consequence to offspring.

Isochromosomes

An isochromosome is an abnormal chromosome that has a deletion of one arm with duplication of the other. It may arise from transverse division of the centromere during cell division (Fig. 7.18a) or from an isochromatid break and fusion above the centromere (in which case it is dicentric). The commonest isochromosome in live births is an isochromosome of the long arm of X, or i(Xq). This results in clinical abnormality (Turner syndrome; see Chapter 6) due to short-arm monosomy and long-arm trisomy. Isochromosomes of Y are also seen in live births, but for other chromosomes an isochromosome usually

Fig. 7.14 (a) Two examples of paracentric inversions of chromosome 12. (b) Pericentric inversion of chromosome 9; this inversion is present in 1% of the normal population (this patient coincidentally has trisomy 21).

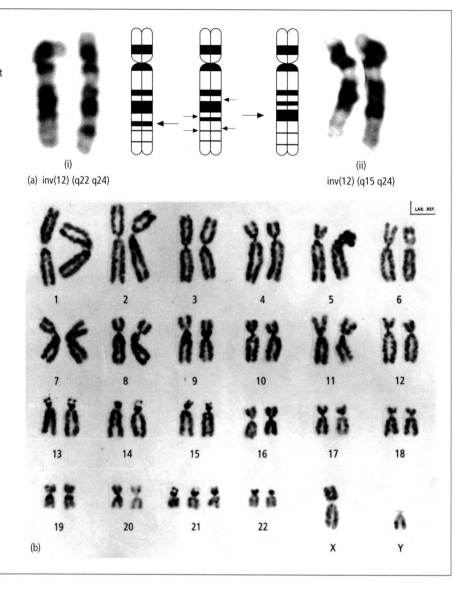

(i)

(a) inv(12) (q22 q24)

(ii)

inv(12) (q15 q24)

(b)

results in an early spontaneous abortion; rare exceptions are isochromosomes of the short arms of chromosomes 9 and 12 (Fig. 7.18b). In many instances, isochromosomes are dicentric, but one centromere becomes non-functional so that the chromosome segregates normally during cell division.

Marker chromosomes

Additional small, usually metacentric, fragments are sometimes detected during routine karyotyping. Some are familial and have resulted from a Robertsonian translocation between satellite chromosomes (often involving the short arm of chromosome 15) arising in meiosis in a parent or ancestor. Provided the marker chromosome (or centric fragment) contains only repetitive and ribosomal DNA, there will be no clinical consequences. Occasionally, transcribed genes are also included, in which case there may be associated disability. An example is the cat-eye syndrome due to inv dup(22), and cases of inv

dup(15) that include the Prader–Willi syndrome/Angelman syndrome critical region.

Cytogenetic and molecular methods for the detection of chromosomal aberrations

A number of different methods can now be used to detect chromosomal abnormalities. These include various cytogenetic methods as well as molecular methods, some of which have become available only recently.

Cytogenetic methods

The cytogenetic methods include routine karyotyping (see Chapter 5) using, in an increasing number of laboratories, computerised systems for image capture, manipulation and

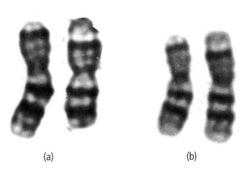

(a) (b)

Fig. 7.16 Large pericentric inversion of chromosome 7. The normal chromosome in each case os shown on the left. (a) Parent with balanced inversion. (b) Abnormal child with duplication (7q32-qter) and deficiency (7p22-pter) resulting from a cross-over within the paternal inversion.

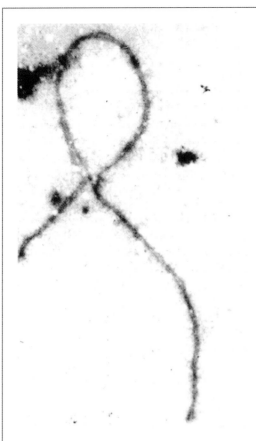

Fig. 7.15 Electron micrograph of the synaptonemal complex of a 46,XY,inv(2)(p13;q25) carrier. Homologous pairing has been achieved by one homologue forming an inversion loop.

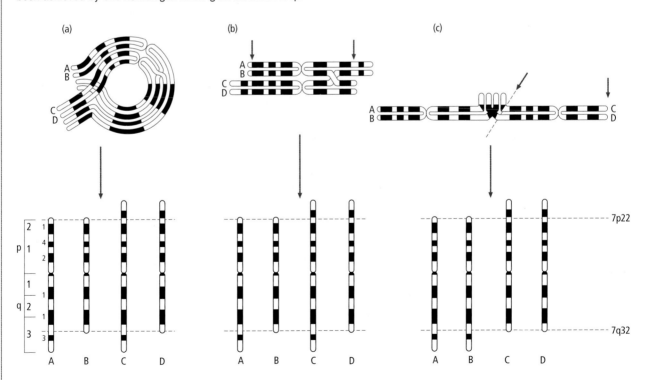

Fig. 7.17 The results of crossing-over at meiosis (a, b) within and (c) outside the pericentric inversion of chromosome 7, as shown in Fig. 7.16. A is the normal chromosome 7 and D has the pericentric inversion. In (a) and (b), two types of abnormal recombinant chromosome are formed (B and C, each with a duplication deficiency). In (c), crossing-over outside the inversion produces no abnormal recombinant.

Fig. 7.18 (a) Dicentric isochromosome for the long arm of the X. Staining by G-banding (left pair) and C-banding (right pair). The dicentric is the chromosome on the right in each pair. (b) Dicentric isochromosome for the short arm of chromosome 9 in a patient with the features of trisomy 9p syndrome. Only one centromere (the top one) is functional.

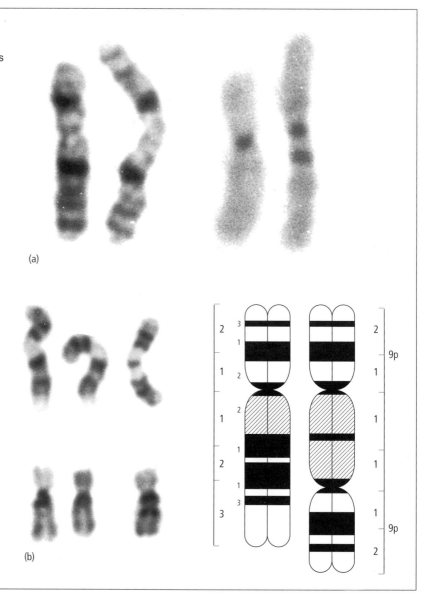

(a)

(b)

analysis. In addition, some laboratories use specialised staining techniques such as R-banding (reverse banding), in which the bands stain in the opposite fashion from that seen with G-banding. This is achieved by heating the chromosomes in a saline buffer before staining with Giemsa and may be useful if the telomeres are involved in aberrations.

Fluorescence *in situ hybridisation*

A particularly useful cytogenetic technique is FISH (mentioned above and described in detail in Chapter 5). This can be used for rapid detection of aneuploidy on interphase chromosomes in prenatal testing (Fig. 7.19), particularly where QF-PCR (see below) is not available. In addition, FISH can be used to detect specific disease-associated chromosomal microdeletions or microduplications (such as the microdele-

tion at 22q11 associated with velocardiofacial syndrome) and to identify the chromosomal origin of chromosomal material in complex rearrangements (see below). As mentioned in chapter 5, FISH is currently being increasingly used clinically in PGD to determine the fetal sex and to detect unbalanced translocation products in situations where there is a family history of an X-linked recessive genetic condition or a known apparently balanced parental chromosome translocation, respectively (see Chapter 12). A clinical research technique is to use bacterial artificial chromosome (BAC) probes to carry out FISH to locate the specific breakpoint in individuals who have a clinical phenotype and an apparently balanced chromosomal translocation. Then, once a breakpoint-spanning BAC is identified, candidates for the probable disrupted causative gene can be identified using online databases. This research technique was, for example, employed (see Fig. 7.20

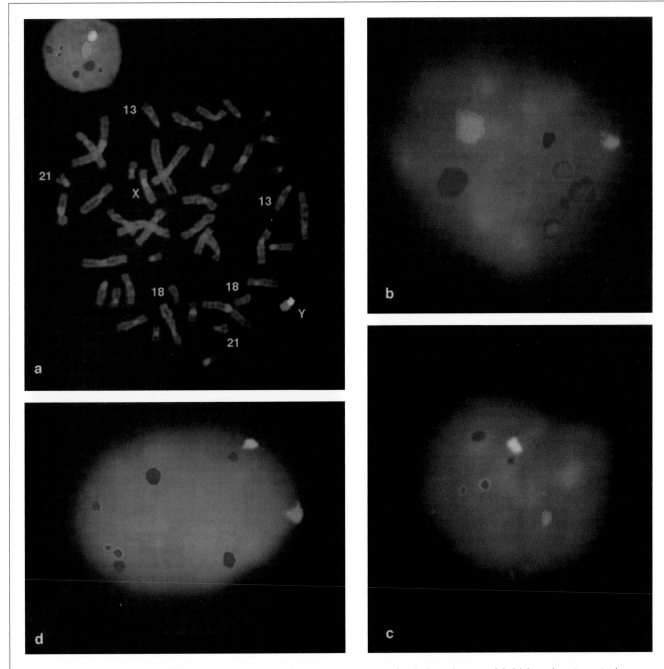

Fig. 7.19 Use of multicolour FISH probes to determine chromosome copy number in interphase nuclei. (a) Lymphocyte metaphase and interphase nuclei showing centromeric probes for the X chromosome (lilac), Y chromosome (yellow) and chromosome 18 (dark blue); a YAC clone marks chromosome 13q (green) and two overlapping cosmid clones mark chromosome 21 (red). (b) Uncultured amniotic fluid cell nucleus from a female fetus hybridized with the above probes, revealing a normal number of each chromosome. (c) As in (b), from a normal male fetus. (d) As in (b), from a male fetus with trisomy 21 (Down syndrome). From Divane *et al.*, Prenatal Diagnosis 1994; 14:1061–69.

and Johnson *et al.*, 2006, in Further reading) to confirm the *CHD7* gene on chromosome 8 as an important cause of CHARGE association, a syndrome comprising colobomata, choanal atresia, developmental delay and malformations of the heart and ear.

DNA-based methods

Several molecular methods using DNA rather than chromosome preparations have proved particularly useful means by which to detect chromosomal aberrations. In particular,

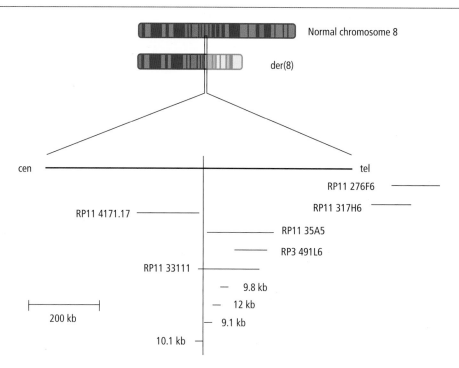

Fig. 7.20 Derivative chromosome 13 resulting from a balanced reciprocal 8;13 translocation identified in a pair of monozygotic twins affected by the CHARGE association. Mapping of the chromosome 8 breakpoint was undertaken using a series of FISH probes, leading to the identification of the causative *CHD7* gene. The relative positions of the chromosome 8-specific FISH probes are indicated. Probe RP11 33111 spanned the breakpoint on chromosome 8. Clones to the right of the long vertical line mapped to the der(13) and normal 8. Probe 10.1 kb (which spanned exons 4 and 5) localised to both the normal and the derivative chromosome 8, while probe 9.1 kb (which spanned exons 6 and 7) localised to both derivative chromosomes 8 and 13. Reproduced from Journal of Medical Genetics, Johnson et al., 43, 280–4. © 2006 with permission from BMJ Publishing Group Ltd.

QF-PCR, multiple ligation-dependent probe amplification (MLPA) and high-resolution array comparative genomic hybridisation (aCGH) are increasingly used for such purposes.

Quantitative fluorescent PCR

In the UK, QF-PCR has generally replaced interphase FISH as the standard method by which prenatal or neonatal testing is carried out, if appropriate, for the rapid detection of aneuploidy involving chromosomes 21, 18 or 13. It can also be used to detect sex chromosome aneuploidy, if required. In QF-PCR, several polymorphic short tandem repeat microsatellite markers distributed over the chromosomes in question are amplified by PCR using primers labelled with one of a range of fluorescent dyes. In fact, typically, multiplex PCR (i.e. a combination of several simultaneous PCR reactions within one tube) for markers on chromosomes 13, 18 and 21 is carried out. This is followed by accurate determination of the size and relative abundance of the DNA products on an automated sequencer (such as an ABI 3130xl). Careful analysis of the resulting peaks, comparing the peak heights or areas, allows the determination of the dosage (i.e. relative amounts) of each of the chromosomes being examined. The diagnosis of a trisomy requires a clear trisomic pattern on a chromosome indicated by either three peaks (representing three alleles) or two peaks (with one peak being of approximately twice the size of the other), for at least two informative markers (see Figs 7.2 and 7.21a and b).

Multiple ligation-dependent probe amplification

The MLPA DNA analysis technique (see Chapter 4) now provides an additional method by which specific deletions (or duplications) can be identified. This technique permits, in a few hours, relative quantification of more than 40 different nucleic acid sequences in a single reaction (Fig. 7.22). A range of kits have now been manufactured that are designed to screen for subtelomeric microdeletions, for microdeletions affecting various regions with a single large gene, such as dystrophin, or for interstitial deletions or duplications known to be responsible for a range of genetic syndromes.

Array comparative genomic hybridisation

Submicroscopic deletions and duplications located anywhere in the genome can be detected using high-resolution aCGH.

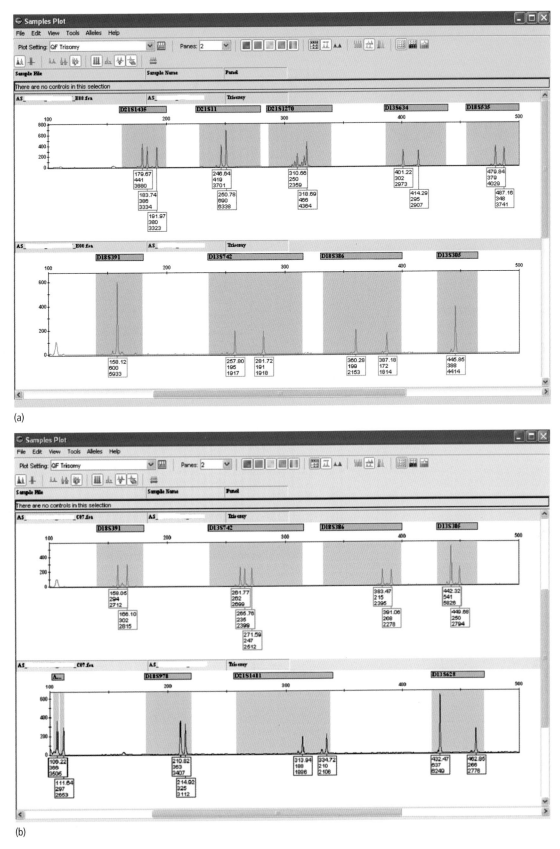

(a)

(b)

Fig. 7.21 (a) QF-PCR result for a pregnancy affected by trisomy 21. The graph shows either trisomic diallelic (two peaks with a 2:1 size ratio) or triallelic patterns for the microsatellite markers on chromosome 21, but normal diallelic peaks of approximately equal sizes for chromosomes 18 and 13. An uninformative homozygous marker (producing a single unhelpful peak) on chromosome 18 and also for chromosome 13 is also visible, resulting from a pair of alleles that possess the same number of repeats. (b) QF-PCR result for a pregnancy affected by trisomy 13.

Fig. 7.22 (a) MLPA result for a patient affected by Williams syndrome. The blood DNA MLPA results (top) are shown together with a chart showing the peak ratios for each probe (bottom). The patient possesses a microdeletion on one chromosome 7, as can be seen from the reduced size of the blue peaks relative to the red control peaks (with a ratio of approximately 0.5 instead of 1.0) for the six DNA probe sequences that are located within the deleted region. The probes are displayed by the analysis software in order of sequence length rather than according to their order along the chromosome. The MLPA kit was obtained from MRC-Holland. (b) MLPA results for the Williams syndrome region on chromosome 7, using DNA from a normal control individual.

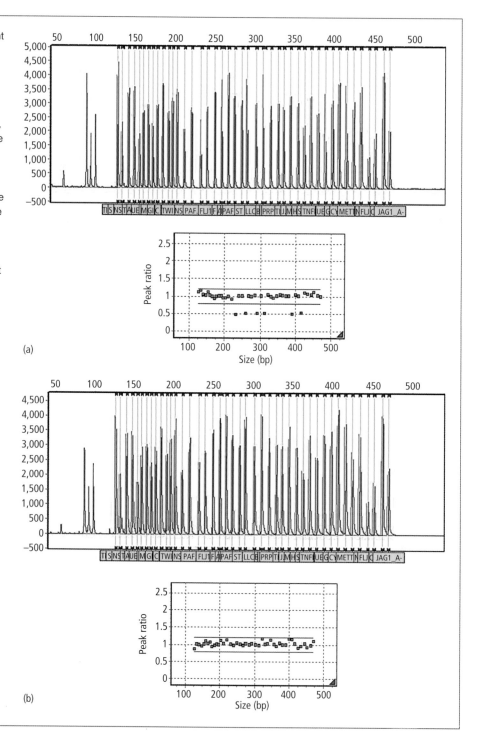

Array CGH is based on sequence and marker data from the Human Genome Project. It utilises microarrays of thousands of DNA sequences, spaced at intervals along the chromosomes, spotted onto slides (Fig. 7.23). Arrays vary in resolution, from 1 Mb between sequences, to tiling path arrays with a resolution of about 1 kb. A subject's test DNA is labelled with a green fluorescent dye and mixed with reference genomic DNA labelled in red. The mixture is hybridised, for example, to a microarray of 3000 (1 Mb resolution) genomic DNA sequences. After washing, the microarray is scanned by a laser. The fluorescence is measured at each spot, with the green:red ratio indicating the relative abundance of subject versus reference DNA. The ratios from all the spots can be plotted against a chromosome map to reveal regions of copy-number variation. The method identifies pathological duplications and deletions, which may be difficult to distinguish from non-pathological

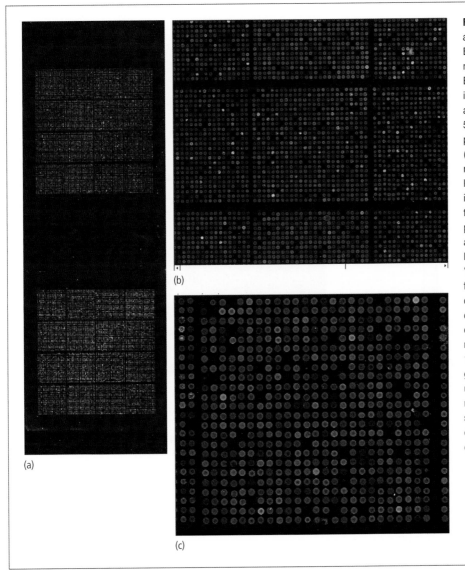

(a)

(b)

(c)

Figs. 7.23 (a–c) Images showing an aCGH slide ('CytoChip' from BlueGnome Ltd) at increasing magnification. The slide shown uses BAC microarrays to permit investigation of genomic copy number at a higher resolution (approximately 500 kb on average) than would be possible by standard karyotyping (approximately 4 Mb). The spots represent different known genomic loci. Intensely red or green signals indicate an excess of patient relative to control DNA or vice versa. The presence of two identical hybridisation areas on each slide (the upper and lower grids in (a)) permit the use of a 'dye-swap' technique, in which the fluorescent labelling of patient and control DNA samples are reversed for one of the hybridisation areas, in order to allow confirmation of the results. Even higher resolution (e.g. 11–14 kb in clinically important genomic regions) can be obtained using oligo-array CGH (greater numbers of spots are present on the slide, each spot containing an oligonucleotide, rather than a BAC clone).

copy-number variation without testing parental samples or reference to population control data, available from databases such as DECIPHER (http://decipher.sanger.ac.uk).

Regions of deletion or duplication detected by aCGH (see Fig. 7.24 for an example) can, if appropriate, be confirmed by FISH (Fig. 7.25). aCGH is increasingly being used to identify pathogenic regions of copy-number alteration in patients with unexplained learning disability and dysmorphic features (Fig. 7.26). It can also be used to detect such alterations at chromosome breakpoints in patients with apparently balanced reciprocal chromosome translocations.

Identification of the chromosomal origin of complex structural rearrangements

Identification of the chromosomes involved in numerical and gross structural rearrangements is usually obvious using standard G-banding procedures. The origin of smaller duplications

and deletions may be more difficult to determine, particularly if the aberration is unbalanced and has arisen *de novo*. Complex rearrangements involving several chromosomes, for example as found in some malignant tissues, may prove impossible to resolve by chromosome banding alone. In these situations, DNA probes may be used in molecular *in situ* hybridisation procedures to label the specific components of an abnormal chromosome and so identify their origins. In addition, DNA probes can be used to help to determine the precise position of a breakpoint in a chromosome translocation, and this can occasionally be invaluable in the identification of genes underlying specific conditions, such as the CHARGE association, as mentioned above (Fig. 7.20). There are many types of chromosome-specific probes that can be used for such investigations, including repetitive (alphoid) probes, which are centromere-specific, and cosmid or yeast artificial chromosome (YAC) probes, which contain an insert large enough to provide a clear signal in the majority of metaphases. Commercially

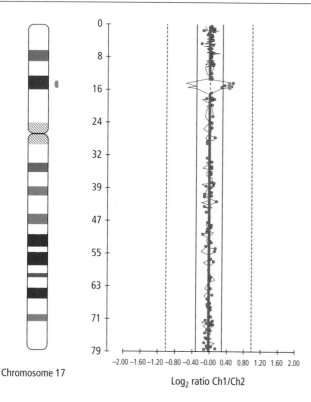

Chromosome 17

Log$_2$ ratio Ch1/Ch2

Fig. 7.24 aCGH results of chromosome 17 in a patient with mild hereditary motor and sensory neuropathy (HMSN). The altered ratio of fluorescence, of patient DNA (Ch1) compared with control (Ch2) is clearly indicated (green line adjacent to the chromosome idiogram) at the region on 17p that is affected by a microduplication. The abnormality is confirmed on the superimposed dye-swap profile showing inverted ratios (red trace). It is known that duplication of the gene encoding peripheral myelin protein-22 (PMP22) in this region (17p11.2) is a common cause of HMSN type 1A (also known as Charcot–Marie–Tooth disease type 1A). When the diagnosis is suspected clinically, the duplications at this site are more usually detected by MLPA.

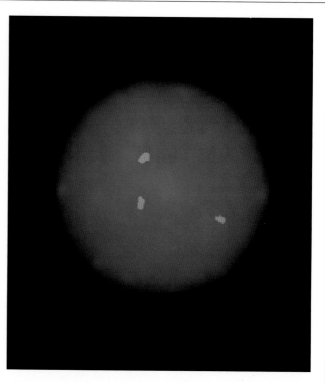

Fig. 7.25 Interphase FISH image showing the presence of three signals instead of the normal two, using a probe hybridising to the region on chromosome 17p11.2 containing the *PMP22* gene. This confirms the presence of the microduplication at this region that was indicated on aCGH (Fig. 7.23). Such duplications would not be clearly visible by FISH on a metaphase spread due to the proximity of the two signals on the same chromosome.

available non-isotopic detection systems that incorporate fluorescently labelled DNA probes are most often used. Figure 7.27 shows alphoid repeat probes for the X chromosome (labelled with Texas red) and chromosome 18 (labelled with fluorescein isothiocyanate) in a FISH procedure that clearly identifies both chromosomes in both metaphase and interphase. Chromosome-specific DNA probes can be made from an entire chromosome and used to 'paint' by FISH those parts of a structural aberration derived from that chromosome (Fig. 7.28). Chromosome paints may be made from chromosome-specific genomic libraries, single-chromosome somatic-cell hybrids or PCR-amplified chromosomes sorted by a fluorescence activated cell sorting (FACS) machine. All these probes require a pre-annealing step to suppress repetitive DNA sequences before application in FISH experiments.

Chromosome paints may also be made from *abnormal* chromosomes, which are sorted by FACS, amplified by PCR and painted onto *normal* metaphase chromosomes. As shown in Fig. 7.29, the paint probe reveals the origin of each chromosome segment present in the abnormal chromosome and, at the same time, identifies the exact breakpoint involved in each chromosome. This technique of 'reverse painting' has revealed that most *de novo* duplications are tandem duplications or other forms of intrachromosomal rearrangement.

Multicolour FISH (M-FISH) is a more recent development that enables several DNA probes to be used simultaneously. When applied to chromosome paints, it is possible, using different combinations of fluorescent dyes, to give each chromosome a distinctive colour and this can be useful in the analysis of complex chromosome rearrangements (Fig. 7.30).

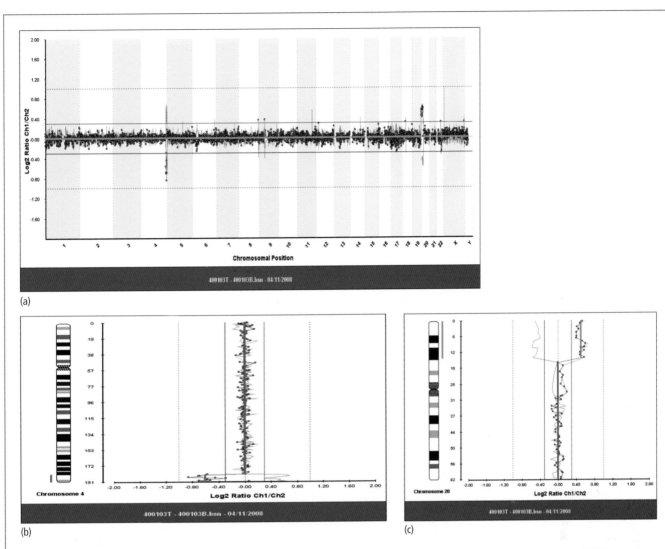

Fig. 7.26 aCGH analysis of a patient with a t(4;20) unbalanced translocation. (a) Chart showing ratio of patient to control DNA across the genome, using aCGH with BAC clones spaced at a median of 565 kb generally, at 250 kb at the subtelomeric regions and at 100 kb at 90 specific known disease loci. Regions of clinically significant abnormality were detected on chromosomes 4 and 20, resulting from the unbalanced translocation. (b, c) Individual aCGH chromosome profiles showing a deletion on the long arm of chromosome 4 and a duplication on the short arm of chromosome 20 in the patient with the unbalanced t(4;20) represented in (a).

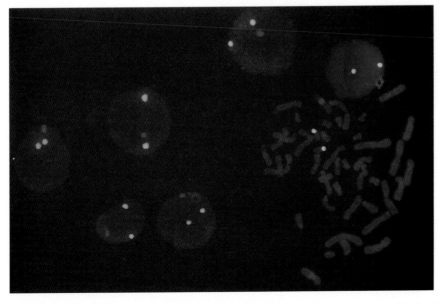

Fig. 7.27 Identification of chromosomes 18 and the X in metaphase and interphase using FISH. Alphoid centromeric repeat probes were detected with FITC (chromosome 18; green) and Texas red (X chromosome; bright red), counterstained with propidium iodide (dark red). Karyotype 46, XY.

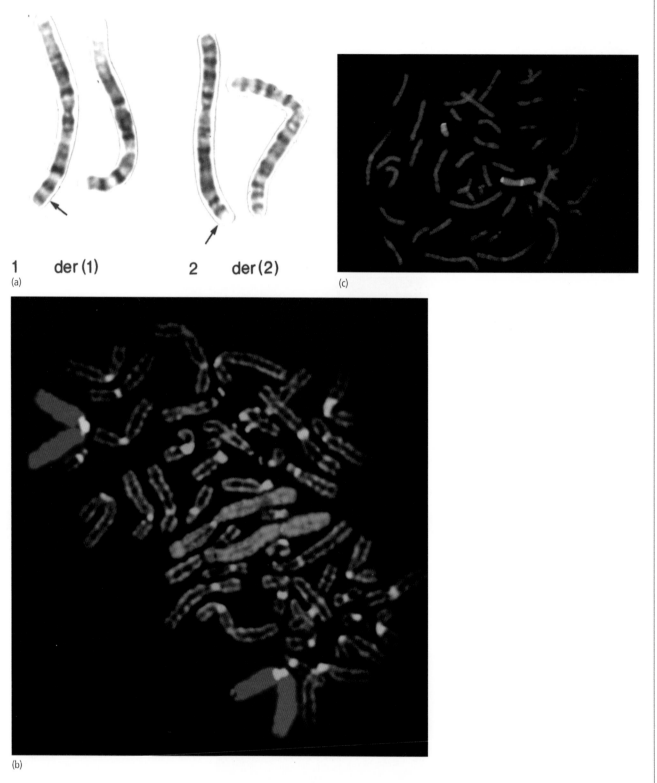

1   der (1)   2   der (2)

(a)

(c)

(b)

Fig. 7.28 Examples of chromosome-specific painting. (a) A small reciprocal translocation involving the distal ends of the long arms of chromosome of chromosomes 1 and 2 is difficult to distinguish by G-banding. (b) The same translocation revealed by hybridization with chromosome 1-specific paint (red) and chromosome 2-specific paint (green). (c) The result following chromosome painting of a male metaphase with a Y chromosome-specific paint (green) and an X chromosome-specific paint (red). Regions of Y homology on the X chromosome (the tip of Xp and the proximal third of Xq) or of X homology on the Y chromosome (the tip of Yp) appear yellow due to the combined red and green fluorescence. Note that the PAR2 region at the tip of Xq (mentioned in Chapter 6) is too small to produce a signal. Also, no green signal is visible in the heterochromatic region of Yq because the DNA repeats are suppressed by the hybridisation method that was used. (d) Example of three-colour forward chromosome painting: chromosome 1 (red), chromosome 2 (green) and chromosome 6 (yellow).

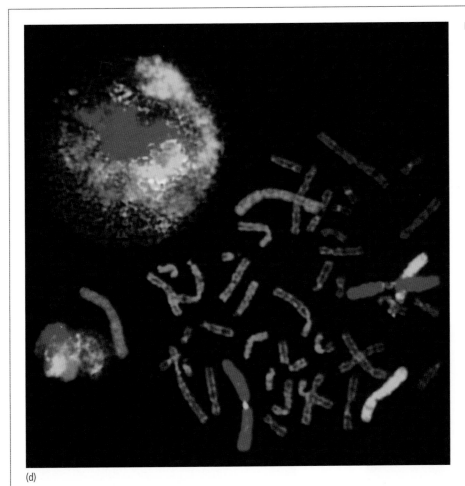

Fig. 7.28 *Continued*

(d)

Other aberrations

Mosaic

A mosaic is an individual with two or more cell lines that were derived from a single zygote. For example, about 1% of patients with trisomy 21 are mosaics with normal and trisomic cell lines. This arises after fertilisation. Usually the initial zygote has trisomy 21 and a normal cell line is produced at a subsequent mitosis by anaphase lag. Less frequently, the initial zygote is normal and a trisomic cell line arises at a subsequent mitosis by non-disjunction. In this event, a cell line with monosomy 21 will also be produced, which will tend to be lost. The presence of the normal cell line tends to ameliorate the clinical picture, and if the abnormal cell line is confined to the gonad (gonadal mosaic), then an outwardly normal parent may have a high risk of producing abnormal children.

Chimaera

A chimaera is an individual with two cell lines that were derived from two separate zygotes. This could arise by the early fusion of fraternal twin zygotes, by double fertilisation of the egg and a polar body or, more commonly, by exchange of haemopoietic stem cells *in utero* by dizygotic twins. Chimaerism is confirmed if a double contribution of maternal and paternal alleles can be demonstrated in the two cell lines.

Uniparental disomy and isodisomy

Normally, each parent contributes one member of each pair of autosomes and one sex chromosome, but occasionally both homologues of an autosome are from one parent with loss of the corresponding homologue from the other parent. This can arise if the conception is trisomic for the homologue and one homologue is lost from the zygote by anaphase lag at an early cell division to leave the two copies of the homologue that came from the same parent (trisomic rescue). If the trisomy resulted from non-disjunction at the *first* meiotic division, the gamete with the extra chromosome will, as mentioned above, have contained both (non-identical) homologues of that chromosome from one parent. If, post-fertilisation, trisomic rescue then occurs by loss of the third copy of that chromosome (the

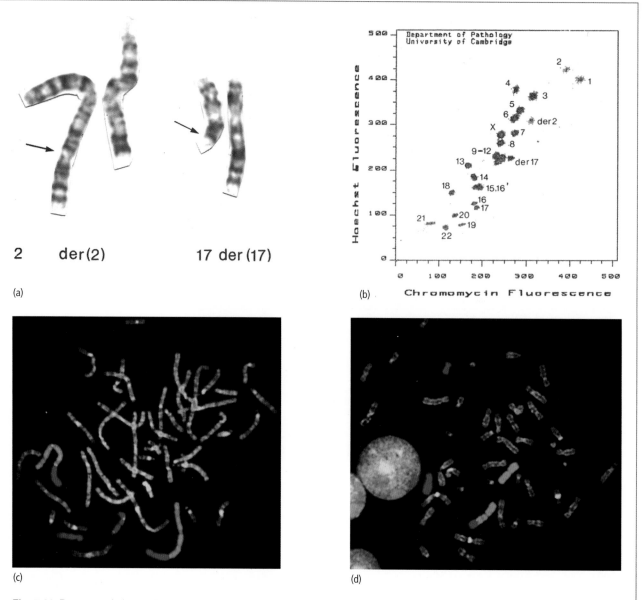

Fig. 7.29 Reverse painting in the analysis of a 46,XX, t(2;17)(q31;q25) translocation. (a) G-banded preparation showing chromosomes 2 and 17 and their derivatives from a balanced translocation carrier. (b) Flow karyotype showing the positions of the two derivative chromosomes from which paint probes were prepared following chromosome sorting and amplification. (c) The der 2 probe (green) and the der 17 probe (red) hybridized to a normal male metaphase to confirm the origin and breakpoints of the translocation. (d) The same der 2 and der 17 paints hybridized to a metaphase from the balanced translocation carrier.

copy that was present in the other parent's gamete), uniparental disomy will result in the patient. In contrast, if the trisomy resulted from non-disjunction at the *second* meiotic division, then the two homologues in the disomic gamete will be identical and uniparental *isodisomy* will be found in the patient after trisomic rescue (see Figs. 7.31 and 9.5).

Uniparental disomy and isodisomy result in a normal karyotype, but can be detected by DNA marker analysis. Their clinical consequences arise from genomic imprinting (see Chapter 6) of certain chromosomal regions with consequent parent-specific expression of alleles in these regions. For example, Prader–Willi syndrome (see Chapter 6) is usually caused by a paternal deletion of the proximal long arm of chromosome 15, but occasional patients with the same clinical appearance have no deletion but have maternal uniparental disomy for chromosome 15. Uniparental isodisomy can also lead to homozygosity for mutant genes on the involved chromosome and so result in an autosomal recessive single-gene disorder in a child with only one parent being a carrier.

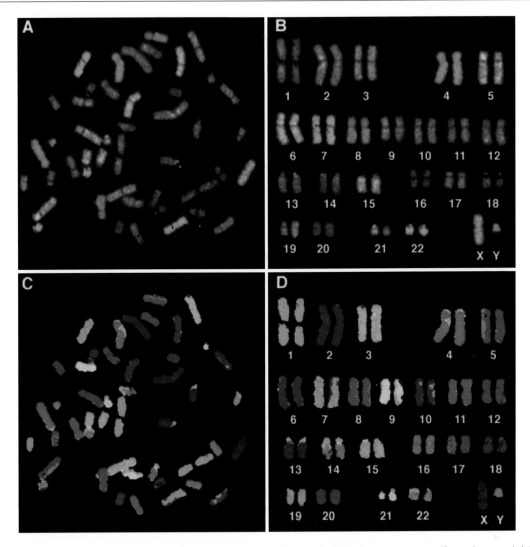

Fig. 7.30 Multicolour FISH using a paint probe composed of a combination of all 24 chromosome-specific probes, each labelled with a different combination of five fluorochromes and analysed by spectral imaging. Reprinted with permission from Schröck *et al.*, Science, 1996; 273:494–497. ©1996 American Association for the Advancement of Science.

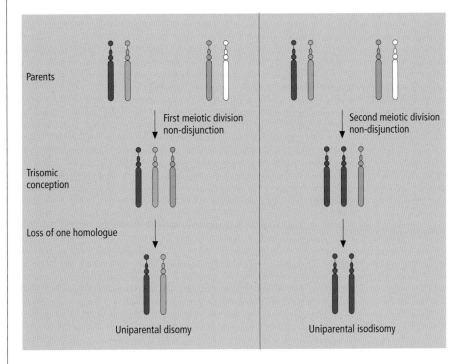

Fig. 7.31 Diagram of the mechanism of origin of uniparental disomy and isodisomy.

SUMMARY

- With light microscopy, the smallest visible chromosomal addition or deletion is around 4 Mb in size and typically contains many genes.
- Polyploidy refers to an abnormal number of chromosomes that (in contrast to aneuploidy) is an exact multiple of the haploid number, which in humans is 23.
- Mosaicism (for an aneuploid cell line) can arise from non-disjunction at a mitotic cell division.
- A carrier of a balanced translocation is usually clinically normal but may produce chromosomally unbalanced offspring.
- The investigation of complex chromosomal structural rearrangements can be facilitated by the use of chromosome-specific fluorescent DNA probes, either alone or in combination.

- Uniparental disomy refers to the situation where the two homologues of an autosome have come from just one parent, e.g. the mother. If both of the homologues originated in the same grandparent, then the appropriate term is uniparental isodisomy. The clinical consequences of uniparental disomy can include imprinting disorders and, in the case of uniparental isodisomy, autosomal recessive conditions.
- MLPA and aCGH are two different DNA analysis methods that can detect submicroscopic regions of deletion or duplication.
- QF-PCR is a modern DNA-based means by which chromosomal aneuploidies (e.g. trisomy 21, 18 or 13) can rapidly be detected prenatally or neonatally.

FURTHER READING

Bugge M, Collins A, Hertz JM, Eiberg H, Lundsteen C, Brandt CA, Bak M, Hansen C, Delozier CD, *et al.* (2007) Non-disjunction of chromosome 13. *Hum Mol Genet* **16**:2004–10.

Cimini D, Degrassi F (2005) Aneuploidy: a matter of bad connections. *Trends Cell Biol* **15**:442–51.

Ferguson-Smith MA, Trifonov V (2007) Mammalian karyotype evolution. *Nat Rev Genet* **8**:950–62.

Gardner RJM, Sutherland GR (2003) *Chromosome Abnormalities and Genetic Counseling*. Oxford Monographs on Medical Genetics. Oxford University Press: Oxford.

Johnson D, Morrison N, Grant L, Turner T, Fantes J, Connor JM, Murday V (2006) Confirmation of CHD7 as a cause of CHARGE association identified by mapping a balanced chromosome translocation in affected monozygotic twins. *J Med Genet* **43**:280–4.

King RW (2008) When 2 + 2 = 5: the origins and fates of aneuploid and tetraploid cells. *Biochim Biophys Acta* 1786:4–14.

Tolmie JL, MacFadyen U (2006) Down syndrome and other autosomal trisomies. In *Emery & Rimoin's Principles and Practice of Medical Genetics*, 5th edn, pp. 1015–37. Churchill Livingstone: Edinburgh.

Self-assessment

1. Which of the following are correct with regard to human chromosomes?

A. Modern light microscopes can detect deletions that are 4kb of DNA in size

B. A visible chromosomal abnormality usually involves many genes

C. Triploidy refers to the presence of an additional haploid number of chromosomes, i.e. a total of 69 in humans

D. Aneuploidy refers to the situation in which the total number of chromosomes is an exact multiple of the haploid number and also exceeds the diploid number

E. Monosomy for a chromosome can result either from non-disjunction or from delayed chromosomal movement in anaphase

2. With regard to chromosomal breaks, which of the following are correct?

A. They can result in structural aberrations such as translocations

B. They result in unstable sticky ends

C. Their repair involves the BRCA1 protein

D. Their frequency is increased by ionising radiation and in Fanconi anaemia

E. They are randomly distributed

3. Which of the following are true statements regarding balanced reciprocal chromosome translocations?

A. Carriers usually have significant learning difficulties

B. Some carriers have a risk of over 10% of having chromosomally unbalanced offspring

C. They may involve either the short arm or the long arm

D. They do not involve the X chromosome

E. During gametogenesis in carriers, chromosomes pair to form quadrivalents, from which two chromosomes always pass to each daughter cell

4. With regard to Robertsonian (centric fusion) translocations, which of the following are true?

A. They occur in acrocentric chromosomes

B. They usually occur as a result of chromosome breaks through the centromeres

C. Carriers of Robertsonian translocations typically have a total of 46 chromosomes

D. During gametogenesis, a quadrivalent forms at meiosis

E. Centric fusion of chromosomes 13 and 14 is the most common chromosomal translocation in humans.

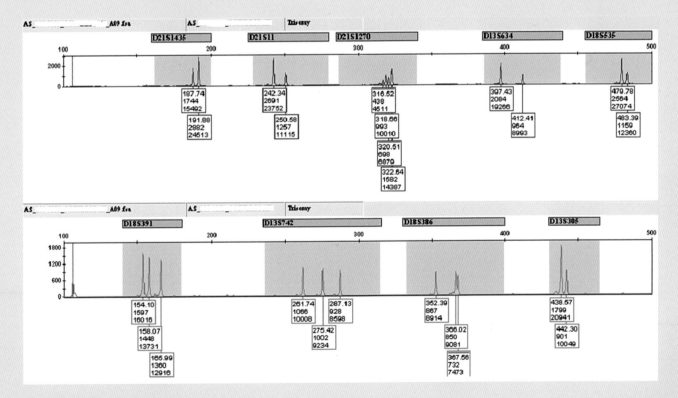

Fig. 7.32 See Question 7.

5. Which of the following statements are correct with regard to chromosomal submicroscopic deletions?

A. They may be detected by FISH, MLPA or aCGH
B. DNA sequencing is a useful means by which they can be detected
C. They may result from unequal crossing-over between two repeat sequences on the same arm of a chromosome
D. Breaks in both arms of a chromosome can result in a ring chromosome containing a centromere
E. They are more common than duplications in human chromosomes

6. Which of the following statements are true of uniparental disomy?

A. It results where two homologues of an autosome have originated in the same parent
B. It results in a total of 47 chromosomes
C. It can cause an imprinting disorder
D. Uniparental isodisomy can only result in an autosomal recessive condition if both parents are carriers
E. Uniparental isodisomy refers to the situation where both chromosomal homologues originated in the same grandparent

7. What is likely to be the chromosomal abnormality affecting the pregnancy for which the results are shown in Fig. 7.32?

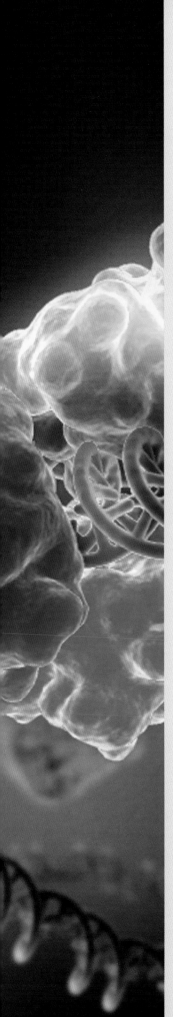

CHAPTER 8
Typical Mendelian inheritance

Key Topics

Introduction

Single-gene disorders (Mendelian disorders) are due to mutations in one or both members of a pair of autosomal genes or to mutations in genes on the X or Y chromosome (sex-linked inheritance). These disorders show characteristic patterns of inheritance in family pedigrees. Figure 8.1 shows some of the more commonly used symbols for constructing family trees (see Fig. 12.1 for other symbols).

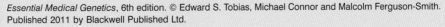

Essential Medical Genetics, 6th edition. © Edward S. Tobias, Michael Connor and Malcolm Ferguson-Smith.
Published 2011 by Blackwell Published Ltd.

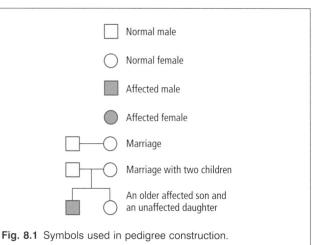

Fig. 8.1 Symbols used in pedigree construction.

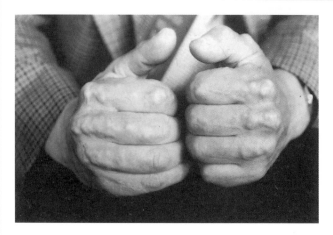

Fig. 8.2 Tendon xanthomata in familial hypercholesterolaemia.

Introduction to autosomal single-gene inheritance

The 44 autosomes comprise 22 homologous pairs of chromosomes. Within each chromosome, the genes have a strict order, each gene occupying a specific location or locus. Thus, the autosomal genes are present in pairs, one member being of maternal and one member of paternal origin. If both members of a gene pair (i.e. alleles) are identical, then the individual is homozygous for that locus. If different, then the individual is heterozygous for that locus. Alternative forms of a gene arise by mutation of the normal allele and may or may not have an altered function.

Any gene-determined characteristic is called a trait. If a trait is expressed in the heterozygote, then the trait is dominant, whereas if it is only expressed in the homozygote, it is recessive. In some instances, the effects of both alleles may be seen in the heterozygote, and these are called codominant traits.

Autosomal dominant inheritance

Autosomal dominant inheritance is most easily demonstrated by considering an example. The patient in Fig. 8.2 has cholesterol deposits (xanthomata) over his extensor tendons and also has premature coronary artery disease. His pedigree (Fig. 8.3) shows the typical features of autosomal dominant inheritance. Both males and females are affected in approximately equal numbers. Persons are affected in each generation and males can transmit the condition to males or females and vice versa. Unaffected persons do not transmit the condition. This condition, familial hypercholesterolaemia (FH), is due to a single mutant gene on the short arm of chromosome 19. Thus, each of the affected persons in this family is a heterozygote, and as each has married an unaffected person (normal homozygote) the expected ratio of affected to unaffected offspring is as seen in Fig. 8.4.

It is equally likely that a child will receive the mutant or the normal allele from the affected parent, and so on average

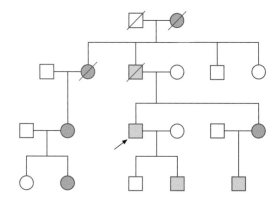

Fig. 8.3 Pedigree of a family with familial hypercholesterolaemia. The patient in Fig. 8.2 is indicated by an arrow.

there is a 1 in 2 or 50% chance that each child of a heterozygous parent will be affected. Although each affected individual has the same mutant gene, there is variation in the time of onset and severity of xanthomata and vascular disease. This variable expression (variable expressivity) is typical of an autosomal dominant trait. Its basis is unclear, but it is likely to be at least partly due to the effects of other, 'modifier', genes (see Chapter 9).

The most important gene for FH has been cloned and over 800 different mutations identified. It produces a protein that acts as a receptor for apolipoprotein B in circulating low-density-lipoprotein (LDL) particles. These particles, which contain cholesterol, can be bound and then internalised by a wide variety of cells, via clathrin-mediated endocytosis. Defects in this LDL receptor (LDLR) result in defective clearance and hence elevated levels of LDL-cholesterol (see Soutar and Naoumova, 2007, in Further reading). At least two other genes have now been identified that can cause a similar phenotype. Mutations in the gene that encodes proprotein convertase subtilisin/kexin type 9 (*PCSK9*) are a rare cause of severe hypercholesterolaemia, while a less severe phenotype (type B hypercholesterolaemia) results from mutation of the gene that

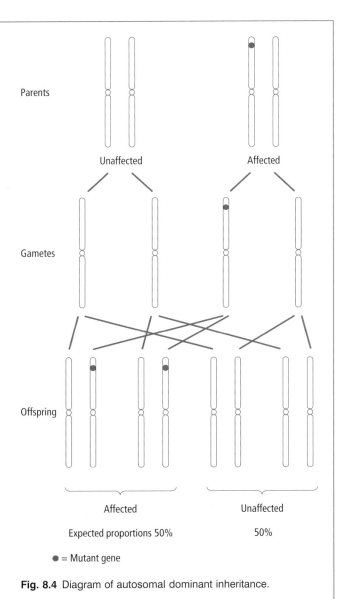

Parents

Unaffected   Affected

Gametes

Offspring

Affected   Unaffected

Expected proportions 50%   50%

● = Mutant gene

Fig. 8.4 Diagram of autosomal dominant inheritance.

encodes the apolipoprotein B-100 protein (*APOB*). However, in contrast to the many different *LDLR* mutations, in European individuals, a single *APOB* mutation predominates.

FH affects 1 in 500 individuals and marriages have occurred between affected heterozygotes. In such marriages, on average one-quarter of the offspring will be unaffected, one-half will be heterozygous affected and one-quarter will be homozygous affected. In the homozygous affected persons, there are no normal LDLRs and the disease shows precocious onset and increased severity with symptoms of coronary heart disease in late childhood. Family members at risk can be counselled on the basis of plasma lipid profiles, mutation analysis or by tracking the defective gene within a family using DNA analysis. Cholesterol-lowering therapies include dietary manipulation, statins (competitive inhibitors of HMG-CoA reductase, an enzyme involved in cholesterol synthesis) and ezetimibe (an inhibitor of intestinal absorption of cholesterol).

Another relatively commonly encountered example of an autosomal dominant condition is hypertrophic cardiomyopathy (HCM). Like FH, it affects around 1 in 500 individuals. The heart muscle enlargement that occurs in HCM results, in affected individuals, in outflow obstruction and a decrease in cardiac chamber size, leading to a reduced ability to pump blood effectively. In most cases, HCM has a strong genetic basis. This is in marked contrast to cases of dilated cardiomyopathy (DCM), only about 30% of which are familial (and include metabolic, mitochondrial and sarcomeric abnormalities in addition to muscular dystrophies). In HCM, the genetic predisposition is due to the inheritance of a single mutation in one of more than 12 autosomal genes that generally encode sarcomeric proteins (see Marian, 2010, in Further reading). Approximately 80% of the mutations reside within just two of these genes: β-myosin heavy chain (*MYH7*) and myosin binding protein C (*MYBPC3*). The penetrance varies among families from 25 to 100%, with the clinical manifestations ranging from progressive heart failure to sudden cardiac death. Those relatives who are at risk can be offered cardiac screening (including electrocardiography and echocardiography) and, if affected, can be treated pharmacologically or surgically including, if there is a high risk of cardiac arrest, the insertion of an implantable cardioverter-defibrillator or ICD.

The invaluable and comprehensive catalogue of human genes and genetic disorders, Online Mendelian Inheritance in Man (OMIM), authored by Victor McKusick and colleagues at Johns Hopkins University, is publicly accessible via the internet (see Further reading). Each entry in OMIM is assigned a six-digit reference number, with the first digit being 1 for an autosomal dominant locus or phenotype, 2 for autosomal recessive, 3 for X-linked, 4 for Y-linked, 5 for mitochondrial and 6 for autosomal entries created after 15th May 1994. At least 4458 autosomal dominant traits are known in humans. Some of the commoner and more clinically important of these are shown in Table 8.1. The pedigree pattern for each is similar to FH. In general, they tend to be less severe than recessive traits, and, whereas recessive traits usually result in defective enzymes, in dominant conditions, structural, carrier, receptor or tumour-suppressor proteins are usually altered. In many dominant traits, such as the form of inherited colon cancer known as familial adenomatous polyposis (FAP), an individual may have the mutant gene and yet have a normal phenotype. This is called non-penetrance and is an important exception to the rule that unaffected persons do not transmit an autosomal dominant trait. These individuals can pass the condition to descendants and so produce a skipped generation. In some other dominant traits, for example Huntington disease, the onset of symptoms (and hence the penetrance) is age-dependent, and reassurance of family members at risk on the basis of clinical examination is not possible until they reach an advanced age. A test for the mutant gene may, however, be available, as in Huntington disease, for example. Variable expression and non-penetrance (total and age-related) are important factors when providing genetic counselling for families with autosomal dominant traits.

Table 8.1 Autosomal dominant diseases

Disease	Frequency per 1000 births
Inherited breast cancer susceptibility	5–10* (for females)
Inherited colon cancer susceptibility	2–5*
Dominant otosclerosis	3
Familial hypercholesterolaemia	2
Familial hypertrophic cardiomyopathy	2
Von Willebrand disease	1
Adult polycystic kidney disease	1
Multiple exostoses	0.5
Neurofibromatosis type 1	0.4
Huntington disease	0.3
Myotonic dystrophy	0.2
Congenital spherocytosis	0.2
Marfan syndrome	0.2
Tuberous sclerosis	0.1
Familial adenomatous polyposis	0.1
Dominant blindness	0.1
Dominant congenital deafness	0.1
Others	0.8
Total (approximate)	18–26

* Estimates, including familial cancer due to low-penetrance cancer genes.

When a condition shows full penetrance (such as achondroplasia), the recurrence risk for the clinically normal parents of an affected child is low but not negligible because of gonadal mosaicism (see Chapter 9). The presence of such mutations confined to the gonad would cause a high recurrence risk (of up to 1 in 2) and can only be proven when unaffected parents have a second affected child. This possibility thus needs to be considered when counselling a family with an apparently new mutation.

Counselling problems can also arise when the mutant gene is unstable. Myotonic dystrophy is a common adult-onset form of muscular dystrophy that is due to an unstable length mutation. Small length mutations may produce few or no symptoms, but expansion in successive generations can result in increasing disease severity (see Chapter 9).

Some autosomal dominant traits are so serious that they usually preclude reproduction (e.g. Apert syndrome and progressive myositis ossificans). In this situation, neither parent will be affected and the affected child will represent a new mutation. If the child fails to reproduce, then the mutant gene is transmitted no further and there will be only one affected individual in the family. For several autosomal dominant traits,

including Apert syndrome, progressive myositis ossificans, Marfan syndrome and achondroplasia, the risk of a new mutation increases with increasing paternal age, and for some dominant traits (e.g. retinoblastoma and neurofibromatosis), DNA analysis has demonstrated a paternal excess of new mutations.

Autosomal recessive inheritance

Sickle-cell disease is an example of an autosomal recessive trait. Figure 8.5 shows the characteristic sickle shaped red blood cells in an affected patient. These distorted red cells have a reduced survival time and this results in a severe chronic haemolytic anaemia with a need for repeated blood transfusions. The distorted red cells may also occlude vessels causing recurrent infarctions, especially of the lungs, bones and spleen.

The predominant haemoglobin in normal adults is haemoglobin A (HbA) which has two α-globin and two β-globin polypeptide chains in each molecule. Sickle-cell disease is caused by a point mutation in each β-globin gene on chromosome 11 at the codon for the sixth amino acid. The resulting haemoglobin S (HbS) has a substitution of valine in place of glutamic acid. This difference causes distortion of red cells, especially at reduced oxygen tension (the basis of the 'sickling test') and also alters the electrophoretic mobility of the protein (Fig. 8.6). Affected patients with sickle-cell disease have two mutant HbS gene copies (HbS/HbS), one having been inherited from each parent.

The pedigree of a family with sickle-cell disease is shown in Fig. 8.7. The parents in this family are clinically normal yet are heterozygotes (carriers) for the mutant β-globin gene (HbA/HbS). Their normal β-globin gene produces sufficient haemoglobin A to prevent symptoms. Apart from the two children, no other individuals are affected in the family, but the relatives' carrier status can be determined by haemoglobin electrophoresis.

Figure 8.8 shows the possible offspring for parents who are both carriers for sickle-cell disease. On average, one-quarter of their children will be homozygous normal, one-half heterozygous and one-quarter homozygous affected. The observed segregation ratio can be compared with that predicted. Two points must be borne in mind, however, when using this approach for a suspected autosomal recessive trait. Firstly, it is unlikely that any single family will have produced sufficient children to give the ratio exactly. Secondly, there is an automatic bias, as families only come to medical attention by virtue of an affected child, and those carrier parents who, by chance, produce only unaffected children will be missed. As shown in Fig. 8.9, when both parents are carriers for a recessive trait, if they have only two children, then the proportions of none to one to both affected will be 9:6:1. Hence, only seven of every 16 couples at risk will come to medical attention. A correction for this bias needs to be made by not counting the first affected child in each family when determining the segregation ratio.

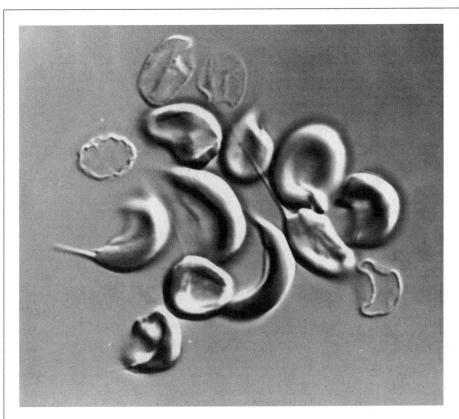

Fig. 8.5 Sickle-shaped red cells in a sickle haemoglobin (HbS) homozygote.

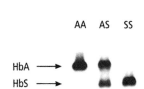

Fig. 8.6 Haemoglobin electrophoresis at alkaline pH to demonstrate individuals who are homozygous for HbS, heterozygous (HbS/HbA) or homozygous normal (HbA/HbA).

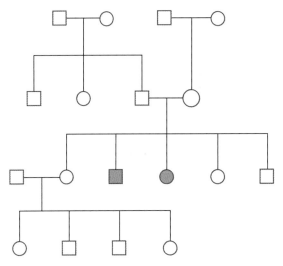

Fig. 8.7 Pedigree of a family with children affected with sickle-cell disease.

For a parent with sickle-cell disease, each child must receive a mutant allele. If the other parent is homozygous normal (HbA/HbA), then only unaffected heterozygote offspring (HbA/HbS) will be produced. If by chance a person with sickle-cell disease marries a heterozygote, then there will be a 1 in 2 chance on average that each child will be affected. If both parents have sickle-cell disease, then only children with sickle-cell disease can be produced.

Family members at risk can be screened by the sickling test or haemoglobin electrophoresis and, where a pregnancy is at risk of homozygous sickle-cell disease, prenatal diagnosis by DNA analysis may be offered.

The majority of parents of children with sickle-cell disease are not blood relatives (consanguineous), but if they are there is an increased risk for this and other autosomal recessive disorders. The increased risk in this situation is caused by the

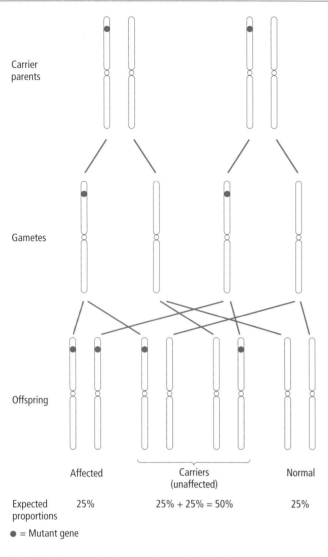

Carrier parents

Gametes

Offspring

Affected | Carriers (unaffected) | Normal

Expected proportions: 25% | 25% + 25% = 50% | 25%

● = Mutant gene

Fig. 8.8 Diagram of autosomal recessive inheritance.

parents sharing one set of grandparents and the chance that each has inherited the same mutant gene from one grandparent (Table 8.2). The proportion of shared genes (coefficient of relationship, *r*) decreases by one-half for each step apart on the pedigree. In highly inbred populations, the affected person has a substantial risk of mating with a carrier, and this may result in a pedigree with apparent vertical transmission of an autosomal recessive trait (pseudodominant inheritance; see Chapter 9). Hence, parental consanguinity, while not a prerequisite, is an important clue that a condition affecting their child is an autosomal recessive trait.

Sickle-cell disease affects up to 1 in 40 black Africans, who have a carrier frequency of up to about 1 in 3. This high frequency is believed to be due to the selective advantage of these carriers with regard to malarial infection (see Chapter 11). Ethnic associations may also arise from the founder effect (see Chapter 11) in genetically isolated populations (Table 8.3). Hence, the ethnic origin of a patient may be an important clue in the diagnosis of an autosomal recessive disorder.

Table 8.2 Proportions of genes in common in different relatives

Degree of relationship	Examples	Proportion of genes in common (*r*)
First	Parents to child, sibling to sibling	1/2
Second	Uncles or aunts to nephews or nieces, grandparents to grandchildren	1/4
Third	First cousins, great-grandparents to great-grandchildren	1/8

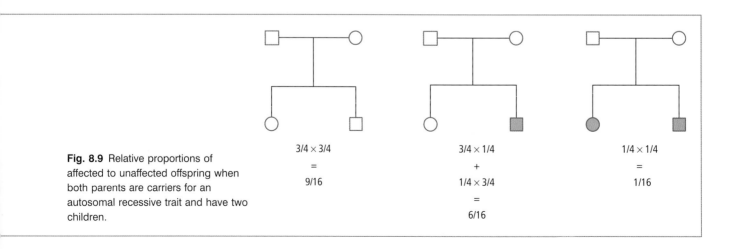

3/4 × 3/4

=

9/16

3/4 × 1/4

+

1/4 × 3/4

=

6/16

1/4 × 1/4

=

1/16

Fig. 8.9 Relative proportions of affected to unaffected offspring when both parents are carriers for an autosomal recessive trait and have two children.

Table 8.3 Ethnic associations with autosomal recessive diseases

Disease	Ethnic group(s)
β-Thalassaemia	Mediterranean, Thai, black African, Middle East, Indian and Chinese populations
Sickle-cell disease	African-American. black African, Asian Indian, Mediterranean (especially Greek) and Middle East populations
Tay–Sachs disease	Ashkenazi Jews
Gaucher disease	Ashkenazi Jews
Meckel–Gruber syndrome	Finnish population
Congenital adrenal hyperplasia	Yupik population of Alaska
Severe combined immunodeficiency	Athabascan-speaking Native Americans including the Navajo and Apache Indians
Cystic fibrosis	Caucasians
Albinism	Hopi Indians (in southwest USA)

Table 8.4 Autosomal recessive diseases

Disease	Frequency per 1000 births
Cystic fibrosis	0.5
Recessive learning disability	0.5
α_1-Antitrypsin deficiency	0.3
Recessive congenital deafness	0.2
Phenylketonuria	0.1
Spinal muscular atrophy	0.1
Recessive blindness	0.1
Congenital adrenal hyperplasia	0.1
Mucopolysaccharidoses	0.1
Others	0.2
Total	2.2

At least 1730 autosomal recessive traits are known in humans. Some of the commoner and more clinically important of these are shown in Table 8.4. In about 15% of autosomal recessive traits, an enzyme defect has already been demonstrated and is to be expected in many of the remainder. For many traits, not just one but multiple different mutant alleles may occur at the locus (*multiple allelism* or *allelic heterogeneity*). Some, but not all, of these alleles result in sufficient reduction of enzyme activity to produce disease in the homozygous state. An individual who has two different mutant alleles at a locus is termed a compound heterozygote or genetic compound.

Many conditions that were believed to be single genetic entities are now known to be genetically heterogeneous (i.e. to have several different genetic causes). This should be suspected if different modes of inheritance are apparent in different fami-lies or if offspring of parents who are autosomal recessive homozygotes are not invariably affected. This *genetic heterogeneity* can be proven by demonstrating that different proteins or their respective genes are involved, or, by complementation studies. In complementation studies, cell lines from two affected individuals are fused *in vitro* to determine whether heterogeneous cross-correction of the phenotype can be demonstrated. The similar term *locus heterogeneity* refers specifically to the related situation in which a single genetic phenotype is known to result from mutations in different genes (i.e. at different loci). For example, tuberous sclerosis is known to result from a mutation in either of two different autosomal genes, and the same is true for another autosomal dominant condition, adult polycystic kidney disease. In contrast, *clinical heterogeneity* refers to the converse correlation, where different mutations at one locus can result in different clinical conditions (e.g. different types of mutations in the same androgen receptor gene can result in either androgen insensitivity or spinal and bulbar muscular atrophy).

Summary of autosomal inheritance

Table 8.5 summarises the important distinguishing features of autosomal recessive and dominant inheritance.

Introduction to sex-linked inheritance

A female has two X chromosomes: one of paternal and one of maternal origin. However, with the exception of several X/Y homologous genes (see Chapter 9), one of these X chromosomes is inactivated in each somatic cell (X inactivation, see Chapter 6). This mechanism ensures that the quantity of most X-linked gene products generated in somatic cells of the female is equivalent to the amount produced in male cells. In the process of inactivation, the selection between the maternal and paternal X homologues is random, although once established,

Table 8.5 Typical features of autosomal dominant and recessive modes of inheritance

Autosomal dominant	Autosomal recessive
Disease expressed in heterozygote	Disease expressed in homozygote
On average half of offspring affected	Low risk to offspring of affected individuals
Equal frequency and severity in each sex	Equal frequency and severity in each sex
Paternal age effect for new mutations	Heterozygote advantage may maintain a relatively high frequency of a disease allele
Incomplete or age-dependent penetrance in several conditions	
Variable expressivity (i.e. severity)	More constant expressivity in a family
Vertical pedigree pattern	Horizontal pedigree pattern Importance of consanguinity

Table 8.6 Comparison of typical features of autosomal dominant with male sex limitation inheritance and X-linked recessive and dominant inheritance

Feature	X-linked recessive	X-linked dominant	Autosomal dominant with male sex limitation
Pedigree pattern	Knight's move	Vertical	Vertical
Sex ratio	M ≫ F	2F:1M	M ≫ F
Male-to-male transmission	Never	Never	up to 50% of sons affected
Male-to-female transmission	All daughters carriers	All daughters affected	≪50% of daughters affected
Female-to-female transmission	50% of daughters carriers	50% of daughters affected	≪50% of daughters affected
Male severity	Uniform	Uniform	Variable (severe)
Female severity	Mild	Variable	Variable (mild)

the same homologue becomes inactivated in each daughter cell. Thus, the female is, in fact, a mosaic with a percentage of cells having the paternal X active, and the maternal X being active in the remainder. Each son or daughter receives one or other X chromosome from their mother.

In contrast, a male has only one X chromosome and hence only one copy of each X-linked gene (and is sometimes called hemizygous). The X chromosome remains active in every somatic cell and so any mutant X allele will always be expressed in a male. Each daughter must receive her father's X chromosome. Each son must receive his father's Y chromosome and not his X chromosome. Hence, fathers cannot transmit X-linked genes to their sons.

During meiosis (Chapter 6), the X and Y chromosomes undergo synapsis only within the small pairing (pseudoautosomal) regions at the distal ends of their chromosome arms (see Fig. 6.8). The rest of the XY bivalent remains condensed in pachytene where crossing-over in the non-pairing regions is normally inhibited. DNA sequences with recognised polymorphisms have been identified in the pairing region. Of these, the Yp sequences which are closest to the (non-pairing) sex

determinants show partial sex linkage, while those that are the most distal show 50% recombination and therefore appear to be transmitted as autosomal sequences.

The genes on the remainder of the sex chromosomes are distributed unequally to males and females within families. This inequality produces characteristic patterns of inheritance of mutant genes with marked discrepancies in the numbers of affected males and females.

The pedigree pattern depends upon which sex chromosome carries the mutant gene and whether the trait is recessive or dominant. Occasionally, these pedigree patterns may be mimicked by autosomal traits that show sex limitation, and the distinguishing features are summarised in Table 8.6. For instance, familial breast cancer is generally autosomal dominant with female sex limitation (see Chapter 13). In particular, if the affected males of an autosomal dominant trait with male sex limitation are infertile, then the pedigree pattern is identical to an X-linked recessive trait in which males do not reproduce. In this event, the demonstration of X inactivation in carrier females is an important clue to the correct mode of inheritance.

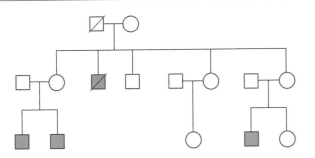

Fig. 8.10 Pedigree of a family with severe X-linked muscular dystrophy (DMD).

X-linked recessive inheritance

Severe sex-linked muscular dystrophy i.e. Duchenne muscular dystrophy (DMD), is an example of an X-linked recessive trait. This condition, which results in progressive proximal muscle weakness with the onset in early childhood, is discussed in more detail in Chapter 15. Figure 8.10 shows a pedigree from an affected family. This pedigree illustrates the typical features of X-linked recessive inheritance. There is a marked discrepancy in the sex ratio, with only males being severely affected, and the affected boys have a similar disease course (little variation in expression). Heterozygous females are usually clinically unaffected (carriers) but transmit the condition to the next generation. This results in a 'knight's move' pedigree pattern of affected males. The condition is not transmitted by an unaffected male.

Figure 8.11 shows the expected proportions of affected to unaffected individuals in the offspring of a carrier female and a normal male. On average, one-half of the daughters will be carriers and one-half of the sons will be affected.

The carrier female is usually clinically normal. A woman with an affected child and an affected brother, or a woman with more than one affected child, is an obligate carrier, as the alternative explanation of multiple new mutations is so unlikely. For each daughter of an obligate carrier there is, on average, a 1 in 2 risk that she too is a carrier. Carrier detection using DNA analysis may be helpful, particularly where a familial DMD gene deletion or duplication is known to be present in the family or where linkage analysis can be performed. Alternatively, creatine kinase (CK) testing can be helpful in determining carrier status. This is because, as a result of X inactivation, a proportion of the muscle cells of a DMD carrier female will have the mutant allele on the active X. These cells will release the muscle enzyme CK, and so in about two-thirds of female carriers, serum CK levels lie outside the normal range (Fig. 8.12). This is helpful in carrier detection, provided precautions are taken to exclude other factors that can raise (exercise, intramuscular injections) or lower (pregnancy) this enzyme level.

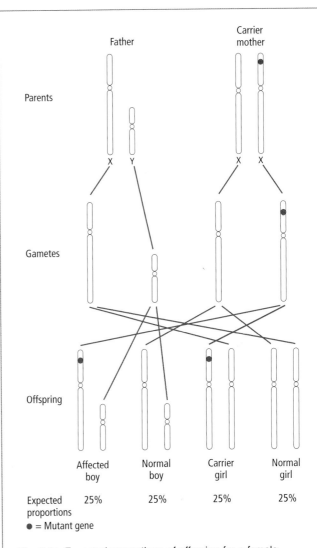

Fig. 8.11 Expected proportions of offspring for a female X-linked recessive heterozygote.

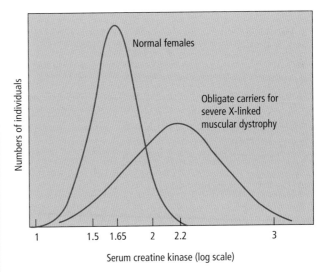

Fig. 8.12 Distribution of serum CK levels in normal females and obligate carriers for DMD. Courtesy of Douglas Wilcox, University of Glasgow.

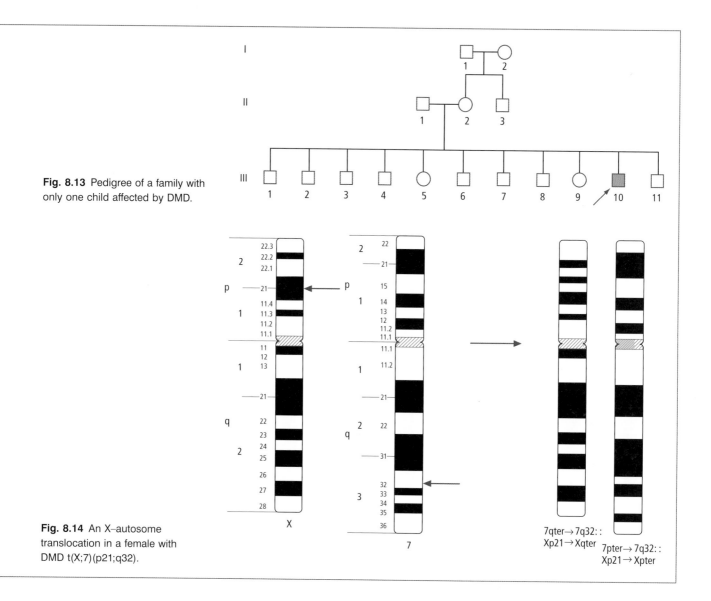

Fig. 8.13 Pedigree of a family with only one child affected by DMD.

Fig. 8.14 An X–autosome translocation in a female with DMD t(X;7)(p21;q32).

Sometimes the child is the only affected individual in the family (Fig. 8.13). In this situation, the mother is not an obligate carrier. In around one-third of cases, the child possesses a new mutation, whereas in the remainder the mother is a carrier. Creatine kinase testing may help to resolve these two possibilities, and the fact that in this example the mother has eight normal sons will diminish (but not eliminate) her chance of being a carrier.

Occasionally a female is affected with this X-linked form of muscular dystrophy. This might arise in a number of ways: skewed X inactivation (resulting in a manifesting heterozygote), a new mutation on the normal X chromosome of a carrier female, a carrier with Turner syndrome (45,X) or an X–autosome translocation. By far the commonest of these possibilities is skewed X inactivation. This arises in a female carrier when, by chance, inactivation of the normal X chromosome occurs in most of her muscle cells. Such a manifesting heterozygote is usually not affected to the same extent as

an affected male. This, incidentally, is also thought to be the mechanism underlying monozygotic female twins where one is affected and the other is asymptomatic. Theoretically, a carrier female might instead have a new mutation at the same locus on her other X chromosome, and she would then be as severely affected as a male. A woman with Turner syndrome cannot inactivate her only X chromosome, which carries the mutant allele, and so she would be as severely affected as a male. Finally, a woman with an X–autosome translocation may be affected if the breakpoint on the X chromosome is at the *DMD* locus (Fig. 8.14). In X–autosome translocations, the karyotypically *normal* X is preferentially inactivated, as otherwise partial monosomy for the involved autosome might occur. This provided an important early clue to the localisation of the gene for X-linked muscular dystrophy, as in each female with muscular dystrophy due to an X–autosome translocation the breakpoint was in the band Xp21. This resulted in damage to the *DMD* gene, with consequent

Table 8.7 Human X-linked recessive traits

Trait	UK frequency per 10000 males
Red–green colour blindness	800
Fragile X syndrome	2.5
Non-specific X-linked mental retardation	5
Duchenne muscular dystrophy	3
Haemophilia A (factor VIII deficiency)	2
X-linked ichthyosis	2
Becker muscular dystrophy	0.5
Haemophilia B (factor IX deficiency)	0.3
X-linked agammaglobulinaemia	0.1

expression of this abnormal gene when the normal X was inactivated.

In addition to the severe form of X-linked muscular dystrophy (DMD), there is a milder X-linked form of muscular dystrophy called Becker muscular dystrophy (BMD). These conditions are due to different mutant alleles of the extremely large 79-exon gene (spanning 2.2 Mb) encoding the protein dystrophin. In about 65% of cases of X-linked muscular dystrophy, DNA analysis reveals a deletion of variable size. This analysis is undertaken using a multiplex polymerase chain reaction (PCR) or the more recently introduced multiplex ligation-dependent probe amplification (MLPA) technique described in Chapter 4 (see Figs 4.11 & 4.12). Such deletions generally lead to a downstream alteration of the reading frame in DMD but not in BMD. Rarely, such a deletion is visible using the light microscope and occasionally other important contiguous genes may be included in the microdeletion. Before counselling a family with muscular dystrophy, it is important to establish the precise type as, in addition to these X-linked forms, autosomal dominant and recessive forms of muscular dystrophy are known (genetic heterogeneity).

So far, 515 X-linked recessive traits are known in humans. Some of the commoner and more clinically important of these are listed in Table 8.7. The frequencies vary in different ethnic groups, for example in certain groups, glucose-6-phosphate dehydrogenase deficiency, particularly where malaria is common, is as frequent as colour blindness is in the UK.

For some X-linked recessive disorders, affected males may reproduce, and in this event all daughters will be carriers (obligate carriers) and all sons will be normal (Fig. 8.15).

Fragile X syndrome (see Chapter 9) provides an important exception to the principle of consistent male severity within a family for an X-linked recessive trait. Fragile X syndrome is caused by an unstable length mutation; small length mutations may produce few or no symptoms in males or females, but subsequent amplification to a larger length mutation may

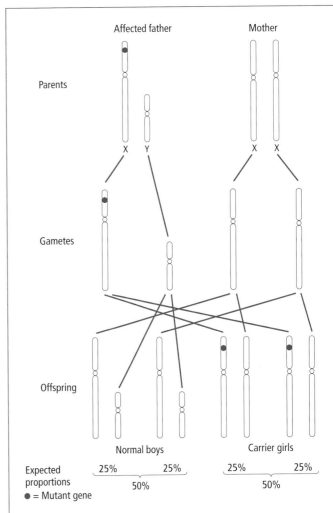

Fig. 8.15 Diagram of the expected proportions of offspring for an affected male with an X-linked recessive trait.

result in offspring with significant learning disability, particularly in males.

X-linked dominant inheritance

Vitamin D-resistant rickets (or X-linked hypophosphataemia) is inherited as an X-linked dominant trait and thus both males and females are usually affected. However, whereas in males the condition is uniformly severe, the female heterozygote is more variably affected because of X inactivation. The pedigree (Fig. 8.16) resembles that of an autosomal dominant trait but the key difference is the lack of male-to-male transmission with an X-linked dominant trait (Table 8.6).

The Xg blood group is also inherited as an X-linked dominant trait, but the other conditions that are inherited in this fashion are rare (Table 8.8). Four others deserve further mention: incontinentia pigmenti (with an early onset of a vesicular skin rash followed by irregular whorled pigmentation

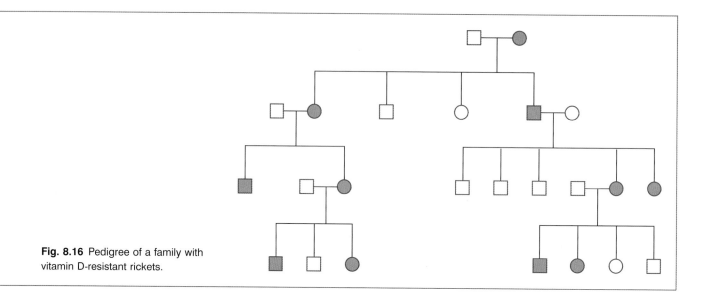

Fig. 8.16 Pedigree of a family with vitamin D-resistant rickets.

Table 8.8 Examples of human X-linked dominant traits
Xg blood group
Vitamin D-resistant rickets
X-linked dominant hereditary motor and sensory neuropathy
Craniofrontonasal dysplasia
X-linked periventricular heterotopia*
Conradi–Hünermann syndrome
Incontinentia pigmenti*
Focal dermal hypoplasia (Goltz syndrome)*
Rett syndrome*

*Lethal in hemizygous males.

in a mosaic pattern, with affected regions representing those in which the normal chromosome has been inactivated; usually due to a partial deletion of the *NEMO* gene), focal dermal hypoplasia (atrophy and linear pigmentation of the skin, together with digital and oral anomalies, learning disability and striated bones), Rett syndrome (developmental arrest at 6–18 months followed by regression, 'hand-washing' automatisms, subsequent seizures and then wheelchair dependency by the age of 10 years; due to *MECP2* gene mutations) and X-linked periventricular heterotopia (epilepsy with multiple uncalcified nodules on the walls of the lateral ventricles; caused by mutations within the *FLNA* gene encoding filamin-A). In these four conditions, the affected males are believed to be so severely affected that spontaneous abortion is usual

and hence generally only affected *females* are seen (also see Chapter 9).

Y-linked inheritance (holandric inheritance)

The inheritance of the sex-determining region Y (*SRY*)/testis determining factor (*TDF*) provides an example of Y-linked inheritance. Males transmit *SRY/TDF* (and their Y chromosome) to all of their sons, but not to their daughters. Mutations in the *SRY* gene at Yp11.3 can result in XY females with gonadal dysgenesis (one type of Swyer syndrome). Such individuals appear to be normal females at birth but at puberty fail to develop secondary sexual characteristics, do not menstruate and have streak gonads. They have a 46,XY chromosome complement. The normal physiological role of *SRY/TDF* was discussed in Chapter 6.

Other human examples of Y-linked diseases are rare, but include submicroscopic Yq11 deletions at the AZoospermia Factor regions (AZFa, AZFb and, most commonly, AZFc), which can result in severe oligospermia and male infertility. The AZFc region contains the 'deleted in azoospermia' (*DAZ*) genes, which encode highly conserved RNA-binding proteins that are essential for normal spermatogenesis and probably regulate the translation of target gene mRNAs. Testicular aspiration of sperm followed by intracytoplasmic sperm injection (ICSI) can be particularly helpful for this and other causes of male subfertility, although it can permit the transmission of a genetic abnormality to the offspring. In the case of a Yq11 deletion, all the sons produced following ICSI will, of course, inherit the abnormality.

- Typical features of autosomal dominant conditions include: (a) a vertical pedigree pattern, (b) a generally equal disease frequency and severity between males and females and (c) variable expressivity.
- In autosomal recessive conditions, heterozygotes are generally clinically unaffected, with affected individuals being either homozygotes or compound heterozygotes.
- A single condition may result from different modes of inheritance (genetic heterogeneity), from mutations in different genes (locus heterogeneity) and often from different mutations in the same gene (allelic heterogeneity). In contrast, clinical heterogeneity refers to the situation in which different mutations at a single locus result in different clinical conditions.
- In X-linked inheritance, male-to-male transmission is absent and, in those females who are affected, the severity is generally more mild and variable than in affected males.
- A few X-linked dominant conditions result in early male lethality with the only living affected individuals being female.
- There are very few Y-linked clinical conditions. Those recognised include: (a) XY females with gonadal dysgenesis (which can result from *SRY* gene mutations) and (b) male infertility resulting from Yq11 microdeletions at the AZF regions).

SUMMARY

FURTHER READING

Harper PS (2010) *Practical Genetic Counselling*, 7th edn. Hodder Arnold: London.

Marian AJ (2010) Hypertrophic cardiomyopathy: from genetics to treatment. *Eur J Clin Invest* **40**:360–9.

Soutar AK, Naoumova RP (2007) Mechanisms of disease: genetic causes of familial hypercholesterolemia. *Nat Clin Pract Cardiovasc Med* **4**:214–25.

WEBSITES

GeneReviews (expert-authored disease reviews; select 'GeneReviews' at this site): **http://www.geneclinics.org**

Online Mendelian Inheritance in Man (OMIM): **http://www.ncbi.nlm.nih.gov/sites/entrez?db=omim**

Self-assessment

1. Which of the following are common features of autosomal dominant conditions?
A. Variable expression and variable age of onset
B. Phenotypic severity influenced by one or more modifier genes or environmental factors
C. A metabolic enzyme defect
D. Parental consanguinity, where the condition affecting the child is extremely rare
E. A maternal age effect is observed in association with new mutations

2. If a man who is affected by autosomal recessive albinism has a partner who is a carrier of the same condition, which of the following is the chance that their second child will be affected?
A. 25%
B. 50%
C. 67%
D. 75%
E. 100%

3. The proportion of genes in common between a woman and her great grandmother's sister is:
A. 1/2
B. 1/4
C. 1/8
D. 1/16
E. 1/32

4–7. Which of the following four terms most closely matches each of the numbered definitions given below?
A. Allelic heterogeneity
B. Clinical heterogeneity
C. Genetic heterogeneity
D. Locus heterogeneity
4. A single condition resulting from different modes of inheritance
5. Multiple different mutant alleles at the same locus, giving rise to a single condition or trait
6. A single genetic phenotype resulting from mutations in different genes or loci
7. Different clinical conditions resulting from different mutations at one locus

8. Which of the following are common features of conditions that are X-linked recessive?
A. Unequal sex ratio for affected individuals
B. Severely affected females
C. Affected boys with an affected father
D. Consanguinity in parents
E. Daughters who are carriers, when the father is affected and able to have children

9. The possible causes of a female being affected by an X-linked recessive condition such as Duchenne muscular dystrophy (DMD) include which of the following?
A. Skewed X-inactivation
B. The individual could be a carrier who also has Turner syndrome
C. X–autosome translocation, with a defective disease-associated gene copy on the translocated X chromosome
D. The presence of a microdeletion on the other, previously normal, X chromosome
E. The presence of a frameshift mutation on the other, previously normal, X chromosome

10. Which of the following conditions are inherited in an X-linked dominant fashion?
A. Vitamin D-resistant rickets
B. Incontinentia pigmenti
C. X-linked ichthyosis
D. Haemophilia B
E. Rett syndrome

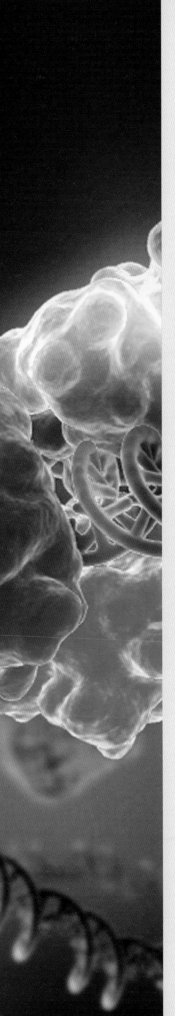

CHAPTER 9
Atypical Mendelian inheritance

Key Topics

Introduction

Although a great many genetic single gene disorders follow typical Mendelian mechanisms of inheritance as described in the previous chapter, there are several genetic conditions that are now recognised as having inheritance mechanisms that, while essentially Mendelian in nature, are atypical, for instance with genetic anticipation or pseudoautosomal inheritance. In addition there are many Mendelian conditions in which the phenotype is a consequence not only of the sequence of the recognised causative gene but also of variations in the sequence of so-called modifier genes. These and other non-classical Mendelian mechanisms are described in this chapter.

Essential Medical Genetics, 6th edition. © Edward S. Tobias, Michael Connor and Malcolm Ferguson-Smith.
Published 2011 by Blackwell Published Ltd.

Genetic anticipation

A few genetic conditions exhibit the phenomenon of genetic anticipation. This refers to the observation that in these diseases, there is a tendency for the age of onset of the condition to decrease and for the severity of the phenotype to increase, in successive generations. The specific conditions that are currently recognised to be associated with this feature all include neurological symptoms. The X-linked recessive condition, fragile X syndrome, exhibits genetic anticipation, as do several autosomal dominant conditions. The latter include myotonic dystrophy, Huntington disease and several forms of spinocerebellar atrophy (SCA): currently SCA types 1, 2, 3, 6, 7, 8, 12, 17 and a complex form known as dentatorubral-pallidoluysian atrophy (DRPLA).

In each of these conditions, there is a common underlying molecular mechanism. This is the presence of a tract of trinucleotide repeat units that lies within or adjacent to a disease-associated gene and a tendency for the tract to become progressively larger by expansion at meiosis once it becomes 'unstable' by reaching a certain threshold size. In addition, while in most individuals the trinucleotide repeat tract is not harmful, expansion of the tract beyond a certain size results in it becoming a pathogenic mutation.

In the genes associated with Huntington disease and SCA (types 1, 2, 3, 6, 7 and 17), the CAG repeat tract is situated within the coding sequence itself, with an expansion therefore resulting in additional glutamine amino acids within the encoded protein. In contrast, in the fragile X syndrome gene, the CGG repeat tract is located in the 5′ untranslated region (UTR) with an expansion resulting in transcriptional repression and loss of function of the protein. In relation to myotonic dystrophy (type 1), however, the underlying CTG repeat expansion at chromosome 19q13 is located within the 3′ UTR of the dystrophia myotonica protein kinase (*DMPK*) gene. The mutant *DMPK* mRNA causes abnormal splicing of several genes (by sequestering important RNA-binding proteins) and thus exerts a toxic gain of function effect. Similarly, a toxic gain of function RNA effect is believed to be involved in SCA8 in which a CUG expansion is present at the 3′ end of a non-coding RNA, in SCA12 in which a CAG tract is present in the 5′ UTR of the associated gene and in the relatively rare myotonic dystrophy type 2, which is now known to result from a tetranucleotide repeat, CCTG, located within the first intron of the zinc finger protein 9 (*ZNF9*) gene at chromosome 3q21 (see the review by Ranum and Cooper, 2006, in Further reading).

Huntington disease

Huntington disease, a cause of progressive chorea and dementia, is inherited as an autosomal dominant trait and is caused by an unstable length mutation in the huntingtin (*HTT*) gene. Normally, 10–35 (most commonly 15–20, with a median of 18) adjacent copies of a CAG repeat are found in the first exon,

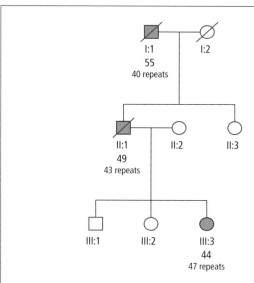

Fig. 9.1 Illustrative pedigree of a family with Huntington disease. The age of onset of symptoms is shown above the number of CAG repeats for each affected individual. The age of onset decreases as the number of repeats increases, in successive generations (i.e. typical genetic anticipation).

within the coding sequence, whereas in affected patients the repeat tract is expanded to 36–120 copies (commonly 40–55). Incomplete penetrance is associated with repeat tracts in the 36–39 range. At the other end of the spectrum, patients with the juvenile form tend to show the largest expansions (usually more than 60 CAG repeat units), but a wide range of age of onset is observed for any specific repeat number. The repeat size is generally stable at maternal transmission but tends to increase at paternal transmission (see Fig. 9.1). Presymptomatic carrier detection and prenatal diagnosis can be offered by direct DNA analysis. The precise mechanism of pathogenesis of the expanded polyglutamine tract is under investigation but may involve the production of toxic insoluble aggregates of HTT protein, due to hydrogen bonding between the expanded polyglutamine stretches of neighbouring HTT protein molecules, or the generation of toxic proteolytic fragments of the mutant HTT. The condition is discussed in more detail in Chapter 14.

Fragile X syndrome

Fragile X syndrome is the commonest inherited form of significant learning disability, with a prevalence of approximately 1 in 5000 males. It is caused by an expansion of a triplet repeat sequence that is located within the 5′ UTR of the *FMR1* gene at Xq27.3.

DNA analysis usually shows an unstable length mutation in the CGG trinucleotide repeat (normally 6–54 repeats, median 30 repeats) in the 5′ UTR of the *FMR1* gene. In the full mutation, *FMR1* becomes hypermethylated (due to cytosine methylation, in a manner similar to the formation of

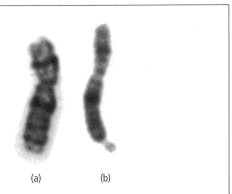

Fig. 9.2 Fragile site at Xq27.3. (a) Normal X chromosome (G-banding). (b) Fragile site visible as a 'gap'.

heterochromatin at centromeric DNA), transcription is suppressed and no FMR protein (FMRP) is generated. The normal physiological role of FMRP is believed to be the regulation, by mRNA binding, of local neuronal protein translation. Such regulation is necessary for the normal development of neuronal dendritic spines and synapses in learning and memory. Paradoxically, however, with premutations (consisting of 55–200 repeats), the long-term clinical effects (see below and Chapter 16) may result from a toxic effect of the *FMR1* transcript rather than its absence (see Garber *et al.*, 2008, in Further reading).

The name of the syndrome resulted from the observation that, under specialised culture conditions (thymidine or deoxycytidine starvation), cytogenetic analysis in males or females who have learning disability and the full fragile X mutation usually reveals a 'fragile site' (an uncondensed region that appears as an apparent gap or unstained region in the chromosome) at Xq27.3 in 10–40% of cells (see Fig. 9.2). One-half of unaffected female carriers of the full mutation also show the fragile site, but the remainder and carriers (male or female) of the premutation have a normal cytogenetic analysis.

Male and female carriers of the premutation (small length mutations) usually have an IQ within the normal range. Potential long-term effects have been reported, however, including, in males, progressive fragile X tremor/ataxia syndrome (FXTAS) and, in females, a premature menopause. Females with the full mutation may be normal or may show mild (approximately 50%) or moderate (1%) learning disability. Males with the full mutation have significant learning disability and 50% have enlarged testes after puberty.

The instability of the length mutation results in atypical X-linked inheritance for fragile X syndrome. For instance, the daughters of those clinically normal males who possess the premutation ('normal transmitting males') will inherit the premutation, which may then be passed on either intact or with expansion to the full mutation. For mothers with the full mutation, one-half of their sons will be affected and one-half of their daughters will receive the full mutation (with about

one-half of these daughters having learning disabilities to some extent). For mothers with the premutation, the risk of expansion to the full mutation at meiosis depends upon the size of the mother's premutation. The condition is discussed in more detail in Chapter 16.

Spinocerebellar ataxia type I

Spinocerebellar ataxia type 1 (SCA1) is an inherited progressive neurodegenerative disorder characterised by ataxia, dysarthria and progressive bulbar dysfunction. The onset is usually in the third or fourth decade with progressive cerebellar ataxia and spastic paraparesis. The rate of progression of the clinical phenotype is variable. DNA analysis for specific length mutations for SCA1 (and other SCA types including 2, 3, 6 and 7) can be undertaken when the diagnosis is suspected.

This disorder is inherited as an autosomal dominant trait due to unstable length mutations in a CAG polyglutamine repeat within the coding sequence of the gene *ATXN1* at 6p23. Normal individuals show a stable inheritance of 19–36 repeats, whereas in affected patients the repeat length is expanded to 42–81 units and is unstable, with a strong tendency for further expansion at paternal transmission. The size of the repeat is inversely correlated to the age of onset (i.e. earlier onset with larger repeats). Presymptomatic and prenatal diagnosis can be offered by direct DNA analysis.

Type I is the commonest form of SCA (50% of cases) but at least 27 other variants with autosomal dominant inheritance are known. As mentioned above, SCA types 1, 2, 3, 6, 7 and 17, at least, are all caused by expansion of a $(CAG)_n$ repeat within the coding sequences of the respective genes, resulting in expanded polyglutamine tracts.

Myotonic dystrophy

Myotonic dystrophy (dystrophia myotonica or DM) is an autosomal dominantly inherited condition with a frequency of around 1 in 7500 and is the most common inherited neuromuscular condition. It typically involves progressive muscle weakness, myotonia and cataracts, in addition to a tendency to cardiac conduction defects and risks associated with general anaesthesia. Genetic anticipation is a feature of the condition, and the genetic basis is an unstable length mutation of a CTG repeat tract within the 3′ UTR of the *DMPK* gene. It is believed that the resulting abnormal *DMPK* mRNA indirectly exerts a toxic intracellular effect on the splicing of other genes such as the chloride channel 1 (*CLCN1*) gene, which appears to be responsible for the myotonia. The expression levels of genes adjacent to *DMPK* also appear to be reduced by the presence of the expanded repeat tract. Normal individuals show stable minor length variations of this region (with 4–37 CTG repeats), whereas, in DM, large expansions (usually over 100 repeats but may be over 2000) are seen and these larger repeat tracts are unstable. There is a general (but incomplete) correlation between the size of the repeat sequence and the clinical severity, with congenitally affected infants usually possessing more than 1000 CTG repeats.

For the offspring of an affected male, half will be affected and half will be unaffected. In contrast to affected females, however, the risk of a neonatal affected case is minimal. Presymptomatic carrier detection and prenatal diagnosis are possible by DNA analysis. The condition is discussed in more detail in Chapter 16 and the molecular pathogenesis has been reviewed by Cho and Tapscott (2007; see Further reading).

Pseudoautosomal inheritance

An unusual phenomenon known as pseudoautosomal inheritance is observed with a sex chromosome-linked condition, Léri–Weill dyschondrosteosis, for which the underlying gene is located within the pseudoautosomal region of the short arm of the X chromosome, as described in Chapter 6. Recombination between the X and Y chromosomes can take place only within a limited area, corresponding to the pseudoautosomal regions (PARs) 1 and 2 at the tips of the Xp and Xq arms, respectively, in which there is close homology between the X and Y chromosomes. As the 29 genes located within the PARs escape X inactivation (with the exception of the two most proximal PAR2 genes) and are present on both the X and Y chromosomes, mutations within these genes are inherited in an autosomal-like fashion, termed 'pseudoautosomal'. Only one PAR gene has been clearly associated with a clinical condition, the *SHOX* gene, located within PAR1 on Xp and Yp. Mutational inactivation or deletion of one copy of this gene results in Léri–Weill dyschondrosteosis syndrome, in which there is short stature and a characteristic Madelung deformity at the wrist that includes bowing of the radius and dorsal dislocation of the distal ulna. A more severe condition, known as Langer mesomelic dysplasia, results in individuals who are homozygous for inactivating mutations of the *SHOX* gene. Interestingly, haploinsufficiency of the same gene is believed to be responsible for the short stature and skeletal anomalies that occur in Turner syndrome. It is not known why the skeletal features that occur in Léri–Weill dyschondrosteosis are not the same as those in Turner syndrome. It is possible that haploinsufficiency of other X chromosome genes in Turner syndrome partly alleviates the effects of the *SHOX* deficiency or that, in girls with *SHOX* deficiency alone (and therefore normal gonadal function), the oestrogen action at the growth plate may exacerbate the effects of *SHOX* haploinsufficiency. An excellent review of the PAR regions is provided by Blaschke and Rappold (2006; see Further reading).

Autosomal dominant inheritance with sex limitation

In certain genetic conditions, the inheritance is autosomal dominant, but the phenotype may be expressed only in males or in females. For example, in familial breast/ovarian cancer resulting from the inheritance of a mutation in *BRCA1* or *BRCA2* (see Chapter 13), typically only females are affected, while the males can carry the mutation but usually remain unaffected. The inheritance mechanism is then strictly regarded as autosomal dominant with female sex limitation. The converse would be true for the inheritance of prostate cancer in some families.

Pseudodominant inheritance

Gilbert syndrome, one of the commonest inherited conditions, exhibits so-called pseudodominant inheritance. It results in a mild intermittent unconjugated hyperbilirubinaemia, often precipitated by an intercurrent illness. The underlying molecular basis in affected individuals is homozygosity for an insertion (A(TA)$_7$TAA) within the promoter region of the *UGT1A1* gene on chromosome 2. As the carrier frequency for this insertion in the population of Europe and North America is around 50%, a relatively high proportion of the population are homozygous. Moreover, as the partner of an affected individual has a high chance of being a carrier of the insertion, it is common for affected individuals to have affected children (Fig. 9.3). Not surprisingly, therefore, the mechanism of inheritance was previously regarded as being autosomal dominant. Now that the molecular genetic basis has been elucidated and affected individuals identified as being homozygotes, however, the true mechanism of inheritance has been revealed as being autosomal recessive. The term 'pseudodominant' has therefore

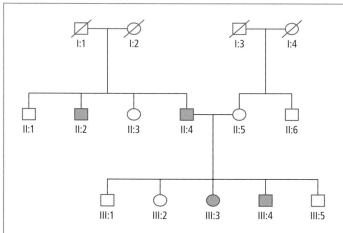

Fig. 9.3 Pedigree illustrating Gilbert syndrome inheritance. The occurrence of the condition in two generations of the family, together with apparent male-to-male transmission, might suggest autosomal dominant inheritance. The condition is now known, however, to be inherited in an autosomal recessive manner but with such a high carrier frequency that affected individuals may be found in more than one generation. Mutation analysis, if performed, would reveal the presence of two *UGT1A1* mutant alleles in individuals II:2, II:4, III:3 and III:4 as well as a single mutant *UGT1A1* allele in individual II:5 (a carrier).

been used to describe this and other similar situations. Interestingly, mutations within the coding region of the same gene, *UGT1A1*, that cause inactivation of the protein rather than merely reducing promoter activity can give rise to the rarer and much more severe autosomal recessive condition known as Crigler–Najjar syndrome type 1, in which there is a severe unconjugated hyperbilirubinaemia.

Pseudodominant inheritance has also been observed (albeit much less frequently) in other conditions such as Friedreich ataxia and, very recently, pseudoxanthoma elasticum. It is more likely to be seen in families in which there is consanguinity.

X-linked dominant inheritance with male lethality

In a few syndromes such as incontinentia pigmenti (associated with the *NEMO* gene), Rett syndrome (*MECP2* gene), X-linked periventricular heterotopia (*FLNA* gene) and focal dermal hypoplasia, the individuals diagnosed with the condition are almost always females (who will be heterozygous), the affected males having died *in utero* resulting in an early miscarriage. As a result, for an affected female, one-third of the live-born offspring will be affected females, one-third will be unaffected females and one-third will be unaffected males. The birth of an affected child to unaffected parents is most likely to be due to a new mutation with a resulting low risk of recurrence for the couple's future offspring (also see Chapter 8 and the review by Franco and Ballabio, 2006, in Further reading).

Mosaicism

Mosaicism refers to the situation that develops when a genetic abnormality arises during mitosis, post-fertilisation. This results in the individual possessing both a normal cell line and a genetically abnormal cell line. A clinical consequence is that only some of that individual's cells may exhibit the phenotypic characteristics of a particular genetic condition. For instance, in so-called segmental neurofibromatosis type 1 (segmental NF1), the clinical features are visible only in certain parts of the body. The mosaicism may, of course, also be present in the gonads with the consequence that the offspring could inherit the mutation. The mutation would then be present in all of the child's cells.

In addition, mosaicism can appear to affect only the gonads, such that a phenotypically healthy individual may possess a genetic abnormality that is present in a proportion of his or her germ cells. The result of such 'gonadal mosaicism' is that a genetic condition such as tuberous sclerosis or Duchenne muscular dystrophy may occur in more than one of the children of a clinically unaffected individual (Fig. 9.4). Care must therefore be taken when counselling the parents regarding recurrence risks following the birth of a child with an apparently new mutation for an autosomal dominant or X-linked condition.

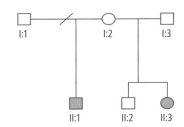

Fig. 9.4 Pedigree illustrating a family with tuberous sclerosis (TS). In this family, a second affected child has been born to the clinically unaffected mother, I:2. Mutation analysis of blood DNA may reveal a TS gene mutation in II:1 but not in either of his parents. The same mutation, however, would be present in the blood DNA of II:3, as a result of gonadal mosaicism in I:2.

Modifier genes and digenic inheritance

Modifier genes

For many apparently monogenic Mendelian conditions, there is only a poor correlation between the genotype at the single gene locus and the phenotype. Additional factors that may contribute to the phenotypic expression of such conditions include environmental factors and modifier genes. Modifier genes are genetic variants that can affect the manifestation of a disorder, for instance its age of onset, the range or severity of symptoms and the rate of disease progression. Susceptibility genes, in contrast, may be regarded as those that alter the liability to develop the condition rather than altering the phenotypic expression of the disease. The products of modifier genes may alter the expression of a distant gene in many ways. These include effects on transcription, splicing and translation, in addition to effects on the encoded protein such as its post-translational modification, transport, secretion, activation and degradation.

It is becoming increasingly recognised that many conditions that were previously regarded as being single-gene disorders are, in fact, actually oligogenic, with the severity or range of the clinical manifestations being the result of a combination of several genetic loci. There are likely to be many genetic conditions that can be described more accurately in this way rather than by the perhaps overly simplistic categorisation into either single-gene disorders or complex/multifactorial disorders.

For example, the age of onset of the autosomal dominant Huntington disease is determined to some extent by the number of CAG triplet repeat units in the polyglutamine-encoding $(CAG)_n$ stretch within the first exon of the gene that encodes the HTT protein. As mentioned above, however, for any given number of repeat units, there is a wide range in the age of onset. It is becoming clear from recent studies that several other genes are likely to be involved in determining the age of onset and that the CAG repeat tract size accounts for only around 70% of the variability. The candidate modifiers for this condition are currently regarded as being the gene encoding a transcriptional repressor known as corepressor C-terminal binding protein (CtBP) that interacts with the HTT protein within the nucleus; the glutamate receptor gene, *GRIK2*; and the *DCHL1* gene, which encodes the ubiquitin carboxyl-terminal hydrolase L1.

Many studies have been undertaken in other predominantly monogenic disorders to identify modifying genes. In the autosomal recessive condition cystic fibrosis, for instance, one of the modifier genes of pulmonary disease severity for which the evidence is greatest, is transforming growth factor β1 (see Drumm *et al.*, 2005, in Further reading). In addition, the risk of developing breast cancer in carriers of a *BRCA2* mutation is now known to be modified by the presence or absence of a *FGFR2* single-nucleotide polymorphism in the germline DNA.

Digenic inheritance

Digenic inheritance refers to the situation in which the clinical condition can arise from the interaction of two different genes. An example of this is autosomal recessive non-syndromic deafness. While this frequently results from mutations in the connexin 26 gene (particularly the 35delG common mutation in Caucasians), the condition can also result from the inheritance of a single mutation in this gene together with a deletion in the connexin 30 gene. Interestingly, both genes lie on the same chromosome, chromosome 13, only 35 kb apart. Perhaps not surprisingly, their protein products functionally interact, together participating in the formation of a multi-subunit hemichannel in the cochlea, necessary for the regulation of potassium in the inner ear.

There has been some debate regarding the possible role of digenic *triallelic* inheritance in the condition known as Bardet-Biedl syndrome (BBS). The phenotype of this condition includes truncal obesity, hypogenitalism, renal dysfunction, polydactyly, retinal dystrophy and learning disability. The underlying cellular defect in BBS lies within the cilia. The defect appears to particularly affect the important intraflagellar transport system that is responsible for the movement of particles from the basal body to the tip of the cilium. At least 12 different BBS-causing genes have been identified to date. In most affected individuals, mutations in both alleles of a single gene (usually *BBS1*) appear to be sufficient to cause the disease. However, in a minority (probably <10%) of cases, the presence of three mutant BBS alleles (with the additional mutant allele most frequently involving *BBS2* or *BBS6*) is detected in affected patients. This apparent digenic triallelic inheritance may alternatively be regarded, however, as autosomal recessive inheritance with a modifier of penetrance.

Uniparental disomy

As mentioned in Chapter 6, a child can, rarely, inherit both copies of a chromosome from one parent. This is termed

Table 9.1 Examples of syndromes that may result from UPD

Syndrome	Causative UPD
Angelman syndrome	Paternal UPD15
Prader–Willi syndrome	Maternal UPD15
Beckwith–Wiedemann syndrome	Paternal UPD11
Russell–Silver syndrome	Maternal UPD7

uniparental disomy (UPD). Trisomy is avoided by the loss of the other parent's homologue of that chromosome from the fetus at an early stage by the process known as 'trisomic rescue'. When both inherited copies of the chromosome are not only from the same parent, but have actually originated in the *same* grandparent (i.e. two copies of the same homologue), then the term used is uniparental isodisomy. Alternatively, when the two copies of the chromosome are inherited from the same parent but have originated in *different* grandparents, the appropriate term is uniparental heterodisomy (Fig. 9.5). One consequence of uniparental disomy is that a child may be affected by an imprinting disorder such as Prader–Willi syndrome, Angelman syndrome, Beckwith–Wiedemann syndrome (see below and Table 9.1), as, for a few specific genes, the parent of origin determines whether or not the genes are expressed. In addition, in uniparental isodisomy, an autosomal recessive condition may arise in a child even though only one of the child's parents is a carrier of the mutation. For instance, cystic fibrosis may rarely occur as a consequence of uniparental isodisomy of chromosome 7.

Imprinting disorders

A few genetic conditions result from alterations in genes that, despite being autosomal, are usually expressed from just one allele, representing either the maternal or the paternal copy of the gene. The transcriptional repression of one allele is the result of imprinting, i.e. a differential methylation of the two gene copies that is dependent upon the parent of origin of each allele. This is the case in Angelman and Prader–Willi syndromes (both of which are discussed in detail in Chapter 6), and in Beckwith–Wiedemann syndrome, which is a fetal overgrowth syndrome with minor dysmorphisms and an increased susceptibility to certain tumours including Wilms tumour. In Angelman and Prader–Willi syndromes, the condition arises from the loss of gene expression from the normally active maternal or paternal gene copy, respectively. Further details regarding the Angelman/Prader–Willi syndrome locus are given in Chapter 16. In theory, a female with Prader–Willi syndrome resulting from a paternally inherited deletion affecting the Prader–Willi syndrome/Angelman syndrome critical region on 15q could have a child with Angelman syn-

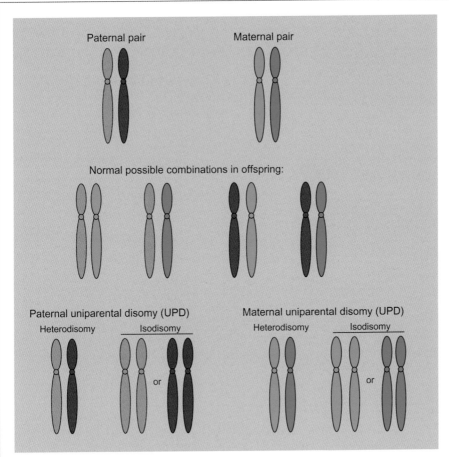

Fig. 9.5 Diagram showing how paternal or maternal UPD can arise by the inheritance of both members of a chromosome pair from either the father or the mother, respectively. Uniparental heterodisomy refers to the inheritance of both chromosomes from the parent, whereas uniparental isodisomy refers to the inheritance of two identical copies of just one parental chromosome.

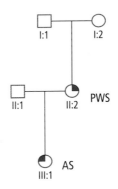

Fig. 9.6 Pedigree of the family reported by Schulze *et al.* (2001) in which the individual II:2 inherited a deletion at 15q11-q13 from her father and thus developed Prader–Willi syndrome (PWS). The daughter of II:2 subsequently inherited the deletion from her and thus was affected by Angelman syndrome (AS).

drome if that child inherited the deletion from her. This has, in fact, been reported (see Fig. 9.6 and Schulze *et al.*, 2001, in Further reading) although fertility is rare in Prader–Willi syndrome.

In Beckwith–Wiedemann syndrome, the various molecular disease mechanisms are especially complex, and usually involve the biallelic expression of one or more genes that are normally expressed from a single allele. Two such genes are the insulin-like growth factor 2 (*IGF2*) gene and the non-translated *KCNQ1OT1* gene, which is a transcriptional inhibitor of other neighbouring genes, including cyclin-dependent kinase inhibitor 1C (*CDKN1C/p57KIP2*). Thus, in Beckwith–Wiedemann syndrome, the important molecular outcome at the protein level is generally the abnormally increased expression of a growth factor, IGF2, or the abnormally reduced expression of a cell-cycle inhibitor, CDKN1C/P57(KIP2).

SUMMARY

- Genetic anticipation refers to the increasing severity and decreasing age of onset of certain conditions in successive generations. It may result from the increasing size, at meiosis, of a tract of trinucleotide repeats, which may lie outside the coding sequence.

- A number of genes located at the ends of the X chromosome are present also on the Y chromosome. These genes escape X inactivation, and a mutation in such a gene may result in a condition (particularly Léri–Weill dyschondrosteosis) that is inherited in an autosomal dominant-like (i.e. 'pseudoautosomal') manner.

- Certain autosomal recessive conditions (e.g. Gilbert syndrome) have such a high carrier frequency that the conditions initially appeared to be inherited in an autosomal dominant fashion. The true 'pseudodominant' inheritance was subsequently revealed by the demonstration, on DNA sequencing, of two mutant alleles in affected individuals.

- X-linked dominant inheritance with male lethality, seen in incontinentia pigmenti and Rett syndrome for instance, results in the only living affected children

being female and, if the parents are unaffected, most likely being the result of a new mutation.

- Mosaicism, arising from a post-fertilisation genetic abnormality, results in a condition affecting only a proportion of the cells of an individual and may affect the gonads without detectable phenotypic effects somatically. Care must therefore be taken in the genetic counselling of parents of a child who appears to represent a new mutation.

- Genetic variation in modifier genes is likely to contribute to the relatively poor correlation between phenotype and genotype (at a particular locus) that is observed for many apparently monogenic Mendelian conditions.

- UPD refers to the situation where a child has inherited both copies of a chromosome from just one parent. Its consequences may include imprinting disorders if the chromosome contains clinically important genes whose parent of origin determines whether or not they are transcriptionally active. In addition, in the form known as uniparental isodisomy, an autosomal recessive condition may be manifested.

FURTHER READING

Blaschke RJ, Rappold G (2006) The pseudoautosomal regions, SHOX and disease. *Curr Opin Genet Dev* **16**:233–9.

Cho DH, Tapscott SJ (2007) Myotonic dystrophy: emerging mechanisms for DM1 and DM2. *Biochim Biophys Acta* **1772**:195–204.

Drumm ML, Konstan MW, Schluchter MD, Handler A, Pace R, Zou F, Zariwala M, Fargo D, Xu A, *et al.* (2005) Genetic modifiers of lung disease in cystic fibrosis. *N Engl J Med* **353**:1443–53.

Franco B, Ballabio A (2006) X-inactivation and human disease: X-linked dominant male-lethal disorders. *Curr Opin Genet Dev* **16**:254–9.

Garber KB, Visootsak J, Warren ST (2008) Fragile X syndrome. *Eur J Hum Genet* **16**:666–72.

Gropman AL, Adams DR (2007) Atypical patterns of inheritance. *Semin Pediatr Neurol* **14**:34–45.

Harper PS (2010) *Practical Genetic Counselling*, 7th edn. Hodder Arnold: London.

Ranum LP, Cooper TA (2006) RNA-mediated neuromuscular disorders. *Annu Rev Neurosci* **29**:259–77.

Rappold G, Blum WF, Shavrikova EP, Crowe BJ, Roeth R, Quigley CA, Ross JL, Niesler B (2007) Genotypes and phenotypes in children with short stature: clinical indicators of SHOX haploinsufficiency. *J Med Genet* **44**:306–13.

Schulze A, Mogensen H, Hamborg-Petersen B, Graem N, Ostergaard JR, Brøndum-Nielsen K (2001) Fertility in Prader–Willi syndrome: a case report with Angelman syndrome in the offspring. *Acta Paediatr* **90**:455–9.

WEBSITE

Online Mendelian Inheritance in Man (OMIM):
http://www.ncbi.nlm.nih.gov/sites/entrez?db=omim

Self-assessment

1. In which of the following conditions is genetic anticipation a common feature?
A. Myotonic dystrophy (DM) type 1
B. Spinocerebellar atrophy type 2 (SCA2)
C. Dentatorubral-pallidoluysian atrophy (DRPLA)
D. Friedreich ataxia
E. Fragile X syndrome

2. Pseudoautosomal inheritance is observed for which one of the following conditions?
A. Duchenne muscular dystrophy
B. Becker muscular dystrophy
C. Léri–Weill dyschondrosteosis
D. Glycerol kinase deficiency
E. Haemophilia A

3. Which of the following are true statements regarding pseudodominant inheritance?
A. It is observed in families affected by Gilbert syndrome
B. It typically occurs when the inheritance of just one mutation is sufficient to cause an individual to be affected
C. It is commonly observed in families affected by Crigler–Najjar syndrome type 1
D. It is more likely when the carrier frequency is high
E. It may be confirmed by molecular genetic investigations using polymorphic DNA markers

4. X-linked dominant inheritance with male lethality is a feature of which of the following conditions?
A. Rett syndrome
B. Vitamin D-resistant rickets
C. Haemophilia B
D. Focal dermal hypoplasia
E. Incontinentia pigmenti

5. Which of the following types of uniparental disomy (UPD) are correctly paired with a genetic condition?
A. Prader–Willi syndrome and paternal UPD of chromosome 15
B. Angelman syndrome and maternal UPD of chromosome 15
C. Beckwith–Wiedemann syndrome and paternal UPD of chromosome 11
D. Russell–Silver syndrome and maternal UPD of chromosome 7
E. Cystic fibrosis (CF) and paternal uniparental isodisomy 7, where the father is a CF carrier

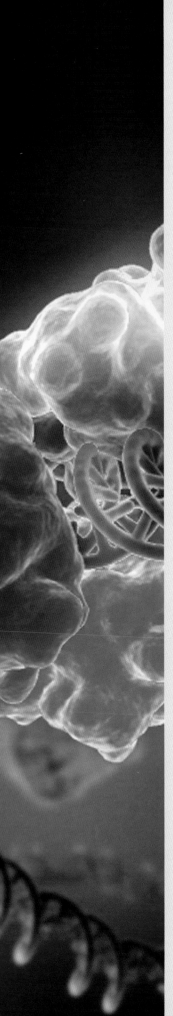

CHAPTER 10
Non-Mendelian inheritance

Key Topics

Introduction

In addition to chromosomal disorders (Chapter 7) and single-gene (Mendelian) disorders (Chapters 8 and 9), there are three further important subgroups of genetic disease, namely multifactorial disorders, somatic cell genetic disorders and mitochondrial disorders.

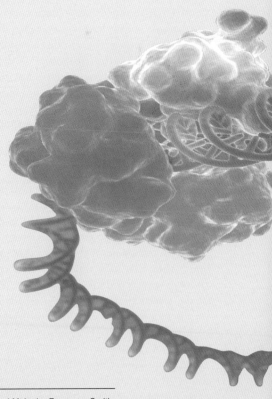

Essential Medical Genetics, 6th edition. © Edward S. Tobias, Michael Connor and Malcolm Ferguson-Smith.
Published 2011 by Blackwell Published Ltd.

Multifactorial disorders

Multifactorial (i.e. complex or part-genetic) traits may be discontinuous (with distinct phenotypes, e.g. diabetes mellitus) or continuous (with a lack of distinct phenotypes, e.g. height), but in each the trait is determined by the interaction of a number of genes at different loci, each with a small but additive effect, together with environmental factors. For discontinuous multifactorial traits, the risk to relatives within an affected family is raised above the general population risk but is low in comparison with Mendelian traits, and rapidly falls towards the general population risk in more distant relatives. Thus, in practice, the proband (the affected individual who draws medical attention to the family) with a discontinuous multifactorial trait is often the only affected person in that family.

Therefore, in contrast to Mendelian disorders, pedigree analysis cannot prove multifactorial inheritance, and studies of twin concordance and family correlation are necessary.

Twin concordance studies

Twins may be identical (monozygotic) or non-identical (dizygotic). Monozygotic twins are genetically identical as they arise from a single zygote that divides into two embryos during the first 13 days of gestation before the primitive streak forms. Monozygotic twinning has no known predisposing factors and occurs with a frequency of 3–4 per 1000 births in all populations. Dizygotic twins result from two ova fertilised by two spermatozoa and so have, on average, one-half of their genes in common and are genetically equivalent to brothers and sisters (siblings). The frequency of dizygotic twinning is increased with increasing maternal age, with increased parity, by a positive family history of twins and is associated with a tall heavy build in the mother. The frequency of dizygotic twins is low in Japan and Asia at 2–7 per 1000 births and high in black Africans at 45–50 per 1000 births (in comparison with 9–20 per 1000 births in Europe and 7–12 per 1000 births in the USA).

For research purposes, the diagnosis of zygosity cannot be based solely upon a similar appearance, and analysis of highly polymorphic DNA markers by DNA fingerprinting (Chapter 4) is the most reliable method. A record of the nature of the placental membranes may also be extremely useful. All dizygotic twins have two amniotic sacs and two chorions. The chorions may secondarily fuse, but the circulations of each part of the placenta normally remain separate. The nature of the membranes for monozygotic twins depends upon the timing of separation. In 75% of monozygotic twins, there is a single chorion with a common placental circulation – this is diagnostic of monozygosity. In the remaining 25%, two chorions are found. These cannot be distinguished from dizygotic twins by examination of placental membranes (Fig. 10.1) and DNA fingerprinting will be required.

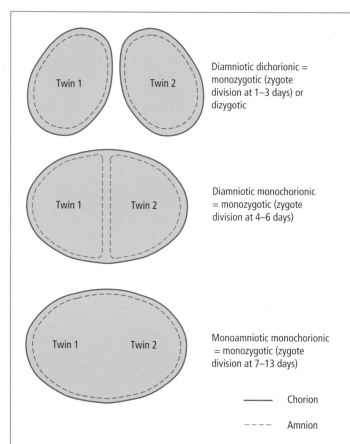

Diamniotic dichorionic = monozygotic (zygote division at 1–3 days) or dizygotic

Diamniotic monochorionic = monozygotic (zygote division at 4–6 days)

Monoamniotic monochorionic = monozygotic (zygote division at 7–13 days)

——— Chorion

- - - - Amnion

Fig. 10.1 Diagnosis of zygosity from the appearance of the placental membranes.

Determination of concordance

Twins are concordant if they both show a discontinuous trait, and discordant if only one shows the trait. There is a tendency to report concordant rather than discordant twin pairs in the medical literature, and this bias needs to be considered in the interpretation of twin studies. For continuous traits the extent of the trait, for example height, is directly compared between the twins. As twins usually share a similar family environment, it may be difficult to separate the relative extent of environmental (nurture) and genetic (nature) contributions to a multifactorial trait. In this respect the concordance of monozygotic twins who have been adopted and reared apart from infancy is of major importance.

Results of twin studies

Monozygotic twins have identical genotypes whereas dizygotic twins are only as alike as siblings (brothers and sisters). If a condition has no genetic component, for example accidental injury, concordance rates are similar for both types of twins. For a single-gene trait or a chromosomal disorder, the monozygotic concordance rate will be 100%, whereas the dizygotic rate will be less than this and equal to the rate in siblings. For

Table 10.1 Concordance rates in twins if a particular inheritance pattern is followed exclusively

Disorder	Concordance	
	Monozygotic	Dizygotic
Single gene	100%	As sibs
Chromosomal	100%	As sibs
Multifactorial	<100% but >siblings	As sibs
Somatic cell genetic	As siblings*	As sibs
Mitochondrial	100%	100%
Non-genetic	As sibs	As sibs

*But >sibs for monozygotic twins if the condition results from a combination of somatic cell events and the inheritance of a single-gene mutation (as in several familial cancer syndromes).

Table 10.2 Degree of similarity of twins for continuous traits

Trait	Degree of similarity	
	Monozygotic (%)	Dizygotic (%)
Height	95	52
IQ	90	60
Finger ridge count	95	49
Diastolic blood pressure	50	27

Table 10.3 Twin concordance for some discontinuous traits

Trait	Concordance	
	Monozygotic (%)	Dizygotic (%)
Atopic disease	50	4
Cancer	17	11
Cleft lip with/without cleft palate	35	5
Cleft palate alone	26	6
Congenital dislocation of the hip	41	3
Diabetes mellitus (insulin-dependent)	30–40	6
Diabetes mellitus (non-insulin-dependent)	100	10
Epilepsy	37	10
Gallstones	27	6
Hypertension	30	10
Hyperthyroidism	47	3
Ischaemic heart disease	19	8
Leprosy	60	20
Manic depression	70	15
Learning disability with IQ <50	60	3
Multiple sclerosis	20–30	6
Psoriasis	61	13
Pyloric stenosis	15	2
Rheumatoid arthritis	30	5
Sarcoidosis	50	8
Schizophrenia	45	12
Senile dementia	42	5
Spina bifida	6	3
Talipes equinovarus	32	3
Tuberculosis	87	26

Table 10.4 Proportion of genes shared by relatives

Degree of relationship	Examples	Proportion of genes in common
First	Parent to child, sibling to sibling	50%
Second	Grandparent to grandchild, nephew or niece to aunt or uncle	25%
Third	First cousins	12.5%

discontinuous multifactorial traits with both genetic and environmental contributions, the rate in monozygotic twins, although less than 100%, will exceed the rate in dizygotic twins (Table 10.1).

Tables 10.2 and 10.3 list the findings in twins for some continuous traits, congenital malformations and common adult disorders. In each multifactorial trait, the concordance rate in monozygotic twins exceeds that in dizygotic twins, although the actual concordance rate in the monozygotic twins ranges from 6 to 100%. This range reflects the heritability of the condition: the higher the monozygotic concordance, the more important the genetic contribution and so the higher the heritability.

Family correlation studies

Relatives share a proportion of their genes (Table 10.4). Thus, if a trait is determined by multifactorial inheritance, relatives should show the trait in proportion to their genetic similarity. This is really only an extension of the twin study technique, and the similarity of different relatives in this respect is known as their correlation. This is measured on a scale of

0–1, where 1 is identical. The more closely related the relatives, the higher the correlation should be for a genetically determined trait.

If parents are not blood relatives, then they would be expected to be as alike genetically as random members of the population. Thus, their correlation for genetically determined traits should only be equal to the general population average. In practice, many slightly exceed this as a result of selective mating for characteristics such as height and intelligence (assortative mating).

Table 10.5 shows the familial correlations for several continuous multifactorial traits. Height, intelligence and total fingertip ridge count provide close family correlations to those predicted from the proportion of genes in common. Table 10.6 shows the frequency of some discontinuous traits in relatives of an affected person. The frequency falls off in proportion to the proportion of genes in common, but is increased in all relatives above the general population frequency.

Hence, twin concordance and family correlation studies can provide support for multifactorial inheritance of a trait, whether discontinuous or continuous. Also, the observed frequencies in relatives provide the basis for genetic counselling for multifactorial disorders (empiric risks).

Continuous multifactorial traits

Many normal human characteristics are determined as continuous multifactorial traits (Table 10.7). These traits, by definition, have a continuously graded distribution. Thus, for height there is a range from the very tall to the markedly short with a mean in English men of 169 cm and a standard deviation of 6.5 cm (Fig. 10.2). As can be seen, the distribution of height in a population is Gaussian, with the majority of individuals centred around the mean. Such a distribution is characteristic (but not diagnostic) of a continuous multifactorial trait.

The interaction of a number of loci to produce such a gradual range can readily be appreciated from the range of shade produced by the interaction of pairs of alleles at one, two and three hypothetical loci for skin colour (Fig. 10.3). Thus, relatively small numbers of loci could, in theory, account for an almost continuous distribution.

Parents of above average height tend to have children who are taller than average but who are not quite as tall as themselves. As a child only receives half of each parent's genes, the expected correlation with the mid-parental height would be 0.71 (i.e. $\sqrt{0.5}$) if height depended only on genetic factors. However, environmental factors are also important, and as the same combination of environmental and genetic factors that operated for each parent is unlikely to occur in the child, this results in a tendency to regress towards the mean. This also operates at the lower end of the normal range of height and tends to be most obvious in families where the degree of parental deviation is extreme. Genome-wide association studies (see below) have in fact now revealed that 18 genetic single-nucleotide polymorphisms (SNPs) account for just 2.6% of variance in adult height, with hundreds of other associated SNPs still to be detected. Similar conclusions are likely to be reached for other continuous complex traits.

Discontinuous multifactorial traits

More than 20 discontinuous multifactorial traits have been described and Table 10.8 lists some of the commoner ones that

Table 10.5 Family correlations for some continuous traits

Trait	Correlation of first-degree relatives	
	Observed	Expected
Height	0.53	0.5
IQ	0.41	0.5
Finger ridge count	0.49	0.5
Diastolic blood pressure	0.18	0.5

Table 10.6 Frequency of discontinuous traits for differing degrees of relationship

Trait	Frequency (%)			
	First-degree relatives	Second-degree relatives	Third-degree relatives	Population frequency
Cleft lip	4	0.6	0.3	0.1
Spina bifida/anencephaly	4	1.5	0.6	0.3
Pyloric stenosis	2	1	0.4	0.3
Epilepsy	5	2.5	1.5	1
Schizophrenia	10	4	2	1
Manic depression	15	5	3.5	1

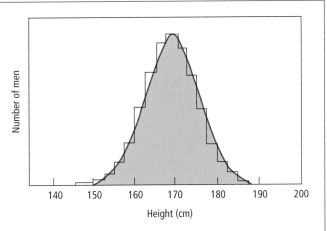

Fig. 10.2 Gaussian distribution of height in English adult males.

Table 10.7 Examples of human continuous multifactorial traits

Height	Red cell size
Weight	Blood pressure
Intelligence	Skin colour
Total ridge count	

Table 10.8 Discontinuous human multifactorial traits

Common adult diseases	Congenital malformations
Rheumatoid arthritis	Cleft lip and palate
Epilepsy	Congenital heart disease
Schizophrenia	Neural tube defect
Manic depression	Pyloric stenosis
Multiple sclerosis	
Diabetes mellitus	
Premature vascular disease	
Hyperthyroidism	

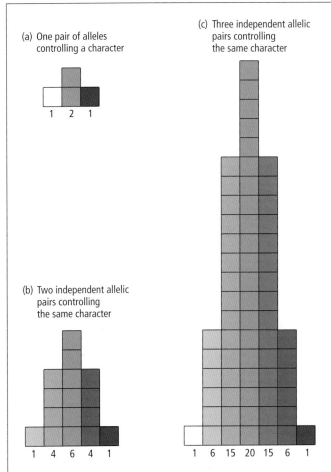

Fig. 10.3 Expected distribution of colour in offspring if the trait is due to (a) a single locus with two alleles, (b) two loci each with two alleles and (c) three loci each with two alleles. Note the approach towards a Gaussian distribution.

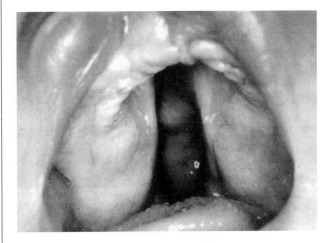

Fig. 10.4 Cleft lip and palate.

are of medical importance. Broadly, these traits can be divided into congenital malformations and common conditions of adult life.

Cleft lip and palate is a congenital malformation that is inherited as a multifactorial trait (Fig. 10.4). In the mildest form, the lip alone is unilaterally cleft, whereas in the most severe form the lip is bilaterally cleft and the palatal cleft is complete. The parents of the child in Fig. 10.4 were unaffected and there was no family history of cleft lip and palate, but by virtue of having produced an affected child, this indicates that

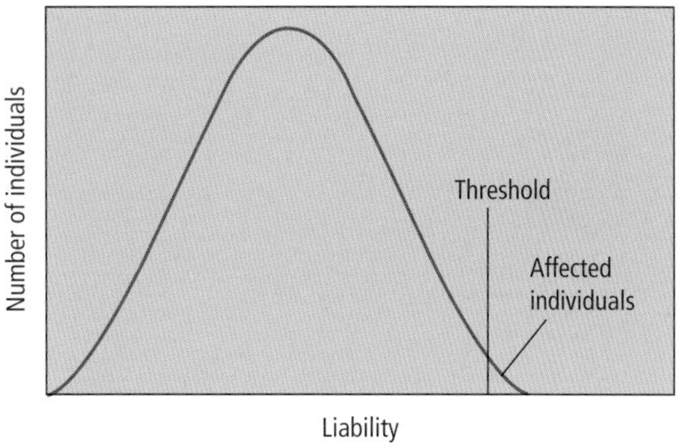

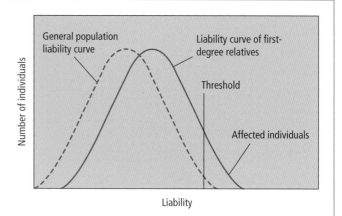

Fig. 10.5 General population liability curve for cleft lip and palate.

Fig. 10.6 Displaced liability curve in first-degree relatives of a proband with cleft lip and palate.

each parent must have some underactive genes for lip and palate formation. However, as they have fully formed lips and palates, they must also have, on balance, sufficient normally active genes. For these discontinuous traits, it is the critical balance between the number of underactive and the number of normally active genes that is important. Only when the balance exceeds a threshold will the malformation occur, and the further the threshold is exceeded, the greater the extent of the malformation. Thus, the liability (including both genetic and environmental factors) can be represented as a Gaussian curve (Fig. 10.5). The threshold is indicated in Fig. 10.5, and the proportion of the population to the right of this threshold (0.1%) equals the general population incidence of cleft lip and palate. For parents (first-degree relatives) of an affected child, the liability curve is shifted to the right, and so we would expect to find an increased frequency (4%) of this malformation among parents and other first-degree relatives (Fig. 10.6). With each further degree of relationship, the liability curve moves back a step towards the general population position, with a corresponding reduction in the incidence (see Table 10.6).

The more severe the malformation in the affected child, the more the parents' liability curve is shifted to the right and the higher the incidence in relatives. Thus, 5% of first-degree relatives are affected if the clefting is bilateral and complete, whereas only 2% are affected if it is unilateral and incomplete.

Some multifactorial traits show an unequal sex ratio (Table 10.9). Thus, while pyloric stenosis affects 5 in 1000 males, only 1 in 1000 females is affected. The incidence is increased in the relatives of affected males, but is even more increased in the relatives of affected females (the Carter effect; Table 10.10). This indicates that the female threshold is higher than the male threshold for this malformation, and so the parents of an affected female need to have a higher proportion of underactive genes and hence a more displaced liability curve.

Table 10.9 Multifactorial conditions with an unequal sex ratio

Condition	Sex ratio (males to females)
Pyloric stenosis	5 : 1
Hirschsprung disease	3 : 1
Congenital dislocation of the hip	1 : 6
Talipes	2 : 1
Rheumatoid arthritis	1 : 3

Table 10.10 Pyloric stenosis frequency in relatives

Relationship	Frequency (%)	Increase on general population risk for same sex
Male relatives of a male patient	5	10-fold
Female relatives of a male patient	2	20-fold
Male relatives of a female patient	17	35-fold
Female relatives of a female patient	7	70-fold

Analysis of the genetic determinants of multifactorial traits

Currently, there is a great deal of interest in analysis of the genetic determinants of multifactorial traits. Several approaches have been utilised including linkage analysis, sibling pair studies, microsatellite marker association analysis with mutational analysis of candidate genes and, most recently, genome-wide association studies using SNPs.

Linkage analysis is a standard approach for the analysis of single-gene disorders but is more difficult in multifactorial traits, especially where these have a continuous distribution. This approach has been more successful when coupled with selective breeding in experimental animals.

Siblings have approximately one-half of their genes in common and thus, at a particular locus, one-quarter of siblings will share two alleles, one-half will have one allele in common and one-quarter will have different alleles. Affected sibling pairs are studied to detect distortions from this expected $1:2:1$ ratio as such distortion with an excess of sharing is a clue that the locus is involved in the causation of the disorder.

Association analysis can be carried out by comparing the frequency of particular alleles (using microsatellite markers for instance) at a locus between an affected group and an unaffected control group. Differences may be clues to genetic determinants that reflect linkage disequilibrium between the genetic marker under study and the causative mutation. A more recent development is a genome-wide association study comparing the genotype frequency, for each of at least 500,000 recognised SNPs, between thousands of cases and thousands of controls. These increasingly reported studies utilise the data generated by the Human Genome Project and HapMap projects (see Chapters 2 and 11). Several such studies have recently been published, including analyses of conditions such as coronary artery disease, type 2 diabetes, breast cancer, rheumatoid arthritis, osteoarthritis, vitiligo and Crohn's disease (see Further reading for examples of such studies and the review by Hunter and Kraft, 2007, for a discussion of the statistical aspects of such analyses). The results indicate which inherited DNA sequence variants are most significantly associated with particular traits and diseases, but generally do not provide information on the precise mechanism by which these variants are associated with the development of the conditions. Such a variant may directly change an amino acid within a protein. Alternatively, it may lie in a non-coding region of a gene and affect the gene's transcription or splicing, or it may be tightly linked to another variant located nearby that is causally associated with the trait.

The preceding approaches identify chromosomal regions of interest and these can be analysed further by mutational analysis in candidate genes from these regions in affected patients.

Somatic cell genetic disorders

When a mutation is present in the fertilised egg, then this mutation will be transmitted to all daughter cells. If, however, a mutation arises after the first cell division, then this mutation will be found only in a proportion of cells and the individual is mosaic (two or more different genotypes in one individual). The mutation may be confined to the gonadal cells (gonadal mosaic) or to the somatic cells (somatic mosaic) or occur in a proportion of both. Irrespective of the distribution of the initial mutation within the individual, there would be no preceding family history but if the gonad includes the mutation there would be a risk to offspring.

Most, if not all, cancers are now known to be (at least partly) somatic cell genetic disorders. Some familial cancers have germ-line mutations but in the remainder a succession of mutations occurs in the somatic cell(s), which progress to malignancy (Chapter 13). In fact, even when a germline mutation is inherited, additional genetic alterations, affecting other cancer genes must usually occur somatically prior to the development of an invasive cancer. In addition, when a mutation is inherited in one allele of a tumour suppressor gene (TSG), the normal (wild-type) copy of the gene must be inactivated by a somatic event for the tumorigenic effect of the gene to be manifest. This is due to the fact that the effect of mutations in TSGs is generally a loss of function (or inactivation) of the protein encoded by that gene with the result that a remaining normal copy of the gene can still function sufficiently to prevent oncogenesis. The loss of the second copy of such a TSG (for instance by deletion or recombination) is often detectable upon DNA analysis as a loss of heterozygosity in the tumour DNA compared with the blood DNA of that individual.

Mitochondrial disorders

Each cell has hundreds of mitochondria in the cytoplasm, and each mitochondrion contains about ten copies of the circular mitochondrial chromosome (Chapter 5). The mitochondria (and their chromosomes) are virtually all derived from the mother and hence mitochondrial disorders due to mutations in these chromosomes show characteristic patterns of inheritance with transmission to all children of an affected mother but no risk to the offspring of an affected man (Fig. 10.7). The mitochondrial DNA has a high mutation rate, and both point and length mutations occur at a tenfold higher rate than in nuclear DNA. The phenotypic effect depends on the location and type of mutation and also on the proportion of mitochondrial chromosomes that are involved. Heteroplasmy with some

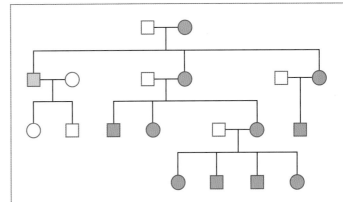

Fig. 10.7 Pedigree from a family with Leber hereditary optic neuropathy showing mutation carriers, not all of whom were symptomatic.

Table 10.11 Examples of conditions with mitochondrial inheritance

DIDMOAD (diabetes insipidus, diabetes mellitus, optic atrophy and deafness – mitochondrial form)

Kearns–Sayre syndrome (chronic progressive external ophthalmoplegia with myopathy)

LHON (Leber hereditary optic neuropathy; Leber optic atrophy)

MELAS (mitochondrial myopathy, encephalopathy, lactic acidosis and stroke-like episodes)

MERRF (myoclonic epilepsy associated with ragged-red fibres)

Pearson marrow/pancreas syndrome (pancytopenia, lactic acidosis and exocrine pancreatic insufficiency)

normal and some affected mitochondrial chromosomes in each mitochondrion is common in mitochondrial disorders and, as cells and tissues can accumulate variable proportions of mutant and normal mitochondrial DNAs through subsequent cell divisions, this can result in a wide phenotypic range in a single family. The process of replicative segregation of mitochondrial DNA tends to cause cells to drift towards having all mutant or all normal mitochondrial DNA (homoplasmy). The high mutation rate for mitochondrial DNA means that the presence of somatic mutations is normally associated with ageing and may be responsible for its somatic effects. In addition, the high mutation rate can contribute to disease expression in a patient with inherited heteroplasmy for a mitochondrial mutation.

Mitochondria are important for energy production, and different tissues vary in the extent to which they rely on this process. The central nervous system, heart, skeletal muscle, kidney and endocrine glands are particularly reliant and hence are the main organs and tissues that are involved in mitochondrial diseases (Table 10.11). At least 59 mitochondrial diseases have been identified and all are rare. An example is Leber hereditary optic neuropathy (LHON). In this condition, there is acute or subacute visual loss at any age but most commonly in the second or third decade. Loss of central vision is usually progressive and bilateral. In addition, cardiac conduction defects may also occur. The condition displays mitochondrial inheritance and specific mutations can be detected in the mitochondrial DNA in the genes encoding subunits of the respiratory chain complex I. In about 95% of patients with LHON, one of three specific point mutations can be found in the mitochondrial DNA. Patients are usually homoplasmic for these mutations, but not all individuals with the mutations develop symptoms. The most important factors affecting penetrance are gender and age. Thus, the lifetime risks of developing symptoms in homoplasmic carriers are around 40% in males and 10% in females and the penetrance is age dependent. In addition, there is a role for as yet unidentified environmental factors.

Many proteins of mitochondria are encoded not by mitochondrial DNA but by nuclear genes. There is, therefore, increasing recognition of mitochondrial disorders that result from inherited mutations within the nuclear genome, with inheritance being autosomal or X-linked rather than mitochondrial. An example of this is the generally autosomal recessive fatal infantile cardioencephalomyopathy (with hypertrophic cardiomyopathy and lactic acidosis) due to deficiency of cytochrome *c* oxidase (complex IV), which represents the terminal enzyme of the respiratory chain. Particularly interesting is a condition causing weakness of the external eye muscles with adult onset, known as progressive external ophthalmoplegia, which can result from mitochondrial DNA deletions. Remarkably, this condition can actually be inherited in an autosomal dominant fashion. This is because the mitochondrial DNA deletions themselves can result from an abnormality in the *nuclear* gene (*POLG*) that encodes the catalytic unit of polymerase γ, the enzyme complex that is responsible for mitochondrial DNA replication (see Hudson and Chinnery, 2006, in Further reading).

Finally, the interesting possibility that some mitochondrial DNA deletions (particularly those that occur somatically) may originate during repair of mitochondrial DNA rather than during its replication has been suggested by Krishnan *et al.* (2008; see Further reading).

SUMMARY

- Multifactorial inheritance implies a contribution of both genetic and environmental factors.
- Twin concordance and family correlation studies can provide support for the multifactorial inheritance of a trait. The observed frequencies in relatives provide the empiric risks upon which genetic counselling for multifactorial disorders is based.
- Multifactorial traits that are continuous (such as height) have a continuously graded distribution, while those that are discontinuous (i.e. with individuals being either affected or unaffected) are present only when a certain threshold of genetic factors is reached.

- For twins, placental membranes that are monochorionic indicate monozygosity, whereas dichorionic membranes represent either monozygous or dizygous twins. Zygosity is determined most reliably by DNA fingerprinting.
- Monozygotic twins are identical genetically (i.e. at the DNA level), whereas dizygotic twins exhibit the same degree of genetic similarity as siblings.
- Genome-wide analyses of the genetic determinants of multifactorial traits may now be undertaken by association studies of the frequencies of each of hundreds of thousands of SNPs in cases and controls.

- Cancers generally develop through the accumulation of somatic cell genetic alterations. In addition, in familial cases, a strongly predisposing cancer gene alteration may have been inherited from a parent.
- Mitochondrial disorders due to mitochondrial DNA abnormalities are maternally inherited with transmission to all of the children of an affected mother but to none of those of an affected father. A few mitochondrial disorders are, however, now known to result from mutations in the nuclear DNA.

FURTHER READING

Barnholtz-Sloan JS, Shetty PB, Guan X, Nyante SJ, Luo J, Brennan DJ, Millikan RC (2010) *FGFR2* and other loci identified in genome-wide association studies are associated with breast cancer in african american and younger women. *Carcinogenesis* **31**:1417–23.

Frayling TM (2007) Genome-wide association studies provide new insights into type 2 diabetes aetiology. *Nat Rev Genet* **8**: 657–62.

Hudson G, Chinnery PF (2006) Mitochondrial DNA polymerase-γ and human disease. *Hum Mol Genet* **15** (Review issue 2):R244–52.

Humphries SE, Drenos F, Ken-Dror G, Talmud PJ (2010) Coronary heart disease risk prediction in the era of genome-wide association studies: current status and what the future holds. *Circulation* **121**:2235–48.

Hunter DJ, Kraft P (2007) Drinking from the fire hose – statistical issues in genome-wide association studies. *N Engl J Med* **357**:436–9.

Ikegawa S (2007) New gene associations in osteoarthritis: what do they provide, and where are we going? *Curr Opin Rheumatol* **19**:429–34.

Jin Y, Birlea SA, Fain PR, Mailloux CM, Riccardi SL, Gowan K, Holland PJ, Bennett DC, Wallace MR, *et al.* (2010) Common variants in FOXP1 are associated with generalized vitiligo. *Nat Genet* **42**:576–8.

Krishnan KJ, Reeve AK, Samuels DC, Chinnery PF, Blackwood JK, Taylor RW, Wanrooij S, Spelbrink JN, Lightowlers RN, Turnbull DM (2008) What causes mitochondrial DNA deletions in human cells? *Nat Genet* **40**:275–9.

Plant D, Flynn E, Mbarek H, Dieudé P, Cornelis F, Arlestig L, Dahlqvist SR, Goulielmos G, Boumpas DT, *et al* (2010) Investigation of potential non-HLA rheumatoid arthritis susceptibility loci in a European cohort increases the evidence for nine markers. *Ann Rheum Dis* **69**:1548–53.

Steele MP, Brown KK (2007) Genetic predisposition to respiratory diseases: infiltrative lung diseases. *Respiration* **74**:601–8.

Wellcome Trust Case Control Consortium (2007) Genome-wide association study of 14,000 cases of seven common diseases and 3,000 shared controls. *Nature* **447**:661–78.

Self-assessment

1. Which of the following are multifactorial discontinuous traits?
A. Cystic fibrosis
B. Blood pressure
C. Weight
D. Diabetes mellitus
E. Head circumference

2. Which of the following are examples of human multifactorial continuous traits?
A. Intelligence
B. Red blood cell volume
C. Cleft lip
D. Neural tube defect
E. Height

3. Which of the following are true of twinning?
A. Monozygous twins have a single chorion in over 95% of cases
B. The proportion of genes shared on average by dizygous twins is the same as that for siblings
C. Dizygotic twins result from a single ovum fertilised by two spermatozoa
D. Monozygotic twins arise from a single zygote that divides into two embryos prior to the formation of the primitive streak
E. The diagnosis of zygosity can be undertaken by the analysis of highly polymorphic DNA markers by DNA fingerprinting

4. For which of the following conditions is autosomal inheritance observed?
A. Fatal infantile cardioencephalomyopathy
B. Leber hereditary optic neuropathy (LHON)
C. MELAS
D. MERRF
E. Progressive external ophthalmoplegia

5. What proportion of genes (or alleles) do first cousins have in common, on average?
A. 50%
B. 33%
C. 25%
D. 12.5%
E. 6.7%

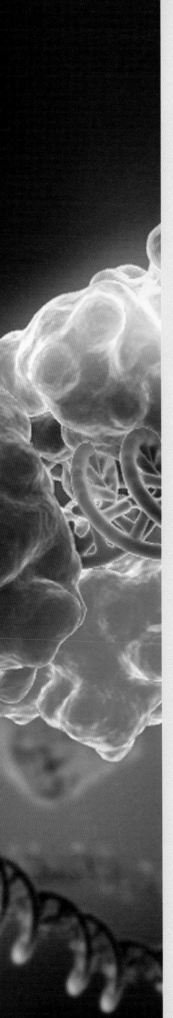

CHAPTER 11

Medical genetics in populations

Key Topics

Introduction

In contrast to the previous chapters, which focused on the different types of genetic diseases at the level of the affected family, this chapter will primarily consider the factors that can influence the population frequencies of genetic disease, as well as the uses of DNA markers in the analysis of human evolution and population migration. The prevalence of a genetic disorder is the number of patients with the condition per 1000 of a defined population at any point in time (e.g. 10 per 1000 births affected), whereas the incidence of a genetic disease is the number of new patients with the condition per 1000 of a defined population in a defined time period (e.g. 10 new patients affected per 1000 adults per annum).

Most information to date on population genetics has related to single-gene disorders, which collectively have a birth prevalence of about 20–30 per 1000 (excluding colour blindness). The population prevalence of individual single-gene disorders may be influenced by three main factors: selection, a founder effect and any alteration to the mutation rate. Other factors that can also play a role are genetic drift (in small populations) and population migration (where the incoming migrants possess different allele frequencies).

Essential Medical Genetics, 6th edition. © Edward S. Tobias, Michael Connor and Malcolm Ferguson-Smith.
Published 2011 by Blackwell Published Ltd.

Selection for single-gene disorders

Prior to Darwin, the different species were held to have been fixed since their outright creation. Darwin challenged this view by showing that traits favoured by the environment tended to increase in frequency, as the favoured animals were more successful at reproduction. Conversely, deleterious traits hindered reproduction and thus fell in frequency. This natural selection operates on the phenotype, which in turn is determined by the genotype, and evolution is simply a change in gene frequencies as a result of selection, with genetic variation thus being a prerequisite for evolution.

Selection is a powerful means of altering gene frequencies for single-gene disorders and it can operate to reduce (by negative selection) or increase (by positive selection) a particular phenotype and hence its genotype. Selection acts on the individual phenotypes and either favours or hinders reproduction and hence the propagation of that individual's genotype. Many populations tend to increase in size over time, but without disturbing factors, such as selection, the relative gene frequencies tend to remain constant. This can be demonstrated mathematically (the Hardy–Weinberg equilibrium; see Appendix 3). With negative selection, the relative frequency of the condition and its gene frequency will decrease, and, conversely, with positive selection, it will increase (Fig. 11.1).

Sickle-cell disease, for example, is inherited as an autosomal recessive trait and, although the carrier parents are asymptomatic, the affected offspring have severe chronic anaemia and

Fig. 11.1 Effect of selection on the frequency of a condition within a population.

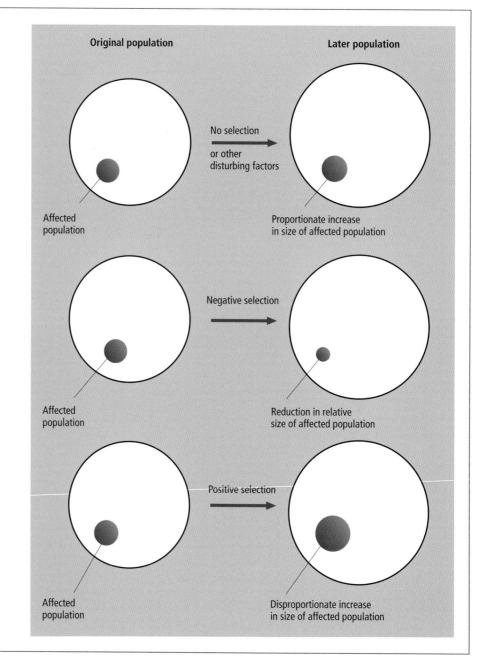

Original population

Later population

No selection or other disturbing factors

Affected population

Proportionate increase in size of affected population

Negative selection

Affected population

Reduction in relative size of affected population

Positive selection

Affected population

Disproportionate increase in size of affected population

in many parts of the world often die before adulthood (and reproduction). With such an effect on the affected homozygote, the birth frequency of carriers would be expected to be low, yet in equatorial Africa, the birth frequency of affected individuals is 1 in 40, and 1 in 3 of the population carry the mutant gene. This high gene frequency has arisen due to a selective advantage for the mutant gene carriers with respect to malaria due to *Plasmodium falciparum*. This is a major cause of death in equatorial Africa and sickle-cell heterozygotes are at an advantage in that their infected red cells undergo more rapid clearance with a better chance of recovery from the malarial infection. This selective advantage no longer operates in regions where malaria has been eradicated and removal of the selective pressure results in a fall in the gene frequency. Thus, the sickle-cell gene frequency has fallen from about 1 in 3 to 1 in 10 in the descendants of black Africans who were transported to America some ten generations ago. Selection for a particular allele also influences the allele frequencies at adjacent closely linked loci due to linkage disequilibrium. This refers to the presence of two or more closely located markers or alleles *together* more often (in a population) than would be predicted by chance.

A selective advantage with respect to malarial infection also operates for heterozygotes for β-thalassaemia (Chapter 17) and glucose-6-phosphate dehydrogenase deficiency, and, as a consequence, these conditions are also prevalent in regions where malaria is (or was) common. A heterozygote advantage is also evident for carriers of congenital adrenal hyperplasia with respect to *Haemophilus influenzae* type B infection, but for the majority of conditions where a natural selective pressure is (or was) operating, its basis is as yet unknown.

Most serious genetic conditions tend to hamper reproduction and so produce negative selection. Advances in treatment can reverse this disadvantage, with the frequency of the condition then rising to a new equilibrium. The rate of change depends on the mode of inheritance. For an autosomal dominant trait where reproduction was previously impossible, restoration to normality would double the frequency of the disorder in a single generation, whereas for an X-linked recessive trait, doubling of the birth frequency would take about four generations. For an autosomal recessive trait, it would take about 50 generations, as most of the mutant alleles in the population would be present in carriers whose reproductive fitness would be unchanged by the availability of treatment. Similarly, enforced eugenic programmes (such as those that led to horrific practices by the Nazis in the mid-20th century) *preventing* reproduction of affected individuals would take similar lengths of time to effect comparable reductions in disease frequencies.

Founder effect and genetic drift for single-gene disorders

For disease-related, religious, geographical or other reasons, a small group of individuals may survive or become genetically

Table 11.1 Examples of genetic isolates with relatively high frequencies of certain single-gene disorders

Isolate	Disorder
Cuna Indians of Panama	Albinism
Hopi Indians	Albinism
Finns	Congenital nephrotic syndrome
Afrikaners	Variegate porphyria, familial hypercholesterolaemia
Old Order Amish of Pennsylvania	Ellis–van Creveld syndrome

isolated from the rest of the population (a genetic isolate), with subsequent expansion of the isolated group after this '*population bottleneck*'.

A founder member of the group may have mutant alleles for some autosomal traits (recessive or late-onset dominant) and so within the population these genes are automatically at a higher frequency than within the general population (Table 11.1). The Afrikaners who settled in South Africa in the 17th century provide several striking examples of this *founder effect*. Thus, for example, in variegate porphyria, which is inherited as an autosomal dominant trait, many current gene carriers are direct descendants of one couple who emigrated from Holland in the 1680s. As a consequence, all will share the same mutation, and a narrow range of causative mutations is thus a characteristic of the founder effect. In addition, it is believed that as a result of a founder, the rare disorder, Ellis–van Creveld syndrome (with extra digits or polydactyly, congenital heart disease and short stature) became unusually frequent in the Old Order Amish community of Pennsylvania. Indeed, it has now been demonstrated from genealogical and molecular studies of the gene copy containing the responsible mutation that the mutant alleles present in all of the affected individuals in that population have a common ancestor. The latter is thought to be one of the original founders of this population who immigrated into the USA in the mid-18th century.

In addition to the founder effect, fluctuations in the frequency of particular genetic disorders can also change by *genetic drift*. This term describes the changes in population gene frequencies that occur on account of random differences, from one generation to the next, in the frequency of transmission of particular alleles. i.e. chance effects of Mendelian segregation. Such fluctuations, usually relatively small, tend to have greater effects in small populations. This is analogous to the greater deviation from the expected 50:50 (heads:tails) ratio that one may observe if a coin is tossed ten times, compared with the deviation that one observes if the coin is tossed 100 times. In practice, it is found that genetic drift generally causes rapid significant differences in disease frequencies only when the reproductive population size is less than 100 individuals.

Table 11.2 Equations for prediction of birth frequency of single-gene disorders

Autosomal dominant disorders	Birth frequency = $2\mu/(1 - f)$
Autosomal recessive disorders	Birth frequency = $\mu/(1 - f)$
X-linked recessive disorders	Birth frequency = $3\mu/(1 - f)$

Altered mutation rate for single-gene disorders

The mutation rate (μ) is usually expressed as an incidence giving the number of mutations at a locus per million gametes produced per generation. The mutant gene frequency reflects the balance between the introduction of new mutant genes to the population and the loss of mutant genes from the population when an affected individual fails to reproduce. If there is no impairment of reproductive capacity, then the biological fitness (f) is normal (1 or 100%), whereas if reproduction is impossible, the biological fitness is zero. The impact of changes in the mutation rate on the frequency of a single-gene disorder depends upon the mode of inheritance (Table 11.2).

If the condition precludes reproduction ($f = 0$), then the respective birth frequencies for autosomal dominant, autosomal recessive and X-linked recessive conditions can be calculated to be 2μ, μ and 3μ. Hence, any change in the mutation rate will have most effect on an X-linked recessive trait and least on an autosomal recessive trait. The risk of a new mutation for several autosomal dominant traits and for some X-linked recessive traits has been shown to be increased with increasing paternal age and is increased by exposure to mutagenic chemicals. Mutation rates are difficult to determine and most information relates to autosomal dominant traits and X-linked recessive traits with estimates of 1–100 (average 10–20) mutations per million gametes per generation for different loci.

Linkage analysis and the International HapMap Project

Pedigree pattern analysis may confirm that a disorder is inherited as an autosomal or sex-linked trait. In such disorders, when the causative gene has not been identified, the next investigative step is to map the gene locus to a chromosomal region. For single-gene disorders with unknown pathophysiology, this mapping is usually accomplished by family linkage studies to detect cosegregation of a trait with genomic markers of known location. This is often followed by mutation screening of candidate genes that are known from current human genome databases to be located within the defined linked chromosomal region.

In practice, it is difficult to detect linkages using marker loci more than about 25 Mb apart and thus a linkage search of the genome (3280 Mb) requires at least 131 (3280/25) well-spaced polymorphic markers. Fortunately, great advances have

been made in identifying markers that can be used for such analyses. Over 5000 highly polymorphic microsatellite (AC/TG)$_n$ DNA markers were identified and mapped in 1996 (facilitating the subsequent mapping of many undiscovered disease genes using individual families). In addition, several million single-nucleotide polymorphisms (SNPs) have since been identified (http://www.ncbi.nlm.nih.gov/projects/SNP/), thus providing a high density of markers for almost every region of each chromosome. Moreover, as described below, this very high density of identified polymorphisms across the genome has also permitted the identification of many individual gene variants that are associated with susceptibility to various multifactorial diseases, often by studies using very large numbers of cases and controls. SNPs are more useful for genome-wide disease association studies than microsatellite markers because of their high abundance, low mutation rate and the ease of high-throughput SNP genotyping.

In addition, if loci are very close together, then recombination between them is highly unlikely and alleles at such loci will pass together through the family. Such a tract of closely linked alleles is known as a haplotype. On account of linkage disequilibrium, haplotype analysis can be clinically useful in an affected family in which a causative mutation has not yet been identified by predicting the presence or absence of an alteration in a closely associated disease gene. Linkage disequilibrium reflects the background pattern of adjacent DNA markers at the time the original mutation occurred: due to their proximity to the gene and hence lack of intervening recombination, adjacent markers will tend to remain in association as a mutation-specific haplotype. Analysis of specific adjacent marker sequences may therefore serve as a useful indirect means of tracking the gene in question in a particular family.

The International HapMap Project (http://www.hapmap.org) was initiated in October 2002 in order to compare the DNA sequences of different individuals and thus identify regions of similarity in which the genetic variants are shared between individuals. The individuals studied were from four different populations around the world, with African ancestry (in Nigeria), Asian ancestry (in Beijing and in Tokyo) and European ancestry (in the USA). The first phase of the project, completed in 2005, provided data on 1.3 million SNPs, while the second phase, completed in 2007, brought the total number of catalogued SNPs to 3.1 million. There are now over 4 million identified SNPs. The millions of SNP variants together partially account for the 0.1% of the human genome that differs between individuals (also see the website of the SNP-cataloguing 1000 Genomes Project).

Interestingly, as a result of the recombination sites having been at specific regions, rather than evenly distributed throughout the genome, sequence variation within the modern human genome tends to be present in discrete 'haplotype blocks' within which there is high linkage disequilibrium. An important aspect of the HapMap Project, therefore, has been the detection of haplotypes not only by extensive analysis of SNPs, but also by the identification of so-called 'tag' SNPs that can

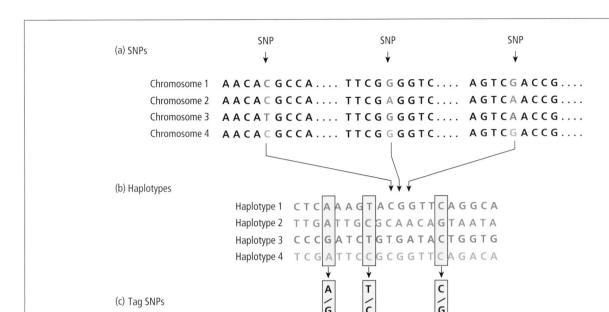

Fig. 11.2 The identification of various haplotypes and the so-called 'tag' SNPs that are selected to represent them uniquely, by the International HapMap Project. In (a), the individual SNPs are shown in colour to differentiate them from the surrounding non-variant chromosomal DNA sequences. These SNPs, together with other surrounding SNPs, can then be grouped and examined as haplotypes, shown in (b). From these haplotypes, individual tag SNPs (c) can then be chosen that can be used to represent the individual haplotypes, their presence or absence thus predicting the surrounding SNP genotypes. Redrawn, with modifications, from International HapMap Consortium (2003) Nature 426:789–796.

be used to uniquely represent each of the haplotype blocks thus detected (see Fig. 11.2 and the illustrated review by Kruglyak, 2008). The analysis of multiple SNPs has also allowed regions of linkage disequilibrium to be defined with higher resolution than previously, and to be displayed automatically online by computers at different levels of magnification (Fig. 11.3). As mentioned above, the information has already enormously facilitated genome-wide association studies, permitting the recent successful identification of gene variants that are associated with several multifactorial common diseases, such as coronary artery disease, type 2 diabetes and rheumatoid arthritis (see Humphries *et al.*, 2010, and Plant *et al.*, 2010, in Further reading, for example). The genetic variants responsible for some multifactorial conditions such as schizophrenia and bipolar disorder have, however, proved far more elusive (see review by Porteous, 2008, in Further reading). In fact, individual alleles can influence one's susceptibility to two or more conditions. For instance, a *TCF2* gene variant that is associated with a reduced susceptibility to type 2 diabetes also confers an increased risk of prostate cancer, perhaps on account of an altered potential for cell degeneration or proliferation (see Gudmundsson *et al.*, 2007, in Further reading).

Human population evolution and migration

As fossil evidence is scarce and often incomplete, an exciting development is the use of polymorphic mitochondrial and Y

chromosome DNA markers to analyse the recent evolution and subsequent migration of human populations. Mitochondrial DNA (mtDNA) is particularly useful as it is non-recombining and is directly inherited through the maternal line (see Chapter 10). Non-recombining Y chromosome sequences, which are inherited through the paternal lineage, have been similarly used. The analysis of such sequences has now been carried out on DNA samples from many modern human populations worldwide. This has permitted 'phylogenetic' trees to be constructed that show the deduced ancestral relationships between different populations. When such data are combined with the calculated mutation rates for the studied sequences, the timing of early events within human pre-history can be estimated. In addition, by taking into account the known geographical distribution of the lineages or populations within the phylogenetic tree or network (generating so-called 'phylogeography'), the past movements of humans between regions can be estimated (see Fig. 11.4). A large privately funded study (the Genographic Project) is currently underway to investigate these population movements from DNA evidence in much greater detail using DNA samples that are being collected from up to 100,000 indigenous people throughout the world (see Behar *et al.*, 2007, in Further reading and the Genographic Project website).

Hundreds of complete mtDNA genome sequences are now available. Such studies of mtDNA from modern human (*Homo sapiens sapiens*) samples from native populations have provided support for the Recent African Origin model of human

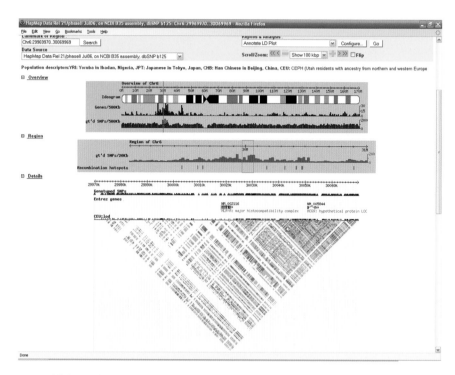

Fig. 11.3 Computer-generated linkage disequilibrium (LD) plot for a 100 kb region of chromosome 6 that contains the HLA-A major histocompatibility gene from the HapMap database (at http://www.hapmap.org). An area of strong linkage disequilibrium can be seen as a dense red triangle in the lower panel that corresponds to a region of approximately 14 kb of chromosome 6, located about 30 Mb from the end of the short arm. International HapMap Consortium (2003) Nature 426:789–796.

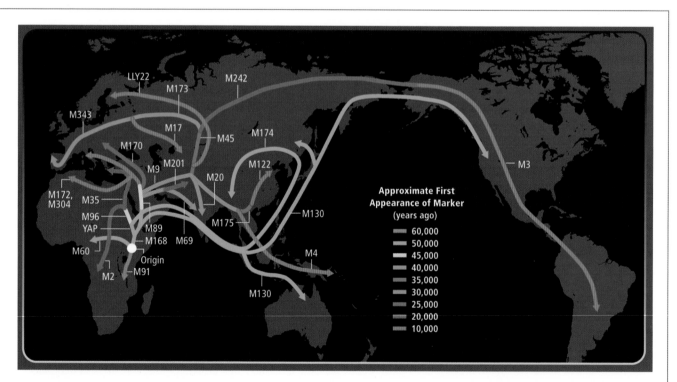

Fig. 11.4 Human migration paths deduced from the analysis of variation at individual Y chromosomal DNA markers in a large number of living individuals. Each marker is numbered (e.g. M343) and can be used to track individual male lineages. The approximate ages of the lineages and where they first appeared are represented by different colours. Reprinted from Stix, 2008 (see Further Reading), with permission from Nature Publishing Group.

evolution. This refers to the hypothesised relatively recent colonisation of the world by modern humans who evolved from *Homo erectus* in sub-Saharan Africa and then, beginning between 50 and 60 thousand years ago, migrated through the rest of the world. *Homo erectus* itself first appeared around 1.8 million years ago. This 'Out-of-Africa' uniregional model (see Fig. 11.5) differs from an earlier Multiregional model (involving the evolution of *Homo sapiens* from *Homo erectus* in several different regions of the world, independently), which has now become less popular. The studies are limited to some extent by the finite longevity of DNA itself, resulting, for instance, in extreme difficulty in extracting mtDNA from *Homo erectus* specimens, and by variations in mutation rates. The Out-of-Africa model has also now been supported by analysis of Y chromosome markers, by recent whole-genome SNP analyses and even by DNA analyses of microorganisms such as *Helicobacter pylori* bacteria carried by migrating humans. The result of this migration is that genetic diversity is now much greater in native Africans than in distantly migrated populations such as Native Americans. This is because at each stage of the migration only a subgroup broke away from the established population, taking with it only a fraction of the existing genetic diversity.

It has, however, been possible to obtain sufficient nuclear and mtDNA from the bones of Neanderthal specimens to permit genetic analysis. In fact, the latest sequencing methods have recently permitted the determination of the entire mtDNA sequence of a 38,000-year-old Neanderthal specimen (see Clark, 2008, in Further reading). When compared with the DNA sequences of modern humans, the differences were found to be so significant that they suggested that Neanderthals evolved separately (diverging around 660,000±140,000 years ago from the lineage that led to modern humans) and it is believed that they became extinct around 30,000 years ago without having contributed any mitochondrial or Y chromosome DNA to us. The extent of the sequence difference between modern humans and Neanderthals is, in fact, as great as around one-half of that which has been found between us and chimpanzees, a lineage from which we diverged around 6.5 million years ago.

Working backwards through evolution to a common ancestor can be achieved by a technique known as coalescence analysis. The most recent common ancestor (MRCA) for the mtDNA of all the sampled individuals, the 'mitochondrial Eve', has been estimated to have lived around 171,000 years ago in East Africa (see Clark, 2008, in Further reading). This individual, possessing a new genetic alteration in her mtDNA, would have been born among a group of modern humans, a new species (*Homo sapiens*), that had split off from the existing *Homo erectus* in Africa around this time. Similarly, the MRCA of the Y chromosome sequences (the 'Y chromosome Adam') can be determined. In general, calculated MRCAs differ according to which genomic loci are undergoing coalescence

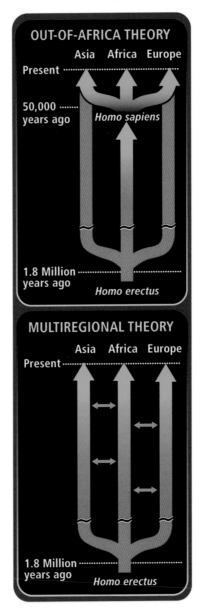

Fig. 11.5 The Out-of-Africa theory has now largely replaced the Multiregional theory as a model of the way in which the world was colonised by modern humans. The Out-of-Africa theory proposes that *Homo sapiens* originated in Africa and then, beginning around 60,000 years ago, migrated out of Africa, replacing earlier hominids such as *Homo erectus*, which had colonised other parts of the world from 1.8 million years ago. Reprinted from Stix, 2008 (see Further Reading), with permission from Nature Publishing Group.

analysis. It is likely, of course, that other individuals will have existed at those times, without transmitting their DNA to any of the present population, i.e. their lineages did not survive.

SUMMARY

- Three important factors that can influence the prevalence of individual single-gene disorders are: selection, a founder effect and mutation rate alteration.
- A founder effect (with a restricted range of causative mutations) results from the possession of one or more mutant alleles by an original 'founder' member of a genetically isolated group of individuals. Disease gene frequencies can also change rapidly in very small populations as a result of genetic drift, i.e. skewed Mendelian segregation.
- The existence of strong linkage disequilibrium between closely linked alleles (as in haplotypes) permits indirect mutation tracking by analysis of adjacent polymorphic markers when the mutation in a specific gene has not yet been identified.
- The detection of millions of SNPs has facilitated large genome-wide association studies, leading to the identification of gene variants that are associated with several multifactorial diseases.
- The study of recent human evolution and population migration has been facilitated by the analysis of mitochondrial and non-recombining Y chromosome DNA sequences, which are inherited directly through the maternal and paternal lineages, respectively.
- Such studies have generally supported the 'Out-of-Africa' model by which modern humans evolved from *Homo erectus* in sub-Saharan Africa and then (beginning around 50,000–60,000 years ago) migrated throughout the rest of the world, eventually replacing *Homo erectus* worldwide.
- Coalescence analysis is a technique that, by working backwards through evolution, allows the estimation of the most recent common ancestor (MRCA) for a population group.

FURTHER READING

Behar Dm, Rosset S, Blue-Smith J, Balanovsky O, Tzur S, Comas D, Mitchell RJ, Quintana-Murci L, Tyler-Smith C, *et al.* (2007) The Genographic Project Public Participation Mitochondrial DNA Database. *PLoS Genet* **3**:e104.

Clark AG (2008) Genome sequences from extinct relatives. *Cell* **134**:388–9.

Gudmundsson J, Sulem P, Steinthorsdottir V, Bergthorsson JT, Thorleifsson G, Manolescu A, Rafnar T, Gudbjartsson D, Agnarsson BA, *et al.* (2007) Two variants on chromosome 17 confer prostate cancer risk, and the one in TCF2 protects against type 2 diabetes. *Nat Genet* **39**:977–83.

Humphries SE, Drenos F, Ken-Dror G, Talmud PJ (2010) Coronary heart disease risk prediction in the era of genome-wide association studies: current status and what the future holds. *Circulation* **121**:2235–48.

Kruglyak L (2008) The road to genome-wide association studies. *Nat Rev Genet* **9**:314–8.

Plant D, Flynn E, Mbarek H, Dieudé P, Cornelis F, Arlestig L, Dahlqvist SR, Goulielmos G, Boumpas DT, *et al.* (2010) Investigation of potential non-HLA rheumatoid arthritis susceptibility loci in a European cohort increases the evidence for nine markers. *Ann Rheum Dis* **69**:1548–63.

Porteous D (2008) Genetic causality in schizophrenia and bipolar disorder: out with the old and in with the new. *Curr Opin Genet Dev* **18**:229–34.

Stix G (2008) Traces of a distant past. *Scientific American* **299**(1):56–63. [A highly readable, well-illustrated and entertaining description of the study of human migration.]

Strachan T, Read AP (2011) *Human Molecular Genetics*, 4th edn. Garland Science: London.

WEBSITES

1000 Genomes Project:
http://www.1000genomes.org/

International HapMap Project:
http://www.hapmap.org/

Genographic Project:
https://genographic.nationalgeographic.com/genographic/index.html

NCBI SNP database homepage:
http://www.ncbi.nlm.nih.gov/projects/SNP/

Wellcome Trust Sanger Institute web site for human genetics and bioinformatics:
http://www.sanger.ac.uk/

US Department of Energy Human Genome Project Information:
http://www.ornl.gov/sci/techresources/Human_Genome/home.shtml

Self-assessment

1. Which of the following are factors that significantly alter the prevalence of an individual single-gene disorder in a population?
A. Selection
B. A founder effect
C. A change in the mutation rate
D. An increase in size of the population
E. A change in the effect of the disorder on fertility

2. Which of the following are correct with regard to single-nucleotide polymorphisms (SNPs)?
A. They may affect the level of gene expression
B. They can affect the amino acid sequence of the protein
C. They almost always vary independently of each other
D. They may facilitate genome-wide association studies
E. They may have no detectable effect on a gene's function

3. Analyses of polymorphic markers are particularly useful in the analysis of:
A. Population migration
B. Determination of the precise location of a rare high-penetrance pathogenic mutation within the *FGFR3* gene
C. Human evolution
D. Distribution of regions of linkage disequilibrium along a chromosome
E. Genes associated with type 2 diabetes

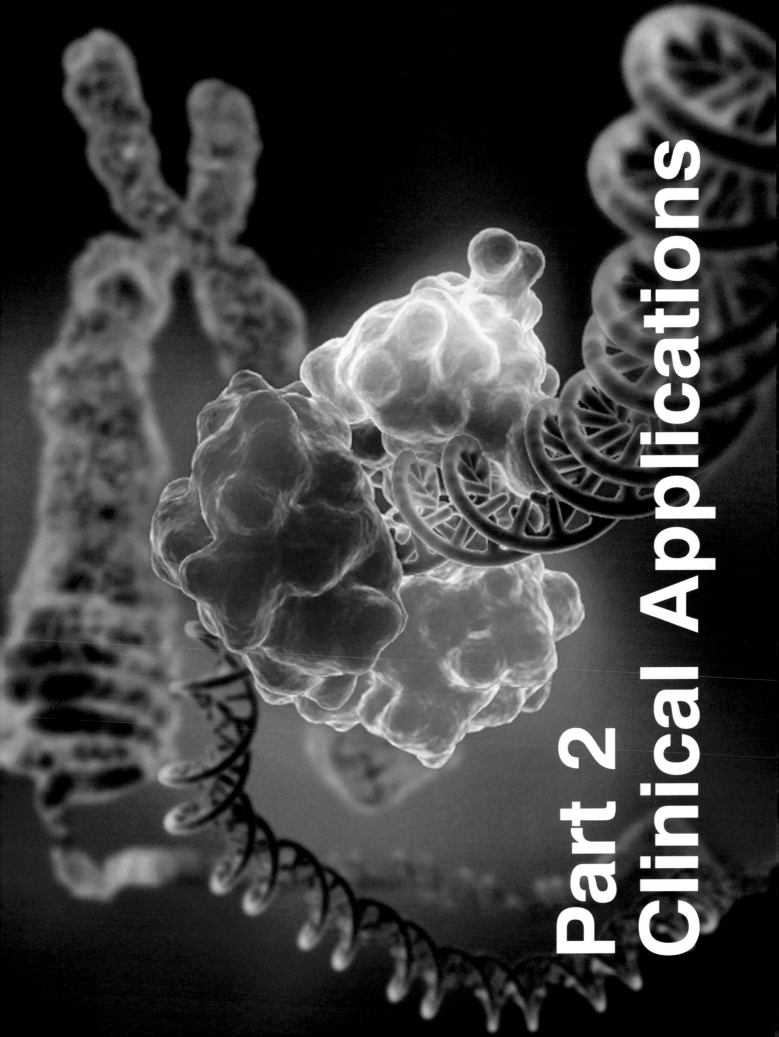

Part 2
Clinical Applications

CHAPTER 12

Genetic assessment, genetic counselling and reproductive options

Key Topics

Introduction

Genetic counselling is the provision of appropriate information and advice about inherited conditions in order to allow informed reproductive choices to be made. In this chapter, the way in which, in the clinic, the relevant genetic information is obtained, recorded and interpreted is described, together with important aspects of genetic counselling. In addition, the various types of invasive and non-invasive techniques for prenatal diagnosis are discussed. These techniques include not only chorionic villus sampling (CVS), amniocentesis and ultrasound scanning but also preimplantation genetic diagnosis and the more recently developed technique of cell-free nucleic acid detection.

Essential Medical Genetics, 6th edition. © Edward S. Tobias, Michael Connor and Malcolm Ferguson-Smith.
Published 2011 by Blackwell Published Ltd.

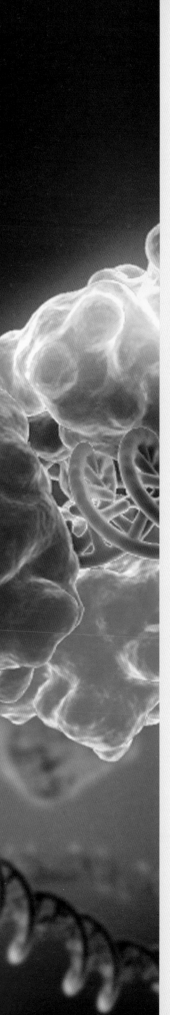

Communication of advice

Genetic counselling is the communication of information and advice about inherited conditions, and a person seeking such advice is called a consultand. This process includes history and pedigree construction, examination, diagnosis, counselling and follow-up.

History and pedigree construction

The affected individual who caused the consultand(s) to seek advice is called the proband. Often the proband is a child, but he or she may also be the consultand or a more distant relative. A standard medical history is required for the proband and for any other affected persons in the family.

Next the pedigree is constructed. A standardised set of symbols is used (Fig. 12.1). The father is conventionally placed on the left, and all members of the same generation are placed on the same horizontal level. Roman numerals are used for each generation, starting with the earliest, and Arabic numerals are used to indicate each individual within a generation (num-

bering from the left). Thus, in Fig. 12.2, III:4 is the proband, and his parents who are seeking advice are II:5 and II:6. When drawing a pedigree, it is advisable to start near the bottom of the page with the most recent generation and work upwards. The offspring of each set of parents are given in birth order with the eldest on the left. For each member of the pedigree, name and age are included. For an extended family study, the full name, age, address and phone number for individuals who need to be contacted should also be recorded. Miscarriages, neonatal deaths, handicapped or malformed children, and parental consanguinity might not be mentioned unless specifically asked about. Enquiries should be made about both sides of the family (not just the side from which the proband's medical condition appears to have been inherited) in order to reveal any additional genetic condition that may be inherited separately within the same family, the existence of which may not have been appreciated previously by the consultand. Finally, as mentioned below, it may be necessary to confirm the diagnosis that affected a relative (particularly for deceased individuals in previous generations) or to ascertain the nature of the condition more precisely.

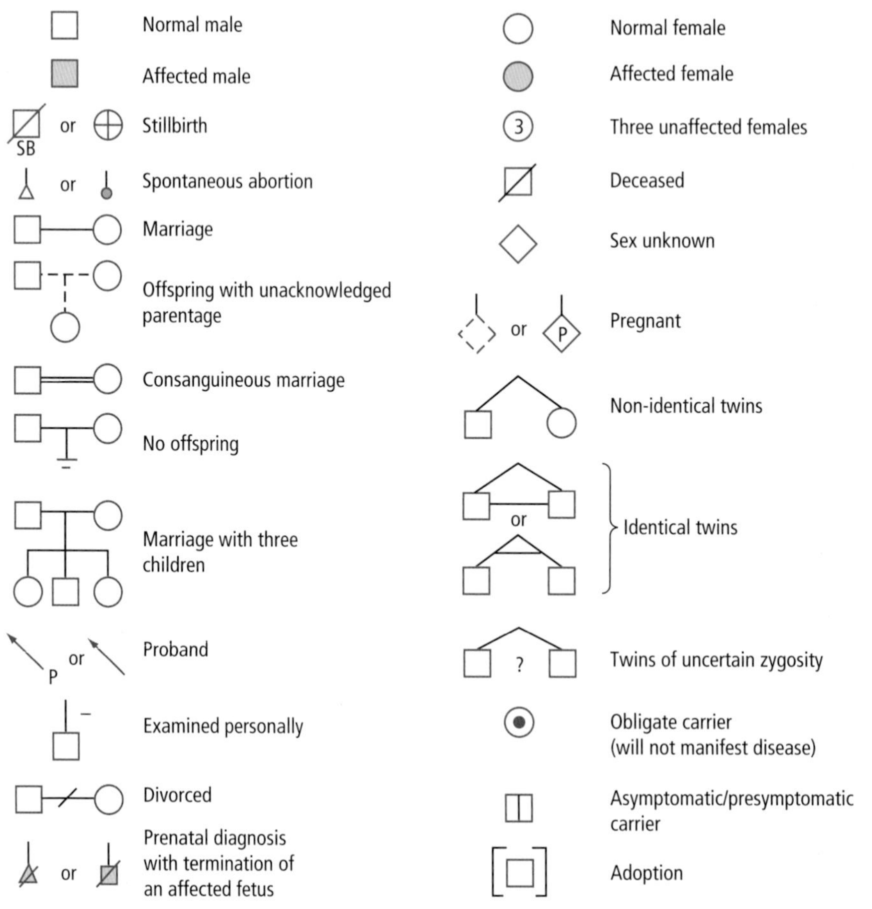

Fig. 12.1 Symbols used in pedigree construction.

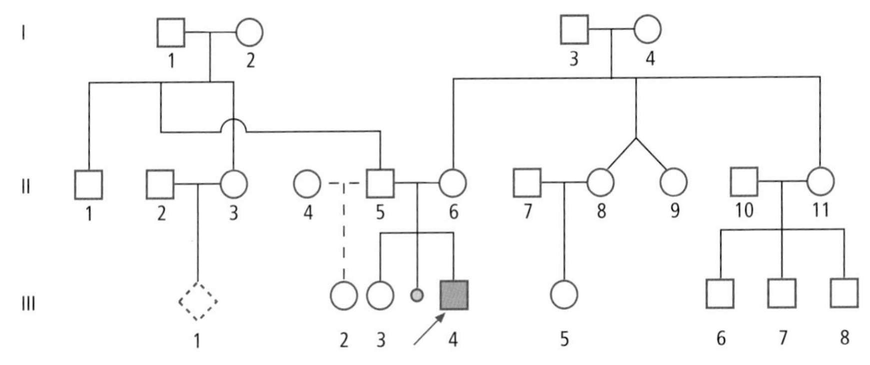

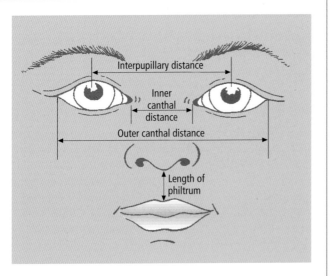

Fig. 12.2 Example of a family pedigree.

Fig. 12.3 Facial landmarks.

Clinical examination

A complete physical examination of the proband is desirable. This examination differs from a routine one, however, in that there is often a need to describe dysmorphic features accurately. A dysmorphic feature is, by definition, some characteristic that is outside the range seen in normal individuals. Table 12.1 and Fig. 12.3 give examples of the terms used for the description of dysmorphic features.

Clinical impressions can be misleading, so it is important to make accurate measurements to confirm features such as widely spaced eyes or disproportionate short stature. Table 12.2 lists some commonly used measurements in this context. The normal ranges of each will vary with age and sex and are provided in standard dysmorphology texts (see Hall *et al.*, 2006, in Further reading). Normally each measurement is close to the same percentile. If not, then the unusual measurements reflect an abnormality. For example, if height and head circumference are on the 10th percentile but interpupillary distance is on the 90th percentile, then relative hypertelorism is present,

Table 12.1 Descriptive terms used in dysmorphology	
Term	**Meaning**
Hypertelorism	Interpupillary distance above expected
Hypotelorism	Interpupillary distance below expected
Telecanthus	Inner canthal distance above expected yet interpupillary distance not increased
Low set ears	Upper border of ear attachment below intercanthal line with head upright
Upslanting palpebral fissures	Outer canthi above inner canthi
Downslanting palpebral fissures	Inner canthi above outer canthi
Brushfield spots	Speckled iris ring (20% of normal babies)
Simian crease	Single transverse palmar crease
Epicanthic folds	Skin folds over inner canthi
Brachycephaly	Short anteroposterior skull length
Dolichocephaly	Long anteroposterior skull length
Clinodactyly	Incurved fifth fingers
Polydactyly	Extra fingers or toes
Syndactyly	Fusion of fingers or toes
Arachnodactyly	Abnormally long and thin digits
Brachydactyly	Abnormally short digits

Table 12.2 Measurements that may be diagnostically useful

Measurement	Comment
Height	
Arm span	
Weight	
Lower segment	Floor to upper border of pubis
Upper segment	Height minus lower segment
Sitting height	
Interpupillary distance	See Fig. 12.3
Inner canthal distance	See Fig. 12.3
Head circumference	Maximum occipitofrontal circumference
Testicular volume	Assessed using Prader orchidometer standards

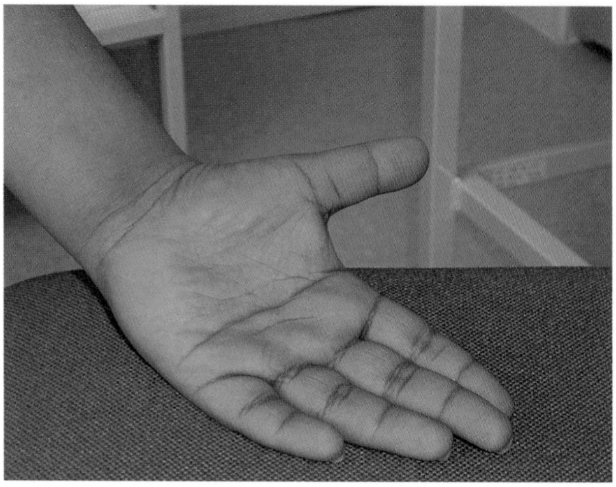

Fig. 12.4. A single transverse palmar crease. Courtesy of Margo Whiteford, Yorkhill Hospital, Glasgow.

although the actual measurement of interpupillary distance is within the normal range.

Examination of the hands is particularly important, not just for the presence of the single transverse palmar crease (Fig. 12.4) that is associated with Down syndrome (and also with many other, albeit rarer, syndromes), but also to detect abnormalities of the fingers. These include fusion of the digits (syndactyly) and abnormalities of their number, length or curvature. It should be borne in mind that a single palmar crease is present on one hand in 4% of the population and bilaterally in 1%.

In patients with multiple dysmorphic features, it is necessary to consider identifiable syndromes. A syndrome (from Greek meaning running together) is the non-random occurrence in the same individual of two or more abnormalities that are aetiologically related. Most syndromes have multiple components, of which few if any are universal or pathognomonic features, and thus the average patient will not have every feature listed for that syndrome in the textbook. Furthermore, some abnormalities are non-specific; for example, reduced height and a high arched palate may be seen in severe learning disability of any cause.

The pattern of dysmorphic or other features is generally more important than a single sign, and, as some dysmorphic features are age related, re-examination at a future date may be helpful. Many syndromes have now been described, and differential diagnosis of these is greatly aided by computerised databases (such as the London (Winter–Baraitser) Dysmorphology Database, POSSUM and the online, freely available, but not expert-curated, Phenomizer) in addition to well-illustrated texts such as *Smith's Recognizable Patterns of Human Malformation* and *The Bedside Dysmorphologist* (see Further reading).

Confirmation of diagnosis

Nowhere in clinical medicine is it more essential to obtain an accurate diagnosis, for without it genetic advice can be totally misleading. The history and physical examination may permit a confident diagnosis or may indicate the need for further investigation. A wide variety of investigations may be required, reflecting the wide spectrum of genetic disease (Table 12.3). Indications for chromosomal and DNA analysis are given in Table 12.4. Chromosomal abnormalities may produce diverse dysmorphic features and malformations, and chromosomal analysis should be considered if these are present, especially if accompanied by learning disability.

Occasionally the affected individuals will have died or be otherwise unavailable for assessment, and an attempt should then be made to obtain hospital or other records that might aid definitive diagnosis. Confirmation of the precise diagnosis is, for instance, often particularly important for relatives who died at a relatively early age of an undefined neurological condition or sudden cardiac event (which might have been secondary to an inherited cardiomyopathy). Similarly, the type of a malignancy may not be reliably known. For example, a 'stomach' or 'abdominal' cancer might, in fact, have been colorectal, gastric, pancreatic or even ovarian in origin. The precise diagnosis may be obtained (with appropriate consent) from hospital records, cancer registries or other reliable genealogical sources.

Counselling

Accurate diagnosis is of paramount importance for meaningful genetic counselling, and thus counselling should never precede the steps involved in diagnosis as outlined above.

Both parents should be counselled and adequate time allowed in an appropriate setting. Few couples can be counselled in under 30 min, and the corner of a hospital ward or a

Table 12.3 Diagnosis of genetic disease

Type	Diagnostic test
Chromosomal disorders	Chromosomal analysis(or quantitative fluorescent polymerase chain reaction for trisomies 13,18 and 21), and increasingly, multiple ligation-dependent probe amplification or array comparative genomic hybridisation for the detection of submicroscopic chromosomal deletions or duplications (see Chapter 7)
Single-gene disorders	Pedigree analysis
	Clinical examination
	Biochemical analysis
	DNA analysis
	Other investigations (imaging, functional studies, etc.)
Multifactorial disorders	Clinical examination
	Biochemical analysis
	DNA analysis (in certain cases)
	Other investigations (imaging, functional studies, etc.)
Mitochondrial disorders	Pedigree analysis
	Clinical examination
	DNA analysis
	Other investigations (imaging, functional studies, etc.)
Somatic cell genetic disorders	Histopathology
	DNA analysis (of a lesion)
	Chromosomal analysis (of a lesion)
	Other investigations (imaging, functional studies, etc.)

Table 12.4 Indications for chromosomal or DNA analysis. Such analyses may also subsequently be carried out as appropriate in the proband's relatives to identify those at risk. This could include the identification of carriers of, for instance, a balanced chromosome rearrangement or a colon cancer-predisposing gene mutation

Chromosomal analysis	DNA analysis/storage
Dysmorphic features suggestive of a chromosomal syndrome	Known or suspected single-gene disorder (patient)
Unexplained learning disability*	Known single-gene disorder (family member if linkage study required)
Family study of structural chromosomal abnormality	Neonatal death with suspected metabolic disorder
Multiple congenital abnormalities	Certain multifactorial disorders
Unexplained stillbirth	Known or suspected mitochondrial disorder
Female with unexplained short stature	
Recurrent miscarriages	
Primary infertility	
Ambiguous sexual development	
Certain types of cancer	
Suspected contiguous gene disorder	

*Also perform DNA analysis to exclude fragile X syndrome and consider multiple ligation-dependent probe amplification (see Chapter 7) and/or possibly array comparative genomic hybridisation to detect microdeletions and microduplications.

crowded clinic room is not adequate. Furthermore, it is inappropriate to counsel too soon after a recent bereavement or after the initial shock of a serious diagnosis.

Counselling needs to include all aspects of the condition and in a manner that can be readily understood by the couple. One might start by outlining the clinical features, complications, natural history, prognosis and treatment/effective management of the condition. Then a simple explanation of the genetic basis of the condition, perhaps with the aid of a diagram, could be given, and a recurrence risk calculated for the consultands. It is often useful to compare this recurrence risk against the general population risk for the condition and for other common birth defects (Table 12.5). Generally, medical geneticists consider a risk of more than 1 in 10 as high and of less than 1 in 20 as low, but risks have to be considered in relation to the degree of disability.

Consultands often feel very guilty or stigmatised, and it is important to recognise and allay this. Common misconceptions about heredity may also need to be dispelled (Table 12.6).

The reproductive options open to the couple may now be discussed (Fig. 12.5). In many consultations, the couples' fears are unjustified and they can undertake a pregnancy with the reassurance that their risk of genetic disease is no different from other couples in the general population. Where there is an increased risk, and especially where the disease burden is significant, then other options need to be considered. In this context, disease burden is the consultand's perception of the cost (physical, emotional and financial) of the disorder. The possibility of prenatal diagnosis for the condition needs to be considered, as, if available, this often encourages a couple to undertake a further pregnancy that otherwise they would be reluctant to contemplate. Where the couple decide not to undertake a further pregnancy, it is necessary for the counsellor to ensure that contraception is adequate and to mention other means of family extension. About 1% of all artificial insemination by donor is performed for genetic indications, such as a husband with an autosomal dominant trait or when both parents are carriers for a serious autosomal recessive disease for which prenatal diagnosis is unavailable. Although this substantially reduces the risk of an autosomal recessive trait, some risk will remain in proportion to the population carrier frequency.

Counselling must be non-judgemental and non-directive. The aim is to deliver a balanced version of the facts that will permit the consultands to reach their own decision with regard to their reproductive future.

For certain conditions, such as balanced chromosomal rearrangements, autosomal dominant traits and X-linked recessive traits, an extended family study will be required, and it is useful to enlist the aid of the consultands in approaching other family members at risk.

Table 12.5 General population risks	
Condition	**Risk**
Spontaneous miscarriage	1 in 6
Perinatal death	1 in 30–100
Neonatal death	1 in 150
Cot death	1 in 500
Major congenital malformation	1 in 33
Serious mental or physical handicap	1 in 50
Adult cancer	1 in 3–4

Table 12.6 Common misconceptions about heredity
Absence of other affected family members means that a disorder is not genetic and vice versa
Any condition present at birth must be inherited
Upsets, mental and physical, of the mother in pregnancy cause malformations
All genetic diseases are untreatable
If only males or females are affected in the family, this indicates sex linkage
A 1 in 4 risk means that, after the birth of an affected child, the next three children will be unaffected
All genetic disorders and their carrier state can be detected by chromosomal analysis
Confusion of odds, fractions and percentage risks

Follow-up

Many consultands can be fully counselled at one sitting, but some will require follow-up sessions. Our policy is to follow the counselling with a letter to the consultands, which summarises the information given and invites them to return if new questions arise. Also, if new opportunities arise (e.g. an improved carrier or prenatal diagnostic test), consultands can be contacted and offered a return appointment through the regional genetic register. The role of the clinical geneticist often also involves organising appropriate clinical surveillance programmes for individuals at risk. This might involve, for instance, regular electrocardiography and/or echocardiography for those at risk of cardiac disease, magnetic resonance imaging scans for those at high risk of developing breast cancer and colonoscopies for those with a bowel cancer predisposition. In addition, it is important to offer those relatives who are at risk genetic testing if available and, if appropriate, clinical screening for early clinical signs.

Special points in counselling

There are several pitfalls for the unwary who practise genetic counselling (Table 12.7). Precision of diagnosis is fundamental

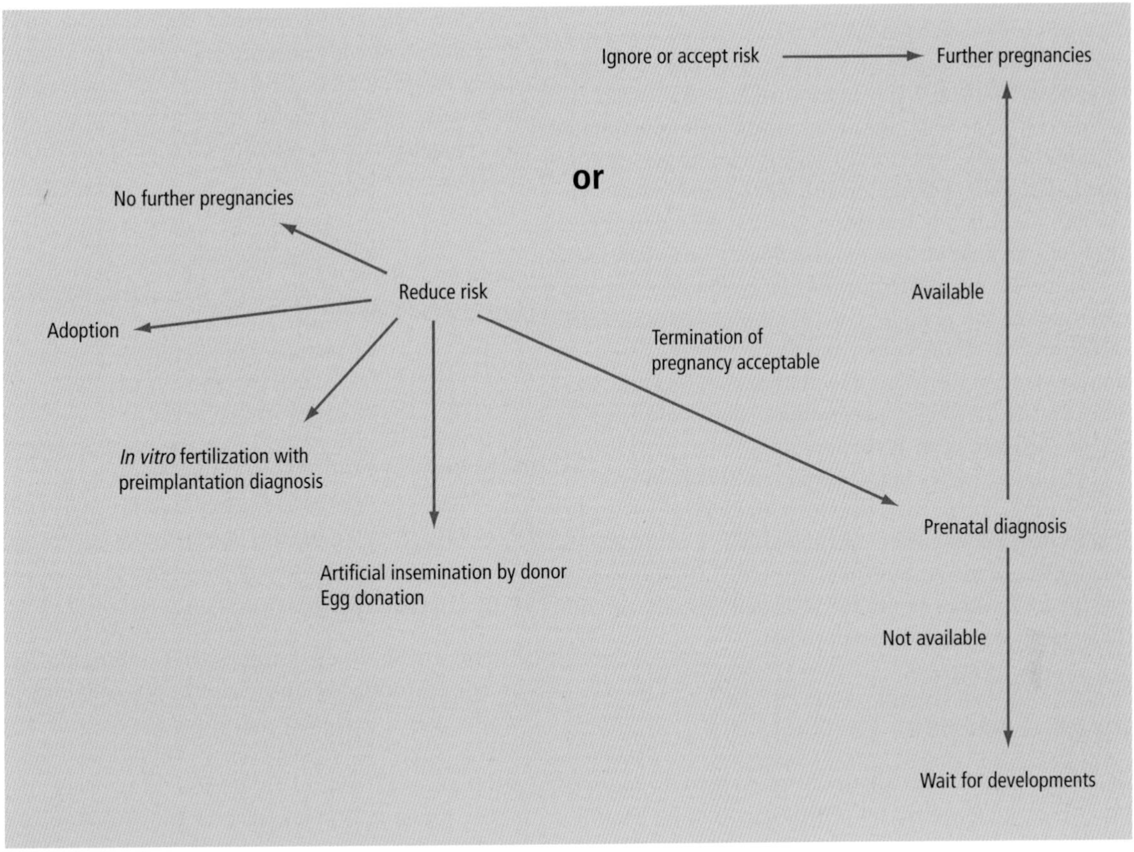

Fig. 12.5 Reproductive options available following diagnosis of a genetically inherited condition.

Table 12.7 Pitfalls and problems in genetic counselling
No diagnosis in the proband
Incorrect or incomplete diagnosis
Genetic heterogeneity
Non-penetrance
Variable expression
Inadequate knowledge of the literature
Previously undescribed disease
Gonadal mosaicism
Unstable mutations

to meaningful genetic counselling, and most mistakes arise from an inaccurate or incomplete diagnosis. Sufficient knowledge of the literature is especially important for syndromic assessment and in relation to genetic heterogeneity.

The counselling details for individual conditions are covered at websites such as GeneReviews and in specific texts such as Firth and Hurst's *Oxford Desk Reference* or Harper's *Practical Genetic Counselling* (see Further reading). These books provide detailed practical advice regarding investigations and counselling (with useful empiric risks) for many clinical problems that have several different genetic causes such as severe childhood deafness, learning difficulties and short stature.

Single-gene disorders

The general principles of genetic counselling for autosomal and X-linked conditions are discussed in Chapters 8, 9 and 15. The important related potential pitfalls are also described in these chapters, including incomplete penetrance, variable expression, genetic anticipation, mosaicism, imprinting, pseudoautosomal inheritance, locus heterogeneity and non-random X inactivation. Additional details are available from the websites and reference books mentioned above.

Multifactorial disorders

For discontinuous multifactorial traits empiric recurrence risks are used. These are the observed (rather than the calculated) recurrence risks for different relatives of an affected individual. Strictly, empiric recurrence risks apply only to the population from which they were collected.

Consanguinity

A consanguineous couple are at increased risk of autosomal recessive and multifactorial traits, including several congenital malformations. If there is no previous consanguinity in the family, the risk of serious disease or major malformations in the offspring of a first-cousin marriage is 1 in 20 (i.e. double the population risk). For the offspring of a first-cousin marriage in an inbred family the risk is 1 in 11 and the risk rises to 1 in 2 for offspring of incestuous unions. Carrier screening to be considered for a consanguineous couple seeking pre-pregnancy advice can include cystic fibrosis and possibly other tests according to ethnic origin and family history. Thus, in addition to cystic fibrosis screening, haemoglobinopathy (thalassaemia and sickle cell) carrier testing could be offered to couples of Mediterranean or Indian/South-East Asian origin, and Tay–Sachs carrier testing to Ashkenazi Jewish couples. In addition, during a pregnancy, detailed ultrasound scanning for fetal malformations might be considered. For a consanguineous relationship with an autosomal recessive condition in a relative, the recurrence risk can be calculated from the proportion of genes in common (see Appendix 2).

Prenatal diagnosis

Prenatal diagnosis includes all aspects of embryonic and fetal diagnosis. Prenatal diagnosis for genetic conditions is presently indicated in about 8% of all pregnancies, and for these couples at increased risk of serious genetic disease, it provides the reassurance without which many would decline to undertake a pregnancy. In practice, 93% of prenatal tests provide reassurance for the couple concerned, and selective termination of pregnancy is undertaken in only 7%. Termination of pregnancy for *fetal* indications that are not associated with a risk of serious fetal abnormality is not permitted by law in the UK. In particular, current practice does not permit the procedure to be used solely for choosing the sex of offspring by terminating pregnancies of the undesired sex.

At-risk pregnancies may be identified prior to or during a pregnancy (Table 12.8). Whatever the reason for the test, it is important to outline to the couple the limitations of the appropriate test or tests and to remind them that no single test or even a combination can exclude all abnormalities. In the event of a positive test resulting in termination of pregnancy, it is important that the *complete* products of conception are sent to the laboratory for diagnostic confirmation.

Prenatal diagnostic techniques may be divided into two broad groups: invasive and non-invasive (Table 12.9).

Amniocentesis

Amniocentesis is the withdrawal of amniotic fluid. This is usually performed at 16–18 weeks of gestation when there is about 180 ml of liquor and the ratio of viable to non-viable cells is maximal. Under aseptic conditions, and after prior placental localisation with ultrasound, a needle is introduced under ultrasound guidance into the amniotic cavity via the maternal abdomen. A volume of 10–20 ml of liquor is withdrawn and this can be used for several different tests (Table 12.10). The chance of maternal cell contamination is greatly

Table 12.8 Identification of at-risk pregnancies	Chromosomal disorders	Single-gene disorders	Multiple congenital malformations
Factors identifiable prior to a pregnancy			
Elevated maternal age	+	–	–
Parental consanguinity	–	+	+
Ethnic origin	–	+	(+)
Positive family history	+	+	+
Maternal illness or medication	–	–	+
Population carrier screening	–	+	–
Factors identifiable during a pregnancy			
Abnormal ultrasound appearance	(+)	(+)	+
α-Fetoprotein screening	(+)	(+)	(+)
Other biochemical screening tests	(+)	–	–
Polyhydramnios/oligohydramnios	(+)	(+)	(+)
Maternal exposure to teratogens	–	–	+

+, Associated; (+), may be associated; –, not associated.

Table 12.9 Techniques for prenatal diagnosis

Invasive	Non-invasive
Amniocentesis*	Ultrasonography*
Chorionic villus sampling*	Other types of imaging
Cordocentesis	Free fetal DNA or RNA in the maternal circulation
Fetal skin biopsy	
Fetal liver biopsy	

*The most commonly used techniques.

Table 12.10 Tests on amniotic fluid cells and supernatant

Fetal sexing*
Fetal karyotyping*
(Fetal enzyme assay)†
Amniotic fluid biochemistry
(Fetal DNA diagnosis)†

*Chorionic villus sampling may be preferred to amniocentesis.
†Chorionic villus sampling is usually preferred to amniocentesis.

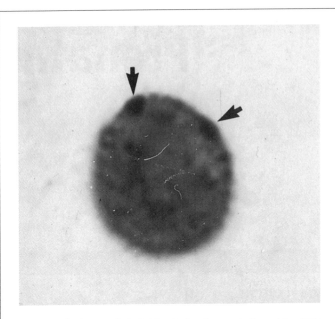

Fig. 12.6 Sexing amniotic fluid cells by demonstration of the Barr body. In this case, two Barr bodies are present (arrows), indicating the presence of three X chromosomes. Full chromosome analysis showed 47,XXX.

reduced if a stilette is used in the needle and if the first few drops of amniotic fluid withdrawn are discarded.

Fetal sexing

This is required for female carriers of serious X-linked disorders, as a preliminary step before using DNA or biochemical analysis to identify the affected males.

Historically, visualisation of the Barr body (in 50–80% of cells) was usually able to permit fetal sexing from amniotic fluid cells within 3 h (Fig. 12.6). Y fluorescence may be confused with fluorescent autosomal heteromorphisms or may be missed in patients with a heteromorphic small Y chromosome. Alternatively, a more recently introduced DNA-based method, quantitative fluorescent polymerase chain reaction (QF-PCR; see below), using X and Y chromosome-specific polymorphic DNA markers permits fetal sexing. This can include an analysis by PCR of intron 3 of the amelogenin (*AMEL*) gene in the X/Y homologous region. In the latter, the presence of a 6 bp deletion in the allele on the X but not the Y chromosome permits determination of the sex of the fetus.

Fetal karyotyping

Fetal karyotyping (or QF-PCR; see below) is indicated for an increased risk of aneuploidy on the basis of maternal age com-

bined with prenatal screening tests (see Chapter 17), a previous child with aneuploidy, pregnancies where one parent has a balanced structural chromosomal rearrangement and to confirm the fetal sex in X-linked conditions.

Maternal age alone should not generally be an indication for fetal karyotyping, as the calculated risk of fetal aneuploidy may be greatly reduced once the results of maternal serum screening and first-trimester ultrasonography are taken into account. These screening procedures reduce the number of pregnancies requiring invasive testing by amniocentesis or CVS (and thus the risk of miscarriage) by around 75%, while significantly increasing the detection rate for Down syndrome (see Chapter 17 for further information).

For fetal karyotyping, the amniotic fluid cells are grown in culture and a result is available in 2–3 weeks. About 1.5% of samples fail to grow, and this is especially likely if the fluid was heavily blood-stained, was less than 5 ml in volume, if transport to the laboratory was delayed or if a local anaesthetic was used. In experienced laboratories, contamination of the fetal amniotic cells with maternal cells is unlikely but should be suspected if the cell cultures take longer than usual to grow and if fibroblasts rather than epithelioid cells predominate.

Chromosomal mosaicism can pose difficult diagnostic problems. In true mosaicism (i.e. mosaicism in the fetus or placenta), the abnormal cell line is usually present in several different cultures set up from the original sample, whereas in pseudomosaicism (i.e. an *in vitro* artefact during cell culture), only one culture is involved. In cases of doubt, fetal blood sampling by cordocentesis or a repeat amniocentesis needs to

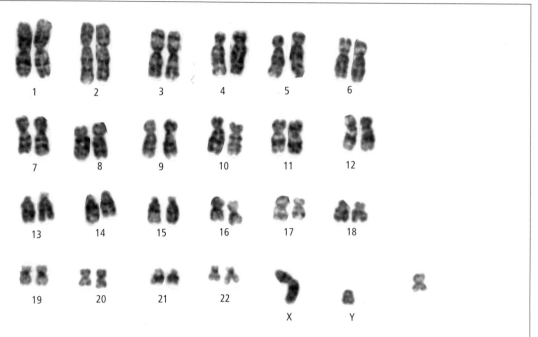

Fig. 12.7 A karyotype from amniotic fluid demonstrating an extra copy of chromosome 20, which was present in 25% of cells from several cultures (true mosaicism).

be considered. Figure 12.7 shows an extra copy of chromosome 20, which was present in 25% of the amniotic fluid cells. Fetal blood sampling showed a normal karyotype and the baby was normal, as in this case the mosaic cell line was confined to the placenta. True mosaicism is found in 0.25% of all amniocenteses and in about one-quarter of these the phenotype is abnormal. 46,XX/46,XY 'mosaicism' is an exception to this as it almost invariably represents maternal cell contamination.

Pseudomosaicism in multiple cells within a single culture is found in about 1% of all amniocenteses. Repeat amniocentesis or fetal blood sampling may be required, especially if few cells were available for analysis and if the abnormality is seen in liveborns. Single-cell pseudomosaicism (excluding single-cell hypodiploidy) is found in about 3% of amniocenteses and, as there is less than a 1% chance that this represents true mosaicism, no further action is generally taken.

Fetal karyotyping is very labour-intensive, and attempts have been made to circumvent this and to shorten the time to diagnosis. One development was the use of interphase cytogenetics involving *in situ* hybridisation with non-radioactively labelled probes (see Fig. 7.19 and 12.8). An efficient and now more commonly used method in UK laboratories for the rapid detection of aneuploidy of chromosomes 13, 18, 21, X and Y is QF-PCR. In QF-PCR, which can be performed on uncultured amniotic fluid samples, four or more microsatellite (commonly tetranucleotide) DNA markers representing each of these chromosomes are amplified by PCR (see Figs 7.2 and

7.20 in Chapter 7). The PCR primers are fluorescently labelled to facilitate detection on an automated DNA sequencer. The ratio of the sizes of allele peaks for each marker on the resulting sequencer output (or electropherogram) should normally be approximately 1 : 1. Aneuploidy is likely if the markers representing one of the chromosomes give peak size ratios of 2 : 1 or result in three peaks instead of two (see Chapter 7). Unfortunately, however, QF-PCR may not detect low-level mosaicism (with less than 20% of the cells being abnormal). As mentioned above, it is also possible to determine the fetal sex using QF-PCR by utilising sex chromosome-specific markers.

Fetal enzyme assay

Prenatal diagnosis is now possible for more than 100 inborn errors of metabolism and is indicated in at-risk pregnancies (Table 12.11). The amniotic fluid cells need to be grown in culture for around 2 weeks in order to provide sufficient cells for the assay of the appropriate enzyme. The enzyme level in these cells is compared with data from known normal and homozygous deficient amniotic fluid cells and with fibroblasts from the proband and parents, if available. Many of these enzymes are expressed in chorionic villi, and, if so, this permits earlier prenatal diagnosis, as not only can the test be carried out in the first trimester but it also yields sufficient material for assay without prior culture.

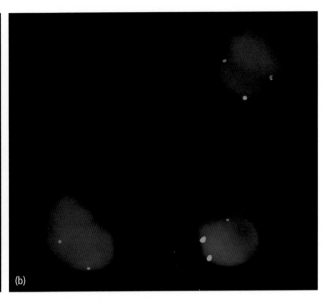

Fig. 12.8 Results of FISH undertaken on uncultured amniocytes: (a) The result after using a commercial 22q11.2-specific probe (designed to detect microdeletions associated with velocardiofacial syndrome), in red, in combination with a 22q-specific control probe in green. The image shows an abnormal signal pattern (one red and two green signals), as observed in the majority of cells scored, suggestive of the presence of the 22q11.2 microdeletion on one chromosome 22. (b) The result following the use of a commercial probe combination consisting of an X centromere-specific probe labelled with a green fluorophore and a Y centromere-specific probe labelled in red. Two nuclei exhibit two green signals and one red signal, while one has one green and one red, suggesting that the fetus is an XXY/XY mosaic. Courtesy of Norma Morrison, Yorkhill Hospital, Glasgow.

Table 12.11 Examples of prenatally diagnosable inborn errors of metabolism (when suspected)

Lipid metabolism

Tay–Sachs disease, Gaucher disease, Niemann–Pick disease, familial hypercholesterolaemia, adrenoleucodystrophy, metachromatic leucodystrophy

Mucopolysaccharidoses

Amino acid metabolism

Methylmalonic acidaemia, homocystinuria, cystinosis, maple syrup urine disease, arginosuccinicaciduria

Carbohydrate metabolism

Galactosaemia, glycogen storage disease (some types)

Others

Lesch–Nyhan syndrome, adenosine deaminase deficiency, xeroderma pigmentosum, urea cycle defects, organic acidurias

Amniotic fluid biochemistry

Two-dimensional electrophoresis of glycosaminoglycans in amniotic fluid (in addition to enzyme testing on cultured amniocytes) can be used for the prenatal diagnosis of some types of mucopolysaccharidosis. In addition, the level of 17α-hydroxyprogesterone in amniotic fluid can be measured in pregnancies at risk of salt-losing, 21-hydroxylase deficient, congenital adrenal hyperplasia (adrenogenital syndrome), particularly if prenatal DNA testing is not feasible.

Assay of α-fetoprotein (AFP) in amniotic fluid may very occasionally be carried out if there is an increased risk of a neural tube defect, indicated by, for example, a previously affected child or a raised maternal serum AFP (see Chapter 17). In practice, however, amniotic fluid AFP analysis is now rarely undertaken in the UK, as fetal ultrasound can usually provide a definitive answer regarding the presence or absence of a neural tube defect.

Fetal DNA diagnosis of single-gene disorders

The current major indications for fetal DNA diagnosis include those listed in Table 12.12 and many rarer single-gene disorders are also diagnosable with this approach. Small quantities of DNA can be extracted from amniotic cells, which may be suitable for targeted PCR and sequencing. However, the amniocytes may need to be cultured for 1–3 weeks in order to obtain sufficient DNA for analysis. The diagnosis may be established through direct demonstration of the molecular defect or, occasionally, by indirect tracking of the mutant gene using intragenic (or closely linked) DNA markers. As sufficient DNA can usually be reliably extracted from a chorionic villus sample without prior culture, and as the test is performed earlier in

Table 12.12 Current major indications for fetal DNA diagnosis of single-gene disorders

Condition
α-Thalassaemia
β-Thalassaemia
Cystic fibrosis
Fragile X syndrome
Haemophilia A
Huntington disease
Muscular dystrophy (Duchenne and Becker)
Myotonic dystrophy
Spinal muscular atrophy

Note: Fetal DNA may also be analysed for the detection of a trisomy (and, if there is a risk of an X-linked condition, for sex determination) by QF-PCR.

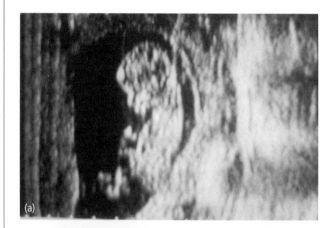

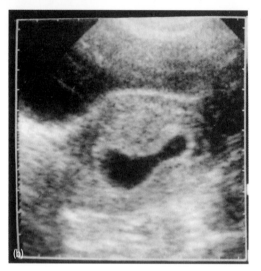

Fig. 12.9 (a) Normal fetus at 10 weeks of gestation. (b) Anembryonic sac at 10 weeks of gestation.

pregnancy, CVS is usually the preferred technique to obtain fetal tissue for DNA analysis.

Risks of amniocentesis

Amniocentesis carries a small additional risk of miscarriage for the pregnancy. In one randomised controlled trial of over 4000 women, this risk was estimated to be 1.0%. In addition, for any pregnancy at 16 weeks of gestation, there is a 2.5% chance of spontaneous miscarriage. If the indication for amniocentesis is raised maternal serum AFP, then a spontaneous abortion rate of 7% is found, as AFP is raised in many non-viable pregnancies. Maternal risks are negligible.

A history of threatened abortion is not a contraindication to amniocentesis but is an added indication. Twenty-six per cent of mothers of babies with trisomy 21 have a history of persistent first-trimester bleeding compared with 1% of controls.

Chorionic villus sampling

Sampling of chorionic villi from the fetus is performed from 10 weeks of gestation onwards and is now available in most major obstetric centres. The biopsy is usually taken under ultrasound guidance via a transabdominal approach. Each biopsy yields about 5–30 mg of tissue, which can be used for fetal sexing, fetal karyotyping, biochemical studies and DNA analysis. A direct fetal chromosomal analysis is possible within 24 h, but, in view of the problem of mosaicism in CVS samples, this should always be followed by chromosomal analysis on cultured cells from the sample 2–3 weeks later (a sample of 5 mg should be adequate for chromosomal analysis). DNA analysis or biochemical tests can be completed in 1–2 weeks, usually without the need to culture the cells and, if termination

of pregnancy is necessary following any of these tests, it can thus be performed in the first trimester. At this stage, the abortion procedure is technically simpler than in the second trimester, there is less parental bonding with the fetus and only the couple and their medical attendants need know about the pregnancy. The spontaneous abortion rate at or beyond 10 weeks of pregnancy is 7%. In most of these pregnancies, which are destined to abort, the ultrasound reveals an anembryonic sac or dead fetus (Fig. 12.9). If the fetus is viable on ultrasound at this stage, the subsequent spontaneous abortion rate is 1–2% if the mother is under 35 years of age. The added rate from the CVS procedure is 2%. Rhesus isoimmunisation should be avoided in rhesus-negative unsensitised mothers by giving anti-rhesus D immunoglobulin.

Where the indication for CVS is increased maternal age alone, a chromosomal abnormality is found in 4–6% compared with 2% for non-chromosomal indications. These figures reflect the high frequency of chromosomal disorders in early gestation (see Table 18.8) and make it prudent to karyotype all CVS samples (if sample size permits) whatever the primary indication.

At the time of CVS, 1 in 65 pregnancies reveal twins. This exceeds the delivery frequency (see Chapter 10) and the discrepancy is believed to reflect spontaneous miscarriage of one or both twins. If one twin is chromosomally abnormal, this twin is liable to die *in utero* ('the vanishing twin') and CVS may reveal 'mosaicism'. Mosaicism is found in 0.66% of CVS cultures and 1.26% of direct analyses (compared with a figure of 0.25% for true mosaicism at amniocentesis). Most of the CVS mosaics are confined to the placenta ('confined placental mosaicism') and do not reflect mosaicism in the fetus, but subsequent amniocentesis will be required to help confirm this in 1–2% of patients who have CVS.

Cordocentesis, fetal skin biopsy and fetal liver biopsy

Under ultrasound guidance, a fine needle can be passed transabdominally into the fetal umbilical cord where it enters the placenta in order to take a fetal blood sample or to perform an *in utero* transfusion. The procedure is possible from 18 weeks of gestation onwards and the procedure-related fetal loss rate is about 1%. There is also a risk of feto-maternal haemorrhage with development or enhancement of rhesus isoimmunisation. Table 12.13 outlines the main indications for fetal blood sampling using this approach.

Some serious skin disorders (e.g. epidermolysis bullosa) can be diagnosed in a fetal skin biopsy taken via a fetoscope, and in occasional metabolic disorders a fetal liver biopsy is necessary for diagnosis.

Ultrasonography

Visualisation of the fetus by ultrasound carries no proven hazard for either mother or fetus. Over 280 different congenital malformations may be diagnosed by an experienced ultrasonographer (Table 12.14). Ultrasound is indicated for a pregnancy at increased risk for any of these disorders. Anencephaly may be detected on ultrasound as early as 10–12 weeks gestation but for most abnormalities 16–18 weeks is the optimal time. Serial scans may be required, especially to detect abnormal growth of, for example, the head or limbs.

Although fetal genitalia can be visualised from 16 weeks of gestation, ultrasonography would not be adequate for fetal sexing for a serious genetic condition.

Fetal cells in the maternal circulation

A non-invasive method of prenatal diagnosis would have obvious advantages over current procedures. There is good evidence that small numbers of nucleated fetal cells enter the maternal circulation throughout pregnancy. These include fetal leucocytes, nucleated red cells and trophoblast cells. Attempts have been made to obtain enrichment of fetal cells in a maternal blood sample with the aim of achieving prenatal diagnosis using DNA analysis (by PCR) or fluorescence *in situ* hybridisation (FISH). The technique has not, however, proved sufficiently reliable for it to be used as a clinical test.

Free fetal DNA and RNA detection

In recent years, it has become clear that, in addition to fetal cells, cell-free fetal DNA can be found in the maternal circulation. The source is most likely to be apoptosis (programmed cell death) of cells in the placenta, and fetal DNA has been found in maternal serum and plasma as early as 7 weeks of gestation.

Table 12.13 Possible indications for fetal blood sampling

Fetal infection

Suspected mosaicism

In utero transfusion for rhesus isoimmunisation

Unexplained hydrops fetalis

Failed amniotic cell culture or late booking

Potentially treatable congenital malformation

Unexplained severe fetal growth retardation

Also, if DNA diagnosis is not available and the fetus is at risk of the following:

   Haemophilia A or B

   β-Thalassaemia

   Sickle-cell disease

   Severe combined immunodeficiency

Table 12.14 Examples of congenital malformations that can usually be diagnosed by ultrasound

System/organ	Malformation
Central nervous system	Anencephaly, spina bifida, hydrocephalus*, microcephaly*, encephalocele
Limb	Severe short-limbed dwarfism, polydactyly, severe osteogenesis imperfecta, limb reduction deformity
Heart	Severe congenital heart disease
Kidney	Renal agenesis, bladder outflow obstruction, infantile polycystic disease
Gastrointestinal tract	Duodenal atresia, anterior abdominal wall defect, diaphragmatic hernia

*May not be detectable in all cases before the last trimester.

There is a great deal of interest in the potential clinical use of this DNA, especially with regard to non-invasive fetal rhesus D blood typing and also fetal gender determination (for instance, using PCR amplification of the *SRY* gene) in pregnancies of carriers of X-linked recessive conditions, and these two tests have proved to be the most useful applications so far. Mutations transmitted from the father to the fetus can also be identified from maternal plasma and this could have practical use in the fetal diagnosis of autosomal dominant disorders such as Huntington disease. More recent research on allele-specific markers in placental mRNA holds out hope for the non-invasive diagnosis of Down syndrome and other aneuploidies. See Wright and Chitty, 2009, in Further reading for a review of this field.

Preimplantation genetic diagnosis

Preimplantation genetic diagnosis (PGD) is increasingly being undertaken in the UK and elsewhere. In this technique, which is discussed in Chapter 1, a single cell can be removed at day 3 post-fertilisation from a 6–10-cell embryo following *in vitro* fertilisation. Using either PCR or FISH, the fetal sex is determined (in cases of sex-linked disease) and the detection of a specific mutation, a mutation-associated haplotype or a chromosomal abnormality can be undertaken. One or two unaffected embryos are then implanted into the uterus and the pregnancy is allowed to continue.

This technique has been used successfully to test many embryos for mutations associated with over 200 different single-gene disorders such as cystic fibrosis, fragile X syndrome, myotonic dystrophy and Huntington disease, and for a variety of unbalanced chromosome abnormalities resulting from parental chromosomal translocations. Although well over 1000 babies have been born following this technique, the chance of a successful birth is currently only around 20% per oocyte retrieval procedure (the figure varying according to the genetic condition and the centre involved). In addition, the procedure is emotionally and physically demanding and is only available at a few centres, and there are still some uncertainties over the theoretical possibility of long-term effects on the offspring. Only a minority of couples currently decide to proceed with PGD rather than other reproductive options. Further information regarding the procedure is available from the website of the Guy's and St Thomas' NHS Foundation Trust (see Websites) which provides a detailed downloadable (PDF-format) guide.

SUMMARY

- Accurate diagnosis of dysmorphic syndromes is important for genetic counselling.
- Syndrome diagnosis is facilitated by the identification of significantly abnormal clinical features and by the use of computerised databases such as the London (Winter–Baraitser) Dysmorphology Database (and POSSUM) or standard reference texts such as *Smith's Recognizable Patterns of Human Malformation* (see Further reading).
- Genetic counselling should be non-directive and non-judgemental.
- Reproductive options that may be discussed in relation to a risk of recurrence include prenatal diagnosis (by CVS, amniocentesis or, if appropriate, ultrasonography), artificial insemination by donor, egg donation, adoption and perhaps PGD.
- With autosomal dominant traits, the genetic counsellor must be aware of variable expression of the phenotype, non-penetrance, conditions showing genetic anticipation and the possibility of gonadal mosaicism in apparently unaffected parents.
- A potentially clinically useful non-invasive method of prenatal determination of fetal sex (and possibly genetic diagnosis) is the analysis of cell-free fetal DNA or RNA in the maternal circulation.

FURTHER READING

Firth HV, Hurst JA (eds). (2005) *Oxford Desk Reference: Clinical Genetics*. Oxford University Press: Oxford.

Hall JG, Allanson JE, Gripp KW, Slavotinek AM (2006) *Handbook of Physical Measurements*. Oxford University Press: Oxford.

Harper PS (2010) *Practical Genetic Counselling*, 7th edn. Hodder Arnold: London.

Jones KL (2006) *Smith's Recognizable Patterns of Human Malformation*, 6th edn. Saunders: London.

London (Winter-Baraitser) Dysmorphology Database and Baraitser-Winter Neurogenetics Database. London Medical Databases Ltd.

POSSUM Database. Murdoch Children's Research Institute, Royal Children's Hospital, Victoria, Australia.

Reardon W (2007) *The Bedside Dysmorphologist: Classic Clinical Signs in Malformation Syndromes and their Diagnostic Significance*. Oxford University Press: London.

Wright CF, Chitty LS (2009) Cell-free fetal DNA and RNA in maternal blood: implications for safer antenatal testing. *BMJ* **339**:161–4.

WEBSITES

GeneReviews:

http://www.genetests.org

Guy's and St Thomas' NHS Foundation Trust: Pre-implantation Genetic Diagnosis (PGD) information:

http://www.guysandstthomas.nhs.uk/services/womensservices/acu/pgd/pgd.aspx

Phenomizer (a new, free, publicly accessible clinical diagnostic database):

http://compbio.charite.de/Phenomizer/Phenomizer.html

Self-assessment

1. The finding of apparent 46,XX/46,XY mosaicism on fetal karyotyping following amniocentesis usually reflects which one of the following?

A. Identical twins
B. Non-identical twins
C. Fetal hermaphroditism
D. Maternal cell contamination
E. Sex chromosome misidentification on karyotyping

2. In the absence of previous consanguinity in a family, the risk of serious disease or major malformations in the child of a first-cousin marriage is:

A. 50%
B. 25%
C. 10%
D. 5%
E. 2%

3. Quantitative fluorescent PCR (QF-PCR) is useful for which of the following?

A. Detection of trisomy of chromosome 13
B. Detection of trisomy 18
C. Detection of trisomy 21
D. Detection of unidentified balanced chromosome translocations
E. Determination of fetal sex

4. Which of the following most closely approximates the added rate of spontaneous abortion that is associated with undergoing a chorionic villus sampling (CVS) procedure?

A. 20%
B. 10%
C. 7%
D. 5%
E. 2%

5. The analysis of fetal-derived DNA is commonly used to detect which of the following?

A. Autosomal trisomy
B. Fetal gender if the mother is a carrier of an X-linked recessive genetic condition
C. Renal agenesis
D. Cystic fibrosis if the parents are both known carriers
E. Anencephaly

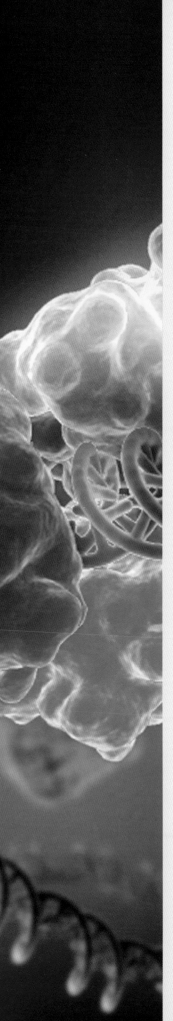

CHAPTER 13
Family history of cancer

Key Topics

Introduction

In this chapter, several important general principles relating to the genetics of cancer predisposition are described, followed by the properties of tumour suppressor genes (TSGs) and oncogenes. Details are also provided regarding the familial cancer predisposition syndromes that are relatively commonly encountered in the genetics clinic. These include the autosomal dominantly inherited breast and ovarian cancer, hereditary non-polyposis colon cancer and familial adenomatous polyposis syndromes, as well as the more recently described autosomal recessive *MUTYH*-associated polyposis.

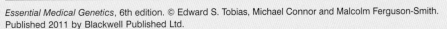

Essential Medical Genetics, 6th edition. © Edward S. Tobias, Michael Connor and Malcolm Ferguson-Smith.
Published 2011 by Blackwell Published Ltd.

General principles

In contrast to many other types of conditions involving genetic alterations, for most cancers the genetic alterations of major effect are generally not inherited and instead arise in somatic cells during adulthood, often as a result of exposure to environmental carcinogens. Multiple mutations are usually involved, and this accumulation is reflected by the histopathological progression. Mutations associated with cancer commonly involve two general types of gene: TSGs and oncogenes. Many TSGs and proto-oncogenes (the normal cellular form of oncogenes) are normally involved in the control of cellular growth and proliferation, and disruption of such control is a consistent feature of cancer. In addition, there is a group of cancer genes that are involved in DNA repair mechanisms (i.e. 'stability genes', such as *MLH1*; see below). These are often regarded as actually representing a subset of TSGs on account of their mutations resulting in loss rather than gain of function of the encoded protein (see below). The involvement of multiple mutations in cancers is probably a result of the necessity in tumorigenesis for cells not only to proliferate but also to overcome several cellular protective mechanisms. These have been described in detail by Hanahan and Weinberg (2000; see Further reading) and include, in particular, apoptosis (programmed cell death) and replicative senescence (the irreversible cell cycle arrest that is responsible for the limited number of cell divisions achievable by non-stem cells).

In a small minority (around 2–5%) of cases of common cancers (e.g. breast cancer and colon cancer, discussed in more detail below), and particularly in certain uncommon cancer syndromes, the inheritance is due to a single gene of major effect. In these families, there can therefore be a high risk of cancer in relatives. The inheritance pattern is, in families where there appears to be Mendelian inheritance, in most cases autosomal dominant with incomplete penetrance (and there can be sex limitation; see Chapter 8). In such cases, the first causative mutation is inherited and is most frequently located in a TSG. For the great majority of cancers occurring in the population, however, there are only fairly weak (although possibly multiple) inherited genetic factors, and the risks to relatives are therefore much lower.

A large proportion of the workload of the clinical genetics service, in partnership with other medical specialties and primary care, is now formed by patients who have a personal or family history of cancer. It is important to identify the minority of families in which there is a significant chance of a mutation being present that confers a high risk of cancer. These are the families in which clinical surveillance of unaffected relatives and possibly extensive mutation analyses would be most beneficial. To this end, guidelines have been devised (see Websites in Further reading) that can assist physicians in selecting those individuals for whom a referral to the clinical genetics service would be most appropriate. Careful history taking is, of course, essential in the evaluation of such families. In addition, it is important to obtain, as far as possible, correct information regarding the age of onset of cancer in relatives and the tumour types. For instance, a 'stomach' cancer might, in fact, prove to have been colorectal (or even ovarian) cancer with significantly different implications for the diagnosis of the condition affecting the family.

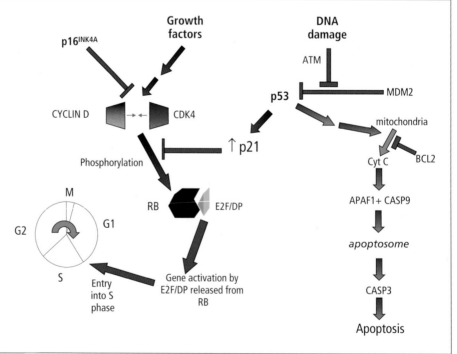

Fig. 13.1 A simplified representation of the roles of RB and p53. These include cell-cycle arrest via transcriptional activation by p53 of the p21 protein. The p21 protein then inhibits the phosphorylation of RB by cyclin/CDK complexes and thus causes loss of transcriptional activation by E2F/DP regulatory proteins. This occurs because, when RB is hypophosphorylated, it can bind to (and thus inhibit) E2F transcriptional regulatory proteins. Another important effect of p53 is programmed cell death (apoptosis), which occurs via the p53-triggered release of cytochrome c from mitochondria and the subsequent activation of a series of proteases known as caspases.

Tumour suppressor genes

Currently, around 90 of these genes have been discovered. The proteins that TSGs encode may, when functioning normally, negatively regulate cell-cycle progression, couple DNA damage recognition to cell-cycle control, promote apoptosis or play a role in cell adhesion (e.g. thus preventing metastasis). TSGs are cancer genes that, when altered, tend to result in a loss of protein function.

TSGs were first discovered as a result of studies on rare inherited forms of cancer as exemplified by retinoblastoma. Although rare, with a worldwide incidence of just 1 in 20,000 live births, retinoblastoma is the commonest malignant eye tumour of childhood and in 20–30% of cases both eyes are affected. In general, all of these bilateral cases and 15% of the unilateral cases result from the inheritance of an autosomal dominant trait. The gene for this trait, *RB1*, is localised to the proximal long arm of chromosome 13 (at 13q14) and in the tumour tissue this gene's functional protein product is absent. The *RB1* gene is now known to encode a protein, RB, that negatively regulates progression through the cell cycle. It achieves this, at least partly, by preventing the activity of the E2F transcription factors (Fig. 13.1). An autosomal dominant trait implies an inherited mutation in only one member of a pair of genes. It was calculated, however, that for such a tumour to occur, an individual who inherits a mutant TSG must also develop an inactivating alteration in the other allele within a retinal cell (Fig. 13.2). This requirement is consistent with the fact that the inherited TSG mutations generally cause inactivation (often as a result of truncation) of the protein and the remaining normal copy of the gene would otherwise still function sufficiently to prevent oncogenesis. The discovery formed the basis for the so-called 'two-hit hypothesis' formulated by Alfred Knudson in 1971.

The inactivating gene alteration may be a missense mutation affecting a functionally important amino acid, a nucleotide sequence change affecting splicing or a protein-truncating mutation (e.g. a stop codon or a frameshift mutation; see Chapter 3). Other types of TSG alteration, especially common as somatic second hits in tumour cells (see below), include methylation of cytosines in CpG dinucleotides around the promoter (causing transcriptional repression or 'silencing') and gene deletions.

As the second 'hit' frequently involves loss of the remaining gene copy through deletion or recombination, comparison of polymorphic markers in the blood and tumour DNA will often reveal loss of heterozygosity (LOH) in the tumour DNA (Figs 13.3 and 13.4). Many tumour types have, in fact, been studied for LOH in order to identify the location of TSGs. Some TSG loci have been identified in this fashion, although more have been found by linkage analysis of large affected families. Many TSGs including *RB1*, *TP53* and *APC* (see below) have now been identified (see Tables 13.1 and 13.2).

In the non-inherited (i.e. sporadic) cases of retinoblastoma, two separate mutations must occur *de novo* in each copy of

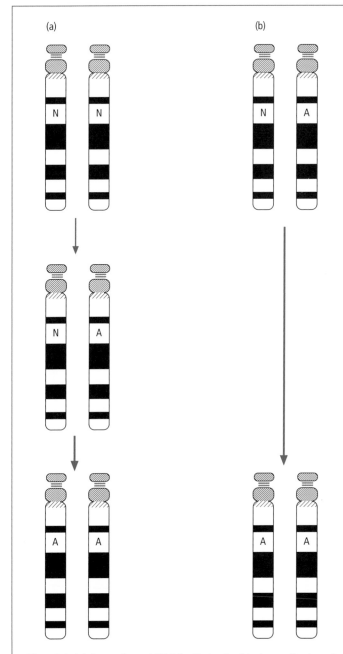

Fig. 13.2 (a) Sporadic and (b) inherited retinoblastoma. Copies of chromosome 13 are shown with either a normal (N) or an abnormal (A) gene.

chromosome 13 somatically (Fig. 13.2). Hence, in contrast to the phenotype in familial cases, bilateral involvement is unlikely and the age at presentation is generally older. The first retinoblastoma mutation in either familial or non-inherited retinoblastoma is usually a point mutation (nonsense, frameshift or splice-site mutation), which may result in a truncated protein or no protein product. Absence of the protein product from an individual allele is, in fact, particularly likely if the abnormal mRNA containing the premature stop codon is degraded by

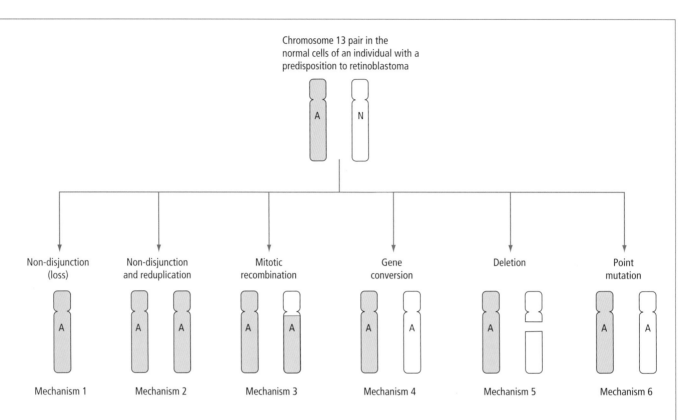

Chromosome 13 pair in the
normal cells of an individual with a
predisposition to retinoblastoma

Non-disjunction (loss) — Mechanism 1

Non-disjunction and reduplication — Mechanism 2

Mitotic recombination — Mechanism 3

Gene conversion — Mechanism 4

Deletion — Mechanism 5

Point mutation — Mechanism 6

Six possible chromosome 13 pairs that might be seen in a retinoblastoma tumour arising in
the individual whose (non-tumour cell) chromosomes are shown at the top of the figure

Fig. 13.3 Mechanisms of loss of a second retinoblastoma allele. N, Normal gene; A, mutant gene.

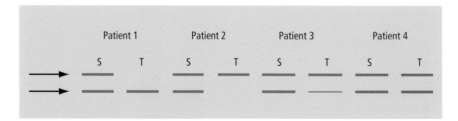

Patient 1   Patient 2   Patient 3   Patient 4

S   T   S   T   S   T   S   T

Fig. 13.4 LOH for a DNA polymorphic marker with two alleles (arrows). Complete loss of one allele in patients 1 and 2, partial loss in patient 3 and no loss indicating another mechanism in patient 4. S, Somatic tissue or blood; T, tumour tissue.

the (now well-recognised) cellular process known as nonsense-mediated decay. In contrast, the second retinoblastoma mutation usually involves loss of chromosome 13 either whole or in part following, for example, mitotic non-disjunction or partial deletion respectively (Fig. 13.3). This second mutation thus often (60%) produces a variable loss of one of the chromosome 13 alleles (mechanisms 1, 2, 3 and 5 in Fig. 13.3) including the retinoblastoma locus, and this can readily be demonstrated by DNA analysis, which shows loss of heterozygosity (LOH) for probes within the deleted region in tumour DNA when compared with the DNA of normal somatic cells such as peripheral blood lymphocytes (Figs 13.4 and 13.5).

Another important TSG that plays an important role in pathways triggering not only cell-cycle arrest (via the *RB1*-encoded protein) but also apoptosis, is the *TP53* gene on chromosome 17p encoding p53 (Fig. 13.1). Perhaps not surprisingly, therefore, mutations in *TP53* appear to be the most common genetic change in cancers. In colon cancer, for example, 75–80% of tumours show LOH for *TP53* and the gene is frequently mutated and/or deleted in other tumours including lung cancer, breast cancer, brain tumours, hepatocellular carcinoma and chronic myeloid leukaemia in blast crisis. Rarely, patients may inherit mutations of *TP53* and, as might be expected, they develop multiple primary cancers at diverse

Table 13.1 Examples of genetic conditions predisposing to tumours, relatively commonly seen in genetics clinics

Syndrome	Tumor	Associated cancers/ traits	Inheritance in familial cases	Chromosome location	Responsible gene	Principal function of encoded protein
Familial breast cancer	Breast cancer	Ovarian cancer (especially with *BRCA1*)	AD	17q21 13q12	*BRCA1* *BRCA2*	Double-strand break repair of DNA Double-strand break repair of DNA
Hereditary non-polyposis colorectal cancer (HNPCC)	Colorectal cancer	Endometrial, ovarian, hepato-biliary, and urinary tract cancer	AD	2p16 3p21 Others	*MSH2* *MLH1* Others	DNA mismatch repair DNA mismatch repair DNA mismatch repair
MutYH (or *MYH*) associated polyposis (MAP)	Colorectal cancer	Intestinal polyposis	AR	1p34.3-1p32.1	*MUTYH*	DNA glycosylase required for base excision repair
Familial adenomatous polyposis (FAP)	Colorectal cancer	Intestinal polyposis, duodenal tumours, desmoid tumours, jaw osteomas & medulloblastoma	AD	5q21	*APC*	Regulation of level of transcriptional activator, beta-catenin. Also a possible role also in mitotic spindle (via interactions with microtubules)
von Hippel-Lindau disease	Renal cancer	Retinal angiomas, cerebellar haemangioblastoma	AD	3p25	*VHL*	Indirect regulator of transcription of hypoxia-inducible genes, via HIF-1α.
Familial melanoma	Melanoma	Pancreatic cancer	AD	9p21	*CDKN2A*	Encodes p16/INK4A, an inhibitor of CDK4 and CDK6 cyclin-dependent kinases. It thus regulates the cell cycle.
Neurofibromatosis type 1	Neurofibromas	Neurofibrosarcoma, brain tumors	AD	17q11	*NF1*	GTPase activating protein, negativley regulating RAS proteins. Cytoskeletal protein interactions.

Table 13.2 Genetic conditions predisposing to tumours, less commonly seen in genetics clinics

Syndrome	Tumor	Associated cancers/traits	Inheritance in familial cases	Chromosome location	Responsible gene	Principal function of encoded protein
Familial retinoblastoma	Retinoblastoma	Osteosarcoma	AD	13q14	RB1	Transcriptional regulation (E2F-mediated) and cell cycle regulation
Li-Fraumeni syndrome	Sarcomas, breast cancer	Brain tumors, leukemia, adrenocortical carcinoma, others	AD	17q13	TP53	Response to DNA damage and other cellular stresses. Transcriptional regulation, cell cycle control and apoptosis.
Familial Wilms tumor	Wilms tumor	WAGR syndrome, aniridia, genitourinary abnormalities, mental retardation & Denys-Drash syndrome.	AD	11p13	WT1	Transcriptional regulation e.g. of apoptotic factors
Gorlin syndrome	Basal cell carcinomas	Jaw cysts, palmar and plantar pits, medulloblastomas, ovarian fibromas	AD	9q22	PTCH	Receptor for sonic hedgehog. Regulation of GLI pathway signaling.
Multiple endocrine neoplasia type 1	MEN1	Parathyroid hyperplasia. Pituitary adenomas. Pancreatic islet cell tumours	AD	11q13	MEN1	Probable roles in transcriptional regulation, genome stability and cell proliferation
Multiple endocrine neoplasia type 2	MEN2	Medullary thyroid cancer plus, in MEN 2A: phaeochromocytoma & parathyroid hyperplasia; and in MEN 2B: phaeochromocytoma & mucosal neuroma	AD	10q11	RET proto-oncogene	Receptor tyrosine kinase

Ataxia telangiectasia	Lymphoma, leukaemia solid tumours	Cerebellar ataxia, immunodeficiency, conjunctival telangiectases	AR	11q22	ATM	Cell cycle arrest (via p53). DNA repair (via BRCA1/MRE11/NBS1).
Blooms syndrome	Solid tumors, leukemia	Immunodeficiency, small stature	AR	15q26	BLM	DNA helicase. Role in DNA repair and/or replication.
Xeroderma pigmentosum	Skin cancer (basal cell or squamous cell carcinomas; malignant melanomas)	Pigmentation abnormalities, hypogonadism	AR	At least eight autosomal loci.	XPA to XPG. XPV	Nucleotide excision repair
Hereditary diffuse gastric cancer	Diffuse gastric cancer	Possibly lobular breast cancer	AD	16q22	CDH1/E-CADHERIN	Cell-cell adhesion ("invasion suppressor"). Also regulates beta-catenin levels.
Neurofibromatosis type 2	Acoustic neuromas	Meningioma, gliomas, ependymomas	AD	22q12	NF2	Links cell membrane proteins to cytoskeleton. Cell adhesion and coordination of growth factor receptor signalling.
Cowden syndrome	Breast cancer, thyroid cancer	Endometrial cancer macrocephaly, mucocutaneous lesions	AD	10q23	PTEN	Lipid and protein phosphatase
Peutz-Jeghers syndrome	Upper and lower intestinal polyps with risk of maligant change.	Melanin spots on lips and peri-oral region	AD	19p13	LKB1/STK11	Serine/threonine kinase

Fig. 13.5 Demonstration, using fluorescent PCR amplification of an intragenic polymorphic marker sequence, of partial loss of one allele of the *NF1* gene in the DNA of an unusual gastric tumour arising in an individual with an inherited *NF1* gene mutation. The tumour DNA PCR products are represented in red while the blood DNA PCR products are shown in blue. The results are consistent with reduced dosage of one allele (or allelic imbalance) in the tumour DNA, representing almost complete LOH.

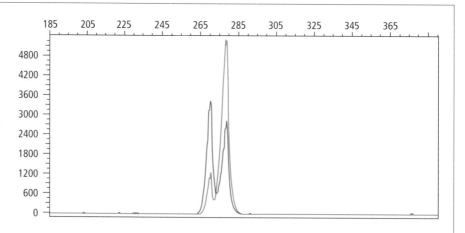

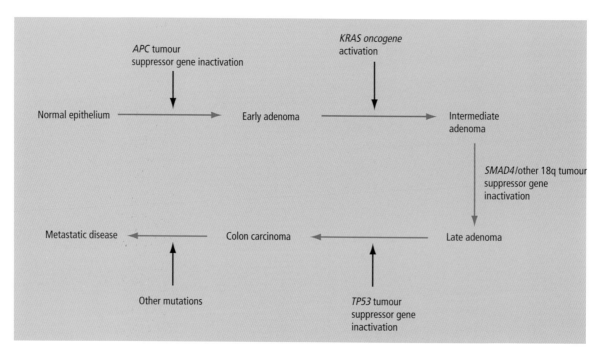

Fig. 13.6 Previously proposed model of stages in progression from normal colonic epithelium to metastatic cancer. More recent evidence suggests that this model is likely to be most applicable to only a minority of colonic carcinomas and would not be applicable to tumours arising in hereditary non-polyposis colon cancer (HNPCC).

sites. Tumours in this autosomal dominantly inherited syndrome, called Li–Fraumeni syndrome, include sarcomas of bone and soft tissues, in addition to leukaemia and tumours of the breast, brain, adrenal, pancreas and stomach.

For retinoblastoma, inactivating mutations at the retinoblastoma locus alone can produce cancer, but, for the majority of tumours, multiple cellular controls must be overcome with the consequent involvement of several loci (see Hanahan and Weinberg, 2000, in Further reading). Such multilocus participation in tumour progression has been clearly described for

colon cancer where at least three TSG loci and one oncogene locus are involved. Although the molecular genetic pathogenesis is undoubtedly more complex and variable than was described in the original linear multistage model proposed by Fearon and Vogelstein in 1990 (Fig. 13.6), the inactivation of the *APC* gene does indeed generally occur at an early stage and the model has provided a very useful basis for many further investigations. In hereditary non-polyposis colon cancer (HNPCC), however, there is a different initiating mechanism (see below).

Genes involved in DNA repair mechanisms

DNA repair systems exist to correct DNA damage due to environmental mutagens and also accidental base misincorporation at the time of DNA replication (see Chapter 3). Inherited defects of either system can result in an increased frequency of cancer.

Defects of the first type of DNA repair lead, for example, to the autosomal recessive disorders xeroderma pigmentosum (in which defective DNA excision repair after exposure to ultraviolet light results in multiple skin cancers and corneal scarring; see Fig. 3.16), *MUTYH*-associated polyposis (described below) and *BRCA1/BRCA2*-related familial breast/ovarian cancer. One of the most important roles of the *BRCA1* and *BRCA2* breast/ovarian cancer predisposition genes is in the accurate repair of double-strand breaks (see below) such as those resulting from ionising radiation or radiomimetic chemicals. If double-strand breaks are not repaired accurately, they can lead to mutations or to larger-scale genomic instability (e.g. with the formation of acrocentric or dicentric chromosome fragments) with consequent tumorigenicity.

For the second type of DNA repair mentioned above, several genes have been identified (e.g. *MSH2*, *MLH1*, *PMS1* and *PMS2*), the gene products of which normally interact to effect mismatch repair (see below). With somatic loss of the second (i.e. normal) allele of such a mismatch repair gene, the cell becomes prone to accumulate genetic mutations. One diagnostically important indicator of this, detectable in a laboratory, is that the pattern of microsatellite repeats at a polymorphic locus can differ from the surrounding normal tissue (an effect known as 'microsatellite instability').

Genes in this subclass of TSG are thus particularly commonly involved, when mutated, as the initiating factor in the more common high-penetrance inherited cancer syndromes (e.g. familial breast/ovarian cancer and hereditary non-polyposis colon cancer, described in more detail below).

Oncogenes

In contrast to TSGs, oncogenes are cancer genes in which mutations cause a gain of function, or overactivity, of the encoded protein. This gain of function is important, as many of these genes encode proteins that normally promote cell-cycle progression. Genetic alteration of one, rather than both, alleles is sufficient to confer a tumorigenic effect on the cell possessing it. While such mutations are common in the cells of tumours, they are much less commonly responsible for familial tumour susceptibility syndromes than inherited TSG alterations, such as those discussed below. The few notable inherited oncogenes that are associated with familial cancer include *RET* (associated with multiple endocrine neoplasia type 2; see Table 13.2) and *MET* (hereditary papillary renal cell carcinoma).

Oncogenes were first discovered by molecular analysis of oncogenic retroviruses that cause cancer in mice, cats and monkeys. For example, the *RAS* oncogene is derived from the Rous avian sarcoma virus, which causes a sarcoma in chickens. Each of these viral oncogenes (the name of which is often prefixed by '*v-*') was actually derived from a normal host gene by recombination between it and the ancestral viral genome. The normal host gene is not normally oncogenic and is usually termed a proto-oncogene (with the gene name sometimes prefixed by '*c-*' e.g. *c-MYC*). The presence of an activated oncogene can be demonstrated experimentally by showing that extracts of tumour DNA have the ability, when artificially introduced (e.g. by 'transfection') into a susceptible rodent cell line *in vitro*, to produce malignant clones.

At least 340 different proto-oncogenes have now been isolated and mapped to human chromosomes (see the Cancer Gene Census under Websites). These genes can be activated to cause cancer by point mutation or by an increase in the number of copies of the gene ('gene amplification'). The latter can occur by the generation of multiple repeats (of an oncogene such as *MYCN*), which are often cytogenetically visible in the form of homogeneously stained chromosomal regions or as a series of tiny fragments called double minutes (small paired extrachromosomal elements lacking centromeres; Fig. 13.7).

Comparison of the DNA sequence in proto-oncogenes in tumour tissue with the other somatic tissues has revealed that specific (somatic) point mutations can be associated with different tumour types. For example, in the *HRAS* gene, a glycine residue is normally present at position 12 but in some patients with bladder cancer, lung cancer or melanoma, the tumour tissue shows a point mutation (GGC to GTC) with substitution of valine at position 12. This change is not inherited but is a somatic mutation within the cells that initiate the cancer. Specific point mutations have also been identified at other critical positions (e.g. 13, 61 and 119) within *HRAS* and at different positions within other proto-oncogenes.

Human proto-oncogenes can also be activated as a result of chromosome rearrangements (which are often characteristic of particular tumour types). A well-known example of the latter mechanism is that observed in chronic myeloid leukaemia (CML) and the Philadelphia chromosome. Approximately 95% of affected patients show this chromosome (a smaller-than-normal chromosome 22) within the malignant bone marrow (but not in the unaffected somatic tissues). It is formed by a reciprocal translocation between chromosomes 9 (usually the paternal copy) and 22 (usually the maternal copy) (Fig. 13.8). As a result of this translocation, the *ABL* (tyrosine kinase-encoding) proto-oncogene is translocated from its normal site at 9q34 to chromosome 22q11. There, it becomes juxtaposed to a specific sequence called the breakpoint cluster region (*BCR*). As a result, the *BCR–ABL* hybrid gene encodes a novel chimaeric protein in CML cells, which, on account of its constitutive (i.e. persistent) activity, is believed to be responsible for the neoplastic transformation. The tumorigenic tyrosine kinase fusion protein is the target of one of the first licensed molecularly targeted drugs, known as STI571,

Fig. 13.7 A metaphase spread showing double minutes (some arrowed).

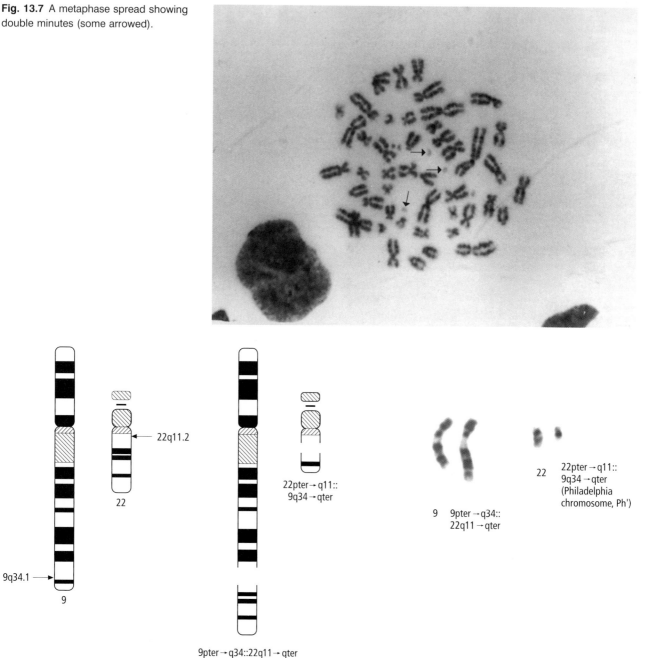

Fig. 13.8 Philadelphia chromosome (Ph') resulting from a reciprocal translocation between chromosomes 9 and 22, specifically t(9;22) (q34;q11).

imatinib mesylate or Glivec (Gleevec in the USA). This compound, which was identified by rapidly testing a very large number of chemical compounds to specifically find a tyrosine kinase inhibitor, therefore represents an exciting major shift in the development of cancer therapeutic agents.

The proteins encoded by many proto-oncogenes are now known to function in pathways regulating cell growth and proliferation by growth factors (see Vogelstein and Kinzler, 2004, in Further reading). Perhaps not surprisingly therefore, cancer genetics and developmental genetics have been linked by the finding that the inheritance of mutations of certain proto-oncogenes can also result in developmental abnormalities. For example, congenital anomalies such as polydactyly can be caused by mutations of different *HOX* (or 'homeobox') genes, a class of transcription factors that are involved in developmental patterning in many species ranging from *Drosophila* to humans. In particular, these genes specify the identity of body segments along the antero-posterior axis (see Hueber and Lohmann, 2008, in Further reading). Mutations in these *HOX* genes can also predispose to leukaemia, as the genes are also regulators of proliferation of haematopoietic cells.

Other cancer-related genes

A large number of other genes (risk 'modifier' genes or genes having individually relatively minor effects on risk) are also involved in the predisposition to cancer by virtue of their roles in processes such as the metabolism of carcinogens. For example, the risk of bladder cancer has for many years been known to be increased in aniline dye workers who are slow metabolisers of isoniazid. This is now known to result from polymorphisms in the *N*-acetyltransferase (*NAT2*) gene. Similarly, carriers of the I1307K polymorphism in the *APC* gene have a 1.5–2-fold increased risk of colorectal cancer. Genome-wide analyses of thousands of cases and controls are now revealing an increasing number of genes in which sequence variants increase the risk of specific cancers. For instance, an increased risk of breast cancer is now known to result from the possession of specific polymorphisms in the *FGFR2*, *TNRC9* or *MAP3K1* gene (see Antoniou *et al.*, 2008, in Further reading).

Genetic counselling aspects of cancer

In the following sections, the key points for genetic counselling of patients with common cancers and their families are summarised and additional information is provided in Further reading. In general, when only one individual is affected in a family and provided that the proband has a unifocal, late-onset tumour that is of a common type, the recurrence risk for other relatives is low. A cancer family syndrome (site-specific or non-specific) should be suspected, however, if there is a positive family history or if the proband has early-onset, multifocal or multiple primary tumours. Although only around 2–5% of cases of the common cancers (e.g. breast and colorectal) follow a Mendelian inheritance pattern, the number of families involved greatly exceeds the total number of families affected by the many different rare tumour predisposition syndromes (such as multiple endocrine neoplasia).

Common familial cancer predisposition syndromes

Over 300 single-gene traits have cancer as a recognised complication, but in this section, only the commoner and clinically most important of these are outlined. Additional information is provided in Tables 13.1 and 13.2 and can be sought from the Further reading references. An excellent further source of clinical information is the book written by Hodgson *et al.* (2006) and the online freely accessible detailed and regularly updated database of GeneReviews (see Further reading). Approximate figures are given below for the risks of individual cancer types in different predisposing syndromes and for the mutation frequencies. It should be noted that the figures stated in the many relevant published research articles and thus in textbooks tend to vary according to how different studies were performed. Penetrance calculations vary, for example, by the precise clinical criteria used, the nature of the population studied and the methods of analysis used.

Breast and ovarian cancer

The female lifetime risk of breast cancer is around 1 in 9 in the UK and the disease is dominantly inherited in around 2–5% of cases overall. Familial (clearly dominantly inherited) breast cancer is most often found to be due to mutations in the *BRCA1* (inherited breast cancer type 1) or *BRCA2* gene. In contrast, a small minority of such families are due to Li–Fraumeni syndrome (see above), Cowden disease (caused by mutations in the *PTEN* gene), Peutz–Jeghers syndrome (with mutations in the *STK11* gene) and other rare single-gene disorders. Inherited breast cancer should be suspected if there is an early age of onset (under 40 years), bilateral disease, coexistent ovarian cancer or a family history of breast cancer or ovarian cancer. As mentioned above, details of the criteria that can be used to identify those patients for whom referral to a clinical genetics centre is appropriate are available online (e.g. see the West of Scotland referral guidelines under Websites).

The female lifetime risk for ovarian cancer is 1 in 60–70 in the UK and North America. Mutations in *BRCA1* or *BRCA2* cause 60 and 25% of hereditary ovarian cancer, respectively (see Hodgson *et al.*, 2006, in Further reading). Such mutations and other hereditary causes should be suspected in the presence of an early age of onset (under 50 years), bilateral disease or a family history of ovarian and/or breast cancer. Alternatively, a mutation in the HNPCC genes *MLH1* or *MSH2* may be found if, in addition to ovarian cancer, there is a family history of colorectal or endometrial tumours (see below). Rare causes include Cowden disease, Peutz–Jeghers syndrome and Gorlin syndrome (with *PTCH* gene mutations).

The *BRCA1* and *BRCA2* genes

Mutations in either of these genes result in a highly penetrant autosomal dominant predisposition to breast cancer and, to a lesser extent, ovarian cancer.

Female carriers of *BRCA1* mutations have a high risk of both breast cancer (reported risk of 65% by 70 years; 95% confidence interval (CI) 44–78%; see the meta-analysis of 22 studies by Antoniou *et al.*, 2003, in Further reading) and ovarian cancer (39% by 70 years; CI 18–54%). Carriers of *BRCA2* mutations also have a high risk of breast cancer in females (45% by 70 years; CI 31–56%) but a lower risk of

Fig. 13.9 Diagram showing selected interactions and functional regions of the BRCA1 protein. The protein is large, comprising 1863 amino acids, and is believed to participate in the repair of double-strand breaks in DNA via its interaction with RAD50, NBS1 and MRE11. Several additional interactions have been described for the protein, a number of which are indicated. The interaction with BRCA2 may occur directly, through the BRCA1 C-terminal (BRCT) domains and/or via RAD51. Following double-strand DNA breaks, ATM protein phosphorylates BRCA1 at its clusters of serines and threonines within the SQ cluster domains.

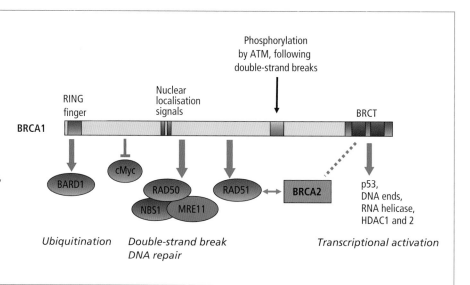

ovarian cancer (11%; CI 2.4–19%; Antoniou *et al.*, 2003), although other studies have reported the latter risk to be as high as 27% (see Antoniou *et al.*, 2009, in Further reading). Generally, these reported penetrances of *BRCA1* and *BRCA2* mutations appear to be significantly lower when calculated using cases that were not selected by family history (Antoniou *et al.*, 2003) than when calculated using families containing only multiple cases of cancer. In such families, the penetrance figures at the upper end of each calculated range are likely to be applicable. This difference is probably at least partly the result of the presence of additional risk-modifying gene alterations in the multiple-case families, as well as shared environmental exposure.

Carriers of mutations in *BRCA2* are at increased risk of developing a wider range of tumours than *BRCA1* mutation carriers. Other cancer types for which the risks are increased in carriers of *BRCA2* mutations include malignant melanoma (2.6-fold increase), prostate (4.6-fold), pancreatic (3.5-fold), gall-bladder and bile duct (5.0-fold) and stomach (2.6-fold) (figures reported by the Breast Cancer Linkage Consortium, 1999). In addition, males possessing *BRCA2* mutations have a risk of breast cancer of around 6% by 70 years.

The BRCA1 *and* BRCA2 *proteins*

BRCA1 and BRCA2 are both very large nuclear proteins that have been found, in the laboratory, to have several biological roles, including DNA repair, transcriptional regulation of other genes and cell-cycle regulation. In relation to tumour predisposition, it appears that the most important function for BRCA1, and probably also for BRCA2, is the maintenance of genomic integrity. This is achieved by the proteins' roles in promoting the potentially error-free form of DNA double-strand break repair known as homologous recombination in preference to error-prone, potentially mutagenic, mechanisms

such as non-homologous end joining and single-strand annealing. Both BRCA1 and BRCA2 facilitate the homologous recombination type of repair by participating in a common pathway and by binding to other proteins, including an important DNA recombinase known as RAD51 (Fig. 13.9). Knowledge of this pathway has led to the development of new molecularly targeted drugs such as PARP1 inhibitors, which promote apoptosis and may prove to be beneficial in the treatment of cancers in *BRCA1* or *BRCA2* mutation carriers (see Rodon *et al.*, 2009, in Further reading).

Mutation detection

A wide variety of different inherited mutations in *BRCA1* and *BRCA2* have been reported, most of which cause truncation (and thus loss of function) of the protein. A limited number have been found recurrently. For instance, several founder mutations have been identified in different populations, including the 185delAG and 5382insC *BRCA1* and the 6174delT *BRCA2* mutations in individuals of Ashkenazi Jewish origin, the 999del15 *BRCA2* mutation in Iceland, and the 5382insC, C61G and 4153delA *BRCA1* mutations in Poland. Mutation analysis to detect a possible mutation in *BRCA1* or *BRCA2* can be carried out by automated DNA sequencing (see Chapter 4) when it is possible to obtain a blood DNA sample from an affected member of the family. Such DNA sequencing of entire gene-coding sequences may be preceded, if appropriate, by DNA analyses targeting specific founder mutations. The selection of families with the most significant family history of breast/ovarian cancer and thus the greatest likelihood of possessing a *BRCA1* or *BRCA2* mutation can be facilitated by the use of computer analysis or more simply by a manual scoring method such as the Manchester scoring system (see Evans *et al.*, 2009, in Further reading for a recent version).

Cancer prevention and early detection

Once such a cancer-predisposing mutation has been identified in a family, asymptomatic gene carriers can be detected, following appropriate counselling, using direct DNA analysis for the specific familial mutation. Individuals who are carriers can then be offered regular clinical screening. Surveillance methods (for those individuals at high risk) for breast cancer currently include regular self-examination, clinical breast examination, mammography and, where available, magnetic resonance imaging (MRI). The latter has now been shown to be a more sensitive means of breast cancer detection than mammography in *BRCA1* or *BRCA2* mutation carriers. For ovarian cancer, trials are underway to evaluate surveillance methods such as serum CA-125 measurement and ultrasound scanning.

Those individuals who are found to possess a pathogenic mutation in *BRCA1* or *BRCA2* can be offered prophylactic surgery, such as bilateral mastectomies, which reduces the cancer risk by at least 90%. Prophylactic removal of the ovaries (usually together with the Fallopian tubes) reduces the risk of ovarian cancer by 80–96% while also reducing the breast cancer risk by 50–55% when undertaken prior to the menopause. Primary peritoneal cancer remains a residual risk, however, despite such surgery. Trials are currently underway to assess the value of risk-reducing drugs, such as those that reduce the synthesis, or the cellular response to, oestrogen. Large studies are also being undertaken to determine the additional factors that may affect an individual's chance of developing breast or ovarian cancer. For instance, a late menarche, having children and breastfeeding each appear to reduce the chance of developing breast cancer, while taking the combined oral contraceptive pill reduces the chance of developing ovarian cancer.

Colorectal cancer

The population risk for colorectal cancer is 1 in 50 in the UK. In most cases, environmental factors play a predominant role in the aetiology, but it has been estimated that genetic susceptibility accounts for 5–10% of colorectal cancers. Only around 2–3% of all colorectal cancers, however, occur as a result of a recognised highly penetrant autosomal dominantly or autosomal recessively inherited syndrome. Most dominantly inherited colorectal cancer is due to hereditary non-polyposis colon cancer (HNPCC), also known as Lynch syndrome (see below). In contrast, familial adenomatous polyposis (FAP) is rarer and accounts for less than 1% of all cases. More recently, an autosomal recessive syndrome, *MUTYH*-associated polyposis (MAP), has been described, with a phenotype like the attenuated form of FAP.

Inherited colon cancer should be suspected if many polyps are present (typical of FAP and MAP; see below), if there is an early age of onset or multifocal cancer, or if there is a family history of colorectal or other related cancers such as endometrial cancer. If no helpful information on the proband is available, the lifetime risk to first-degree relatives is approximately 1 in 17, rising to 1 in 10 if the proband was under 45 years of age at presentation. If a first- and a second-degree relative are affected, the risk is 1 in 12, and if two first-degree relatives are affected the risk is 1 in 6.

Hereditary non-polyposis colon cancer (Lynch syndrome)

The diagnosis of HNPCC syndromes on a clinical basis alone is problematic on account of the fact that there is a likelihood of colorectal cancer clustering within families by chance alone. Various sets of diagnostic criteria for the syndrome have been devised (e.g. see Umar, 2004, in Further reading for a review) and, as for breast and ovarian cancer, less stringent criteria have been formulated (see Websites) to guide the selection of patients for referral to the clinical genetics service.

In HNPCC, there is familial clustering of colorectal and related tumours. Colorectal tumours are common in HNPCC (in 80–90% of males and 40% of females with the condition) and tend to be right-sided (in 65% compared with 25% of sporadic tumours). Another common tumour type in this syndrome is endometrial carcinoma (in 40–60% of affected females). Less common primary tumour sites in HNPCC families are the stomach, pancreas, ovary, kidney and brain. DNA analysis of tumours generally shows microsatellite instability. Despite the name of the condition, polyps (adenomas) may be present, but there are usually less than ten and almost never more than 50, in contrast to FAP (see below) in which there are typically more than 100. Investigation of an individual's tumour material may be helpful, as microsatellite instability (variation in the lengths of microsatellite sequences relative to those in the blood DNA due to a failure to correct replication errors; see below) is a feature that is present in >90% of HNPCC-related tumours but in only 15% of sporadic cases. Furthermore, loss of a mismatch repair protein may be demonstrated in an HNPCC-related tumour using immunohistochemistry with antibodies specific for the individual mismatch repair proteins.

Familial adenomatous polyposis (polyposis coli, Gardner syndrome)

This autosomal dominant syndrome, which has a frequency of 1 in 8000, is characterised by the development of numerous (characteristically more than 100) intestinal polyps (especially in the colon) from early childhood and congenital hyperplasia of the retinal pigment epithelium (CHRPE) (Fig. 13.10). The intestinal polyps are adenomas and, if untreated, almost all affected individuals will develop colorectal cancer by the age of 40 as a result of malignant transformation of the colorectal polyps. There is also an increased risk of upper gastrointestinal tract cancer. Presymptomatic detection is possible by demonstration of CHRPE (in families that show this feature) and, more reliably, by direct DNA analysis to detect a known pathogenic mutation already identified in an affected family member.

Additional abnormalities, particularly in the variant of FAP known as Gardner syndrome, include epidermoid cysts (especially on the scalp) and osteomas on the mandible. In addition, some specific mutations of the *APC* gene can cause a less severe polyposis, known as attenuated FAP (AFAP) in which the number of polyps (15–100 with a mean of 30) aisre intermediate between HNPCC and FAP. There is relatively early-onset colorectal cancer but it occurs later than in classical FAP.

MUTYH-*associated* (MYH-*associated*) *polyposis*

A phenotype similar to AFAP, with 15–200 polyps, is now known to result from mutations in the *MUTYH* gene although this *MUTYH*-associated polyposis (MAP), as mentioned above, is autosomal *recessively* inherited.

Genes and mutations in hereditary colorectal cancer

HNPCC shows locus heterogeneity and can be caused by mutations in one of at least four gene loci (*MSH2* (60%), *MLH1* (30%), *MSH6* and, more rarely, *PMS2*) that were identified predominantly by linkage analysis of large affected families. The function of the proteins encoded by the genes associated with this condition is to form protein complexes at DNA mismatches (following DNA replication) and to trigger the enzymatic repair of the mismatch (Fig. 13.11). Heterozygous mutations in *MSH2*, *MLH1* or *MSH6* give rise to an autosomal dominantly inherited cancer predisposition, with incomplete penetrance (especially in females). As mentioned above, colorectal tumours from affected individuals show microsatellite instability and usually, on immunohistochemistry, loss of staining for a mismatch repair protein. Mutant gene carriers can be identified by DNA analysis and these gene carriers can be offered regular colonoscopy.

A specific nucleotide substitution in exon 15 of the *BRAF* gene, resulting in a valine to glutamate change at amino acid 600 (i.e. a p.V600E mutation) is commonly found as a somatic change in cutaneous malignant melanomas. The same mutation has recently been reported to be a useful indicator of *sporadic* (versus *HNPCC*-related) colorectal cancers when it is detected in tumours that exhibit microsatellite instability.

It is now apparent that *homozygous* mutations in *MSH2*, *MLH1*, *MSH6* or *PMS2* appear to cause an autosomal recessive childhood cancer syndrome rather than classical HNPCC. Affected children may instead develop a brain tumour, leukaemia or lymphoma, together with the café au lait patches that are more typical of neurofibromatosis type 1 (NF1). Supratentorial primitive neuroectodermal tumour (PNET) is a very rare brain tumour that appears to be particularly associated with homozygous mutations in the *PMS2* gene.

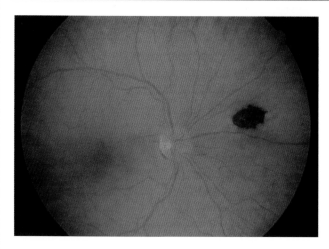

Fig. 13.10 CHRPE in FAP. Reproduced from Tobias, ES, and Connor, JM, 2008. Genetic counselling for childhood tumors and inherited cancer predisposing syndromes. In The Surgery of Childhood Tumors, 2nd edn, pp. 33–48. Edited by Carachi R, Grosfeld JL and Azmy AF. Springer. With kind permission of Springer Science + Business Media.

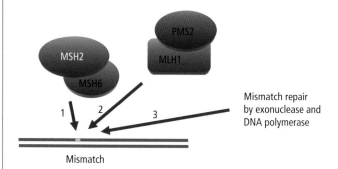

Fig. 13.11 Human mismatch repair system. Repair of mismatched bases following DNA replication involves several proteins and steps. The mismatch is initially bound by the heterodimer composed of MSH2 and MSH6. This is followed by binding of MLH1 and PMS2 to form a complex that then triggers an exonuclease to digest the newly synthesised strand, allowing DNA polymerase to resynthesise the strand with the correct base sequence.

Familial adenomatous coli, in contrast, is caused by mutations in the adenomatous polyposis coli (*APC*) TSG. The APC protein plays an important physiological role in the regulation of the levels of a transcriptional cofactor named β-catenin (Fig. 13.12). Multiple different mutations are found, but commonly they result in protein truncation and a 5 bp deletion of AAAGA at codon 1309 (c.3927_3931delAAAGA) is the most frequent of all the *APC* mutations. *APC* mutations in Gardner syndrome are generally located towards the 3′ end of the gene. Mutant gene carriers require regular colonoscopy and consideration of prophylactic bowel surgery at an early stage.

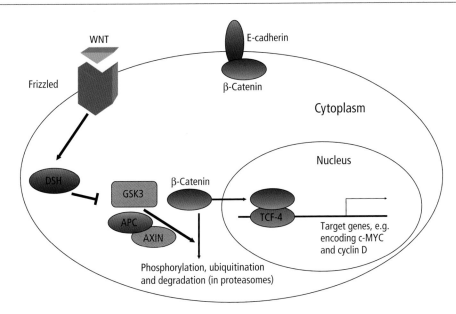

Fig. 13.12 Simplified illustration of the physiological role of APC protein in the WNT pathway. The APC protein, together with AXIN and GSK3, cooperate in preventing overaccumulation of the transcriptional cofactor β-catenin by promoting its phosphorylation, ubiquitination (molecular marking of the protein for subsequent breakdown) and degradation in the proteasome. Physiological WNT signaling or mutational APC (or AXIN) inactivation therefore both lead to inhibition of the phosphorylation of β-catenin, and thus result in increased levels of this transcriptional coactivator. β-Catenin is also bound by the cell–cell adhesion protein, E-cadherin. The inactivation of E-cadherin (as occurs in hereditary diffuse gastric cancer) can therefore lead not only to reduced cell–cell adhesion but also to an increase in free β-catenin.

In attenuated AFAP, mentioned above, the mutations in *APC* are often located towards the 5′ or 3′ ends of the gene and the condition is again autosomal dominantly inherited.

The gene that is mutated in individuals affected by the phenotypically similar but autosomal recessive condition *MUTYH*-associated polyposis (MAP) is the *MUTYH* gene. This gene, which was previously known as *MYH*, encodes a glycosylase that is necessary for base excision repair following oxidative DNA damage, particularly the repair of an A–oxoG pair.

Prevention and early detection

Those individuals with a significantly increased risk of developing colorectal cancer can be offered appropriate screening in order to detect such tumours at an early stage. This may take the form, for instance, of a colonoscopy every 2 years from the age of 25 (for HNPCC), with the frequency of screening taking into account the small risk of adverse effects of screening (such as bowel perforation). Those at increased risk of endometrial cancer (e.g. female carriers of a mismatch repair gene mutation) may be offered screening by annual transvaginal ultrasound scanning and annual endometrial biopsies (aiming to detect the pre-cancerous endometrial lesion known as complex atypical hyperplasia). Currently, a study is underway in the UK to evaluate the possible benefit of an intrauterine device containing progestogen (the Mirena coil) in preventing endometrial cancer in such women. Women with HNPCC may also consider the option of prophylactic hysterectomy, in view of their risk of developing endometrial cancer being even higher than for colorectal cancer.

In individuals at high risk of FAP, genetic testing should be offered if a mutation has been identified in the family, and clinical screening such as annual bowel examination (initially by annual sigmoidoscopy) from the age of 11 may be offered. Prophylactic colectomy is usually undertaken in affected individuals at around the age of 16–20 or when more than 20–30 adenomas have developed. Those with AFAP or MAP may be offered similar bowel surveillance to individuals with HNPCC (2-yearly colonoscopy). Studies of drugs that were suggested to have the potential to reduce the incidence of cancer prophylactically in those with HNPCC or FAP, such as non-steroidal anti-inflammatory drugs (NSAIDs), have been conducted, with recent results suggesting a possible long-term beneficial effect, but no such drug is yet licensed for this purpose in the UK.

SUMMARY

- Mendelian inheritance accounts for only around 2–5% of common cancers such as breast or colorectal cancer. In these cases, the pattern of inheritance is usually autosomal dominant with incomplete penetration and often with sex limitation.
- Careful family history taking is essential in determining which families possess a significant genetic cancer predisposition. Suggestive features include an early age of tumour onset, multiple primary tumours in an individual and multiple affected family members.
- Two principal classes of cancer genes exist: TSGs and oncogenes. Mutations in TSGs result in protein inactivation while mutations in the normal form of oncogenes (proto-oncogenes) typically result in a gain of function or increased activity of the encoded protein.
- Several TSGs that are important in familial cancer encode proteins that normally participate in DNA repair.

- For TSGs to exert their tumorigenic effect, they generally have to sustain inactivation of both alleles. This is the 'two-hit hypothesis'. The first hit may be inherited while the second hit may occur through, for example, deletion, recombination or epigenetic transcriptional repression.
- Pathogenic mutations in *BRCA1* and *BRCA2* cause breast and ovarian cancer. The presence of male breast cancer in an affected family suggests a *BRCA2* mutation.
- Mutations in the mismatch repair genes *MLH1*, *MSH2*, *MSH6* or *PMS2* cause HNPCC.
- FAP is an autosomal dominant condition caused by mutations in the *APC* gene (resulting in overactivity of the WNT signalling pathway). It typically results in the presence of over 100 colorectal polyps and a tendency to develop cancer at an early age.
- The phenotype of MAP is similar to that of attenuated FAP. MAP, however, is autosomal recessively inherited and results from defective base excision repair.

FURTHER READING

Antoniou A, Pharoah PD, Narod S, Risch HA, Eyfjord JE, Hopper JL, Loman N, Olsson H, Johannsson O, *et al.* (2003) Average risks of breast and ovarian cancer associated with *BRCA1* or *BRCA2* mutations detected in case series unselected for family history: a combined analysis of 22 studies. *Am J Hum Genet* **72**:1117–30.

Antoniou AC, Spurdle AB, Sinilnikova OM, Healey S, Pooley KA, Schmutzler RK, Versmold B, Engel C, Meindl A, *et al.* (2008) Common breast cancer-predisposition alleles are associated with breast cancer risk in *BRCA1* and *BRCA2* mutation carriers. *Am J Hum Genet* **82**:937–48.

Antoniou AC, Rookus M, Andrieu N, Brohet R, Chang-Claude J, Peock S, Cook M, Evans DG, Eeles R. *et al.* (2009) Reproductive and hormonal factors, and ovarian cancer risk for *BRCA1* and *BRCA2* mutation carriers: results from the International *BRCA1/2* Carrier Cohort Study. *Cancer Epidemiol Biomarkers Prev* **18**:601–10.

Cuzick J, Otto F, Baron JA, Brown PH, Burn J, Greenwald P, Jankowski J, La Vecchia C, Meyskens F. *et al.* (2009) Aspirin and non-steroidal anti-inflammatory drugs for cancer prevention: an international consensus statement. *Lancet Oncol* **10**:501–7.

Evans DG, Lalloo F, Cramer A (2009) Addition of pathology and biomarker information significantly improves the performance of the Manchester scoring system for *BRCA1* and *BRCA2* testing. *J Med Genet* **46**:811–17.

Fearon ER, Vogelstein B (1990) A genetic model for colorectal tumorigenesis. *Cell* **61**:759–67.

Hanahan D, Weinberg RA (2000) The hallmarks of cancer. *Cell* **100**:57–70.

Hodgson S, Foulkes W, Eng C, Maher E (2006) *A Practical Guide to Human Cancer Genetics*, 3rd edn. Cambridge University Press:Cambridge. [An excellent detailed guide to the clinical aspects of inherited cancer predisposition syndromes.]

Hueber SD, Lohmann I (2008) Shaping segments: *Hox* gene function in the genomic age. *Bioessays* **30**:965–79.

Rodon J, Iniesta MD, Papadopoulos K (2009) Development of PARP inhibitors in oncology. *Expert Opin Investig Drugs* **18**:31–43.

Tobias ES (2006) Molecular biology of cancer. In *Emery and Rimoin's Principles and Practice of Medical Genetics*, 5th ed. Elsevier:London.

Umar A, Risinger JI, Hawk ET, Barrett JC (2004) Testing guidelines for hereditary non-polyposis colorectal cancer. *Nat Rev Cancer* **4**:153–8.

Vogelstein B, Kinzler KW (2004) Cancer genes and the pathways they control. *Nat Med* **10**:789–799. [A well-illustrated overview of the molecular biology underlying cancer syndromes.]

William WN Jr, Heymach JV, Kim ES, Lippman SM (2009) Molecular targets for cancer chemoprevention. *Nat Rev Drug Discov* **8**:213–25.

WEBSITES

Cancer Genetic Services in Scotland – Management of Women with a Family History of Breast Cancer (Guidelines, 2009):

http://www.sehd.scot.nhs.uk/mels/CEL2009_06.pdf

Cancer Gene Census website at the Wellcome Trust Sanger Institute (with a downloadable list of cancer genes and their properties):

(http://www.sanger.ac.uk/genetics/CGP/Census/)

Example referral criteria for breast, colorectal and ovarian cancer family histories for the West of Scotland cancer genetics clinics:

http://www.nhsggc.org.uk/content/default.asp?page=s1154_3

Online Mendelian Inheritance in Man (OMIM) genetics database:

http://www.ncbi.nlm.nih.gov/sites/entrez?db=omim

Scottish Intercollegiate Guidelines Network (SIGN): genetic aspects of management of colorectal cancer:

http://www.sign.ac.uk/guidelines/fulltext/67/section4.html

Self-assessment

1. Which of the following is a true statement regarding proto-oncogenes?
A. They are only expressed in malignant tissues
B. The tumorigenic activity of a proto-oncogene usually requires the loss or mutation of both alleles of the gene
C. They inactivate oncogenes
D. They include *MLH1*
E. They participate in the cellular response to growth factors

2. With regard to tumour suppressor genes (TSGs), which of the following are true statements?
A. Tumorigenic mutations in TSGs usually result in a loss of function
B. TSGs encode proteins that usually suppress apoptosis
C. TSGs encode proteins that, in general, promote mitosis
D. TSGs include the *c-MYC* gene
E. TSGs include the genes responsible for hereditary non-polyposis colon cancer (HNPCC) and neurofibromatosis type 1 (NF1)

3. With regard to p53, which of the following is untrue?
A. It can cause cell-cycle arrest
B. It is a cell-membrane tyrosine kinase
C. Inactivating mutations of the gene promote tumorigenesis
D. It is often activated following DNA damage
E. It induces apoptosis

4. With regard to the scenario in Fig. 13.13, which of the following genes is most likely to be mutated in the blood DNA of the 27-year-old woman's older sister?
A. *NF1*
B. *APC*
C. *BRCA1*
D. *RB1*
E. *MUTYH*

5. In the scenario given in Fig. 13.13, if the elder sister's DNA is tested and found to possess a mutation in this gene, then which of the following most closely approximates the younger sister's risk (up to age 70) of developing breast cancer herself, prior to genetic testing of her own DNA?
A. 100%
B. 80%
C. 50%

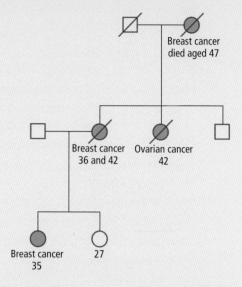

Fig. 13.13 A 27-year-old woman attends the genetics clinic seeking advice. She is the sister of a woman who developed breast cancer at the age of 35. Their mother developed breast cancer aged 36 and again, in the other breast, aged 42. Their maternal aunt was diagnosed with ovarian cancer at the age of 42 and their maternal grandmother died of breast cancer at the age of 47. See Questions 4 and 5 in the Self-assessment.

D. 40%
E. 10%

6. With regard to familial breast cancer, which of the following is true?
A. An inherited mutation in *TP53* is as likely to be the cause as an inherited mutation in *BRCA2*
B. Both alleles of the responsible gene are likely to inactivated in the tumour cells
C. Individuals from families in which one or more males (as well as females) have developed breast cancer have a higher chance of having a *BRCA2* mutation than a *BRCA1* mutation
D. BRCA1 and BRCA2 proteins promote the non-homologous end-joining form of DNA repair
E. *BRCA1* is more frequently associated with pancreatic cancer and malignant melanoma than *BRCA2*

7. In the scenario outlined in Fig. 13.14, which of the following is the most likely underlying family diagnosis?
A. Familial adenomatous polyposis (FAP)
B. Cowden syndrome
C. Gardner syndrome
D. Hereditary non-polyposis colon cancer (HNPCC)
E. Peutz–Jeghers syndrome

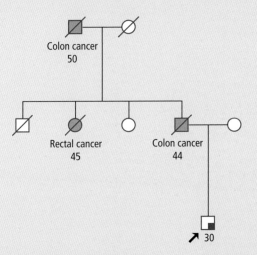

Fig. 13.14 A 30-year-old man is found to have four adenomatous polyps in the sigmoid colon at colonoscopy. He mentions that his father died at the age of 45 with colon cancer (after having been diagnosed at 44), his paternal aunt was treated for rectal cancer at 45 and his paternal grandfather was treated for colon cancer at 50. He asks about the likely underlying cause of the cancers occurring in the family. See Q7 and Q8 in Self-assessment.

8. In the family in Fig. 13.14, if it were possible to test the stored blood DNA from the affected father, which of the following genes would be most likely to contain a mutation?
A. *STK11*
B. *APC*
C. *PTEN*
D. *MUTYH*
E. *MLH1* or *MSH2*

9. Which of the following is true regarding hereditary colorectal cancer?
A. Regular sigmoidoscopy is an effective means of screening for early tumours in HNPCC
B. Congenital hyperplasia of the retinal pigment epithelium (CHRPE) is a retinal lesion that is typically found in HNPCC
C. Women possessing an inherited mutation in a mismatch repair gene possess a significant risk of endometrial cancer
D. Attenuated familial adenomatous polyposis (AFAP) and *MUTYH*-associated polyposis (MAP) are both inherited in an autosomal dominant fashion
E. The presence of microsatellite instability in the tumour tissue DNA suggests that the cause of the bowel tumour is a defect in the base excision repair pathway (e.g. due to a *MUTYH* gene mutation)

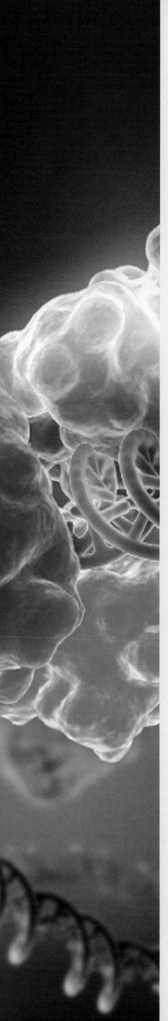

CHAPTER 14
Family history of common adult-onset disorder

Key Topics

Introduction

This chapter will focus on those medical conditions, such as diabetes mellitus and dementia, that commonly occur with an adult onset. Information regarding the predominantly multifactorial aetiology of such conditions is provided, together with details of the much less common subtypes, such as maturity-onset diabetes of the young, in which Mendelian inheritance is observed.

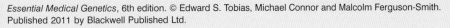

General principles

Common conditions, that is those with a population frequency of greater than 1 in 1000, generally do not follow any clear Mendelian patterns of inheritance. In most cases, they are multifactorial, resulting from a combination of environmental, lifestyle, dietary and genetic factors. There may, as a result of shared genetic or lifestyle/environmental factors, be an apparent familial clustering of cases that can understandably lead to requests for genetic advice. Many specific low-penetrance gene variants that contribute to disease susceptibility are now being identified as a result of enormous research efforts employing large genetic association studies, analysing hundreds of thousands of genome-wide single-nucleotide polymorphisms (SNPs) in thousands of individuals (see Chapter 10). From the resulting data, it has become clear that the genetic contribution to most common adult-onset disorders (and most normal characteristics) is composed of a contribution from several genetic variants that each has a small predisposing effect. As a result, with the exception of a few specific subtypes (examples of which are described below and in Chapter 10), the inheritance of such phenotypic traits and conditions is non-Mendelian. This is despite the fact that the individual genetic variants conferring susceptibility would, if analysed at the DNA level, each be found to be transmitted (generally independently) in a Mendelian fashion.

In a similar manner to congenital malformations (see Chapter 18), in many common conditions of adult life, the threshold model for discontinuous multifactorial traits can be applied. In accordance with this model, the close relatives of an affected individual are at greatest risk, with the risk decreasing rapidly with increasing distance of relationship. Thus, the risks are usually small for second-degree relatives and, for more distantly related relatives, the risks are only rarely elevated significantly. As these conditions are not usually inherited in a dominant or recessive manner, the risks to siblings are often similar to those for offspring for these disorders. The younger the age of onset and the greater the number of affected relatives, the greater the risk to the relatives, due to an increased number of genetic susceptibility variants for that condition in the family. Risk estimation for these common conditions can be based upon published studies of how frequently a particular disease is observed to actually occur in relatives. These so-called 'empiric' risks are invaluable in counselling because calculating such risks would otherwise be very difficult, as the disease predisposition results from a complex combination of both environmental and genetic factors.

The knowledge of which genetic variants are carried by an individual may in the future lead to new ways of subclassifying disease and also to the tailoring of the pharmacological treatment of affected individuals to their genetic profiles. This field, known as pharmacogenetics, is an increasingly important research area for the pharmaceutical industry. For a range of medical conditions, it may ultimately permit the selection of particular drugs that are found to be more efficacious or that have reduced side effects in individuals with specific genetic polymorphisms or particular combinations of them.

In a small proportion of cases of many common disorders, however, the condition results from a mutation in a single gene of major effect. In these cases, which are important to identify, there is typically a lower age of onset and often a family history of similar cases. Depending on the specific gene involved, there may be associated clinical features that can provide diagnostic clues to these relatively rare causes of the common disorder. For instance, an unusual cause of dementia is Huntington disease (HD) (see below). In HD, the unusually early onset of dementia is associated with a movement disorder (chorea). Similarly, in the form of diabetes that results from mitochondrial mutations, there is often early-onset sensorineural deafness.

It is important, therefore, in evaluating the genetic contribution of such cases, to take a full three-generation family history, enquiring about the ages of onset and at death (or rate of progression) in affected relatives and the presence of additional clinical problems. Mendelian risks may be used with caution to counsel relatives in the few families where there is a clear autosomal dominant family history. Genetic testing may be appropriate to identify mutations in single genes of major effect in such cases, but testing for commoner gene variants of small effect is generally regarded in the UK as not appropriate except in specific ethically approved research studies. When requested, genetic testing of clinically unaffected individuals (i.e. presymptomatic testing) for known familial gene mutations should only be undertaken following full genetic counselling, which should include a discussion of possible future difficulties in obtaining medical or life insurance, following established protocols (see Harper, 2004).

Diabetes mellitus: common and monogenic forms

Type 2 diabetes mellitus, formerly known as non-insulin-dependent diabetes mellitus (NIDDM), is becoming increasingly common, affecting 7–10% of individuals in western countries. In contrast to type 1 diabetes (formerly known as insulin-dependent diabetes mellitus), which typically presents in the young between the ages of 10 and 13 years and which results from an autoimmune reaction against the β-cells of the pancreatic islets, type 2 diabetes generally presents in adulthood and results from insufficient insulin secretion together with insulin resistance. Both types of diabetes are multifactorial, with genetic and environmental contributions to their development, particularly obesity in type 2 diabetes. The contribution of genetic factors is, however, relatively more important in type 2 diabetes, for which the concordance rate in monozygotic twins is close to 100%, compared with 10% in dizygotic twins and 10% in other first-degree relatives.

In contrast to type 1 diabetes, there is no significant human leukocyte antigen (HLA) association in type 2 diabetes.

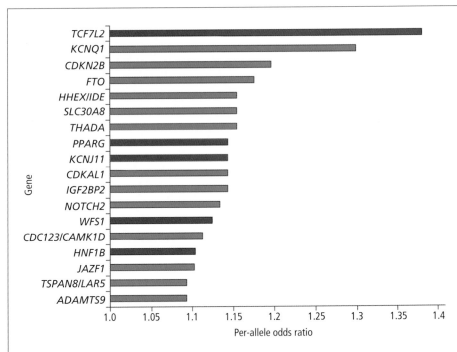

Fig. 14.1 Various loci associated with susceptibility to type 2 diabetes. The relatively small (estimated) effects (calculated as odds ratios) are indicated on the x-axis. Genes shown in blue were identified by genome-wide association studies, whereas those shown in red were found by analysing pre-selected genes. Modified from Prokopenko et al., 2008 Trends Genet. 24(12):613–22, with permission from Elsevier; see Further reading.

Instead, several relatively common predisposing genetic variants (Fig. 14.1) have now been identified, largely from the association studies mentioned above (see Lindgren and McCarthy, 2008, and Prokopenko *et al.*, 2008, in Further reading). The estimated relative effects (reflected in the calculated 'odds ratios') that are associated with the individual variant alleles are small but significant, ranging up to approximately 1.4-fold (Fig. 14.1). The genes involved include, for example, *FTO*, which reduces insulin action as a secondary effect, with the primary effect of its common variants being to influence adiposity. Variants in other genes, such as *TCF7L2*, *CDKAL1* and *KCNJ11*, also increase the risk of type 2 diabetes, but they do so by reducing the ability of the pancreas to secrete insulin. Of these genes, *TCF7L2* confers the highest increase in odds of developing type 2 diabetes (1.37-fold), with the 10% of Europeans who are homozygous for the variant having double the increase (Prokopenko *et al.*, 2008). This gene encodes a transcription factor involved in the WNT signalling pathway. In summary, it appears that the genetic component of type 2 diabetes is formed by the combination of many gene variants, each having a small effect (Fig. 14.2). In total, however, those common gene variants of small effect that have been identified to date account for only approximately 10% of the heritability of type 2 diabetes (see Bonnefond *et al.*, 2010, in Further Reading).

Genes of major effect and associated conditions

In addition to these common variants, a number of mutant genes of major effect have been identified that predispose to monogenic forms of type 2 diabetes. These, however, are indi-

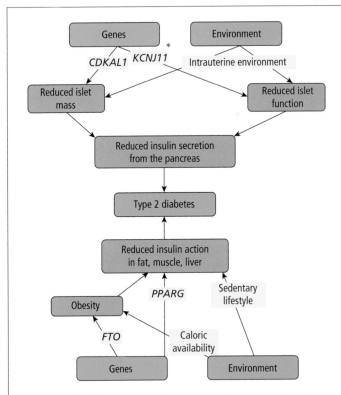

Fig. 14.2 Model for the role of environmental and genetic factors in the development of type 2 diabetes. **KCNJ11* and also *TCF7L2*, are genes whose variants are believed to result in a reduction in insulin secretion by causing diminished islet β-cell function. Modified from Prokopenko et al., 2008 Trends Genet. 24(12):613–22, with permission from Elsevier; see Further reading.

vidually very uncommon. These monogenic forms include maturity-onset diabetes of the young (MODY), mitochondrial diabetes and severe insulin resistance syndromes.

Maturity-onset diabetes of the young

Maturity-onset diabetes of the young (MODY), an autosomal dominant condition, is a form of type 2 diabetes that occurs in the absence of obesity and has an earlier age of onset, typically before the age of 25 years. Although mutations in at least five different genes can cause this condition, the total number of affected individuals together accounts for only 2% or less of patients with diabetes. The most commonly mutated MODY gene is the hepatocyte nuclear factor-1α (*HNF-1α*) gene, mutations in which account for around 70% of individuals affected by MODY. A less common but clinically similar form of MODY results from mutations affecting the *HNF-4α* gene. In contrast, mutations within or large genomic deletions encompassing the *HNF-1β* gene result in a combination of early-onset type 2 diabetes with renal cysts, genital tract malformations and early-onset gout. Mutations in the glucokinase gene can also cause MODY, but result in a mild form that does not require insulin treatment.

Mitochondrial diabetes

A typical maternal inheritance pattern may be observed, with an absence of transmission from the father. Progressive sensorineural deafness is also commonly present and often precedes the diabetes. The A3243G substitution is the most common causative mitochondrial mutation and all offspring of a mother who possesses the mutation will be at risk of developing mitochondrial diabetes, which typically culminates in insulin dependence. Several other mitochondrial DNA mutations are associated with diabetes.

Severe insulin resistance syndromes

In these relatively rare syndromes, in which there is loss of subcutaneous fat, there is typically, in addition to diabetes, severe insulin resistance and hyperlipidaemia. They include the very severe Donohue syndrome (previously known as 'leprechaunism'), an autosomal recessive disorder resulting from insulin receptor mutations, with an onset in infancy. Milder forms include the familial partial lipodystrophy caused by specific mutations in the gene *LMNA*, which encodes lamins A and C (protein components of the protein network that underlie the inner nuclear membrane). In this autosomal dominant condition, there is loss of adipose tissue from the limbs and trunk from puberty, but excess fat accumulation around the neck and face, with hypertriglyceridaemia. Interestingly, *LMNA* mutations can also cause several other quite different conditions, including Emery–Dreifuss muscular dystrophy, premature ageing, axonal neuropathy and myopathy.

Dementia: Alzheimer disease, Huntington disease, prion diseases and other causes

While some cases of dementia result from vascular disease, many are neurodegenerative disorders characterised by intra- and interneuronal aggregates of insoluble protein.

Alzheimer disease

This is the most common dementia (i.e. progressive cognitive impairment) affecting those over the age of 40 years. Other common causes include vascular dementia (due to repeated infarcts) and Lewy body dementia (with fluctuating cognitive impairment and psychiatric symptoms). Less common causes include frontotemporal dementia with Parkinsonism (see below) and Parkinson disease itself.

Alzheimer disease is a dementia that involves a slowly progressive failure of memory and, on neuroimaging, gross cerebral cortical atrophy. Histopathologically, there is neuronal loss, amyloid plaque deposition and the formation of aggregates of intracytoplasmic neurofibrillary tangles. The amyloid plaques are insoluble aggregates of β-amyloid fragments of amyloid precursor protein (see below), while the neurofibrillary tangles represent insoluble twisted fibres that are composed largely of abnormal tau protein. The condition is common in the general population with the lifetime risk being around 1 in 9. As a result of its high frequency, it is not uncommon (25%) by chance alone to have more than one case in a family. However, in only a small proportion of familial cases is there a strong genetic predisposition.

Genetic predisposition

Alzheimer disease is genetically heterogeneous. Approximately 1–3% of cases result from autosomal dominantly inherited single-gene mutations. These typically earlier-onset cases (i.e. before the age of 65) can occur in individuals who have a mutation in a gene of major effect, three of which have been identified. These include *PSEN1* (most commonly) and *PSEN2*, the protein products of which, presenilin 1 and presenilin 2, respectively, are involved in cleavage of the β-amyloid precursor protein. The gene that encodes β-amyloid precursor protein (*APP*) represents the third gene in which a mutation may be found in early-onset familial cases (Fig. 14.3). Mutations in any of these three genes result in excessive quantities of neurotoxic APP cleavage products such as amyloid β_{42} peptide, and subsequently amyloid plaques, deposited throughout the brain.

In contrast, the development of most cases, especially the common late-onset cases, are influenced by combinations of susceptibility gene variants. These include the ε4 allele of the apolipoprotein E (*APOE*) gene (which may determine the rate of clearance of amyloid from the brain and which has three variants, *APOE* ε2, ε3 and ε4). The ε4 allele is much more common in patients with Alzheimer disease than in controls,

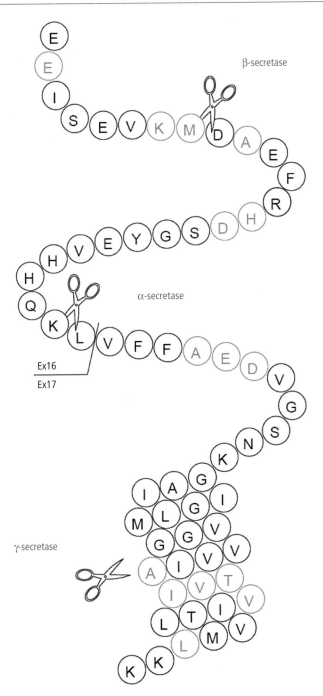

Fig. 14.3 Amino acid sequence encoded by exons 16 and 17 of APP. Red and green amino acids represent those for which there are reported pathogenic and non-pathogenic missense substitutions, respectively. Pathogenic mutations are frequently found close to secretase cleavage sites. Typical Alzheimer disease phenotypes result from mutations that affect the beta and gamma secretase cleavage sites, with the release of amyloid β42 peptide. Modified from Dermaut et al., 2005 Trends Genet. 21:664–72, with permission from Elsevier; see Further Reading.

and the degree of increase in risk of developing Alzheimer disease depends on whether an individual possesses zero, one or (rarely) two ε4 alleles of the gene. The ε2 allele may, in contrast, be protective. The magnitude of the increase in risk (relative risk) associated with different alleles is complex, controversial and can vary according to which population is sampled. The use of *APOE* genotyping is not currently regarded as appropriate in the genetic clinic.

Other forms of dementia

In contrast to the gradual memory loss that is typical of Alzheimer disease, a stepwise progression may indicate vascular dementia. More unusually, a history of stroke or transient ischaemic attacks and a family history may signify a condition known as cerebral autosomal dominant arteriopathy with subcortical infarcts and leukoencephalopathy (CADASIL), which results from mutations in the *NOTCH3* gene. The presence of an associated movement disorder may be indicative of HD (see below and Chapter 9) or of Parkinson disease.

Frontotemporal dementia with parkinsonism-17

Frontotemporal dementia with parkinsonism-17 (FTDP-17) typically manifests between the ages of 40 and 60, affecting principally the frontal and temporal cortex, and progressing over a few years to profound dementia with mutism. After Alzheimer disease, it is the second most common presenile dementia. Its inheritance is autosomal dominant and it is caused by mutations in the gene on chromosome 17 that encodes the microtubule-associated protein, tau, on chromosome 17. The tau protein is the main constituent of the neurofibrillary tangles that are found in Alzheimer disease.

Huntington disease

HD is an autosomal dominant condition with an onset typically between 30 and 50 years of age, and is characterised by progressive chorea (involuntary movements), dementia and psychiatric symptoms. Magnetic resonance imaging may reveal basal ganglia changes such as caudate atrophy. Neuropathological changes tend to lag behind the clinical manifestations but are specific, with atrophy of the small neurones in the caudate and putamen and of the large neurones in the globus pallidus.

The prognosis in HD is progressive disability with death occurring, on average, 17 years from the onset of the condition. In juvenile HD (accounting for 4–5% of cases), the onset is under the age of 20 years, with intellectual decline, seizures, rigidity, myoclonus and dystonia. In around 8% of HD, the onset is over the age of 60 years, with chorea and a slower progression. The diagnosis may be made clinically on the basis of symptoms, signs, family history and neuroimaging, with confirmation by molecular genetic testing.

The mechanism of inheritance of the condition is autosomal dominant with genetic anticipation (see Chapter 9). It

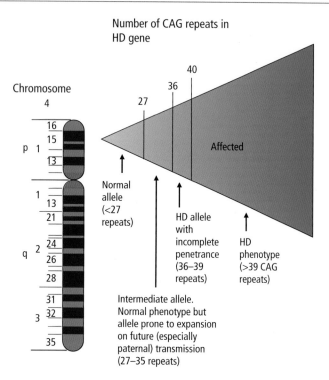

Number of CAG repeats in
HD gene

Fig. 14.4 Clinical effects of different numbers of CAG repeats within the Huntington disease (*HTT*) gene coding region.

is caused by an unstable length mutation in the huntingtin (*HTT*) gene on chromosome 4. In affected patients, the number of CAG trinucleotide repeats is increased from the normal range of 10–35 (median 18) to 36–120 copies (most commonly 40–55). There is a loose inverse correlation between the number of repeats and the age of onset, with this being most apparent for patients with juvenile HD, who typically have more than 60 repeats. Similarly, incomplete penetrance is observed when there are 36–39 repeats, i.e. at the low end of the affected range (see Fig. 14.4). The trinucleotide repeat tract is unstable during meiosis, with its size prone to increase during transmission from the father (see Fig. 9.1). As mentioned in Chapter 9, the CAG repeat region is located within the coding sequence and encodes a polyglutamine tract. It is believed that the neurotoxicity results from the tract's expansion causing the production of insoluble HTT protein aggregates or abnormal proteolytic fragments of the protein. It is now known that the intracellular mechanism for the clearance of the mutant HTT protein involves a process known as autophagy. The finding that this process can be upregulated experimentally by several drugs has suggested the possibility of a future therapy for the condition (see García-Arencibia *et al.*, 2010, in Further reading for a review).

Analysis of the repeat size is technically relatively straightforward by direct DNA analysis. This can be performed as a presymptomatic test in a clinically unaffected individual who has a family history of HD or, alternatively, in prenatal diagnosis. In the case of presymptomatic ('predictive') testing, fully informed written consent must be obtained, generally within a protocol of a series of at least three consultations allowing full discussion of the reasons why the individual is seeking the test and the possible outcomes and implications of such testing.

Prion diseases

Prion diseases also cause dementia. They can be sporadic, can result from infections (e.g. via donor implants) or can be inherited in an autosomal dominant fashion. Creutzfeldt–Jakob disease (CJD), Gerstmann–Sträussler disease and fatal familial insomnia (FFI) are clinically overlapping autosomal dominant conditions that are caused by different specific mutations in the prion protein gene (*PRNP*) gene on chromosome 20. The clinical manifestations are usually cognitive difficulties, ataxia and abrupt jerking movements of the limbs (myoclonus). Death typically occurs 5–7 years after the onset. The pathogenic mechanism is particularly unusual and was discovered by Stanley Prusiner, who consequently won the Nobel Prize for Physiology or Medicine in 1997. Mutations in the *PRNP* gene result in the adoption of an alternative folding pattern ('conformation') by the encoded prion protein, known either as PrP^{Sc} or PrP-res. This altered protein is not only toxic to the cell but appears to act as a conformational template that, by binding to the non-pathogenic normal PrP^C (or PrP-sen) molecule, can cause the latter to adopt the pathogenic conformation. Prion diseases, as mentioned above, can also result from infection with abnormally folded prion proteins. In fact, these prions (which are thus infectious proteins) are the only known infectious pathogens that possess no DNA or RNA. This intriguing pathogenic mechanism is described in more detail in the reviews by Prusiner, 2001, and Moore *et al.*, 2009 (see Further reading).

The bovine spongiform encephalopathy (BSE) epidemic, which occurred in the UK in 1986–2000, was caused and spread by abnormal prions (most likely resulting from a bovine *Prnp* mutation) contaminating cattle feed made from rendered waste from cattle carcases. Over 180,000 cattle were affected and slaughtered, and the disease caused variant CJD in at least 170 patients who were genetically susceptible to the abnormal prion. Blood donors with the infection have spread the disease to recipients, and the long incubation periods associated with CJD (shown to be up to 50 years in the case of kuru) has led to uncertainty about future occurrences. Genes for both susceptibility and resistance to prion diseases have now been identified.

- Common adult-onset conditions generally result from a complex combination of environmental, lifestyle, dietary and genetic factors. The genetic factors are composed of several genetic variants, each having a relatively small predisposing effect.
- Dominant and recessive inheritance mechanisms only apply in a minority of cases of such disorders. Therefore, the risks given to relatives are often based upon observed (i.e. empiric) data and the offspring risks are usually similar to those applicable to siblings.
- Taking a full three-generation family history and recording the ages of onset and associated clinical problems is helpful in identifying the few cases in which there is a strong inherited genetic susceptibility due to a single gene.
- Type 2 diabetes and Alzheimer disease are two common adult-onset conditions that are usually multifactorial, i.e. resulting from a combination of non-genetic factors and several genetic factors, each having a small effect.
- Individually very uncommon forms of type 2 diabetes with a strong genetic component exist. These monogenic forms include MODY (which is autosomal dominant), mitochondrial diabetes and severe insulin resistance syndromes (autosomal dominant or recessive).

- Similarly, regarding dementia, the most common cause, Alzheimer disease, is usually late in onset, with genetic susceptibility being the result of variants of small effect (such as the ε4 allele of *APOE*). Only a small proportion of dementia cases result from the inheritance of a mutation in a single gene of major effect. These types include autosomal dominantly inherited Alzheimer disease (the result of *PSEN1*, *PSEN2* or *APP* mutations), CADASIL, FTDP-17, autosomal dominant prion disease and HD.
- HD is an autosomal dominant neurodegenerative condition. Its inheritance shows genetic anticipation on account of an unstable CAG repeat length mutation in the protein-coding region of the *HTT* gene, with a particular tendency to repeat expansion during paternal transmission. Presymptomatic testing is possible but requires careful genetic counselling according to established protocols.
- Testing for genetic variants of small effect, while appropriate in some research studies, is generally regarded at present in the UK as inappropriate in the genetics clinic. Knowledge of the genetic variants possessed by a patient may, in the future, however, permit the selection of individually tailored drugs. This exciting area, known as pharmacogenetics, is rapidly expanding.

SUMMARY

FURTHER READING

Bertram L, Tanzi RE (2009) Genome-wide association studies in Alzheimer's disease. *Hum Mol Genet* **18**(R2):R137–45.

Bonnefond A, Froguel P, Vaxillaire M. (2010) The emerging genetics of type 2 diabetes. *Trends Mol Med* **16**:407–16.

Capell BC, Collins FS (2006) Human laminopathies: nuclei gone genetically awry. *Nat Rev Genet* **7**:940–52.

Dermaut B, Kumar-Singh S, Rademakers R, Theuns J, Cruts M, Van Broeckhoven C (2005) Tau is central in the genetic Alzheimer-frontotemporal dementia spectrum. *Trends Genet.* **21**:664–72.

García-Arencibia M, Hochfeld WE, Toh PP, Rubinsztein DC (2010) Autophagy, a guardian against neurodegeneration. *Semin Cell Dev Biol* **21**:691–8.

Harper PS (2010) *Practical Genetic Counselling*, 7th edn. Hodder Arnold:London.

Lindgren CM, McCarthy MI (2008) Mechanisms of disease: genetic insights into the etiology of type 2 diabetes and obesity. *Nat Clin Pract Endocrinol Metab* **4**:156–63.

Moore RA, Taubner LM, Priola SA (2009) Prion protein misfolding and disease. *Curr Opin Struct Biol* **19**:14–22.

Prokopenko I, McCarthy MI, Lindgren CM (2008) Type 2 diabetes: new genes, new understanding. *Trends Genet* **24**:613–21.

Prusiner SB (2001) Shattuck lecture – neurodegenerative diseases and prions. *N Engl J Med* **344**:1516–26.

Wellcome Trust Case Control Consortium (2007) Genome-wide association study of 14,000 cases of seven common diseases and 3,000 shared controls. *Nature* **447**:661–78.

Self-assessment

1. With regard to the family described in Fig. 14.5, what is the apparent pattern of inheritance?
A. Autosomal recessive
B. Autosomal dominant
C. Multifactorial
D. X-linked dominant
E. Mitochondrial

2. With regard to the family described in Fig. 14.5, which is the most likely diagnosis?
A. Type 1 diabetes
B. Type 2 diabetes
C. Donohue syndrome
D. Maturity-onset diabetes of the young (MODY)
E. Cerebral autosomal dominant arteriopathy with subcortical infarcts and leukoencephalopathy (CADASIL)

3. With regard to the family described in Fig. 14.5, which of the following statements are correct?
A. A mutation in either *HNF-1α* or *HNF-4α* is a possible underlying basis of the condition affecting this family.
B. The risk to any future offspring of individuals III:1 and III:3 is 25%

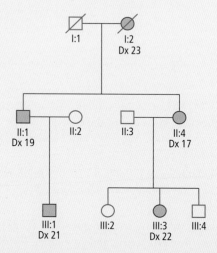

Fig. 14.5 This pedigree shows a family in which several members have been known to be affected by type 2 diabetes from the ages of diagnosis (Dx) shown. Graham (individual III:1) has been feeling unusually tired over the past 4 months and is eventually tested for diabetes. Unfortunately, Graham is also confirmed as having diabetes, at the age of 21, and the family are referred to the genetics department for further advice. See questions 1–3 in Self-assessment.

C. If deafness was also present in the affected individuals shown and if III:1 was not in fact found to be affected, then a mitochondrial DNA mutation is another possible underlying cause of the condition
D. If the situation was as in C, and a mitochondrial DNA mutation were indeed the cause, the risk now to any future offspring of II:1 would be high
E. If a mitochondrial mutation is the underlying cause, then the risk to the future offspring of III:3 would be high

4. With regard to the scenario given in Fig. 14.6, which of the following statements are correct?
A. There is a high likelihood of the condition being inherited by an autosomal dominant mechanism in this family
B. On account of genetic reasons, there a high risk that Billy will develop Alzheimer disease prior to the age of 65
C. Billy has read about *APOE* genetic testing on the internet and is willing to have a blood sample taken for this purpose at the genetics clinic. This would be appropriate
D. Calculation of a precise risk to a relative of a late-onset case of dementia is straightforward after testing for the *APOE* ε4 allele in the family
E. In Alzheimer disease, neurofibrillary tangles are deposited *within* the cell

5. Which of the following are correct statements?
A. Genetic susceptibility variants of individually small effect contribute to only a minority of cases of common adult-onset disorders
B. In most cases of common adult-onset disorders, the risks to siblings are significantly greater than the risks to offspring
C. Both frontotemporal dementia with parkinsonism-17 (FTDP-17) and Huntington disease (HD) are autosomal dominant conditions.
D. In families affected by HD, a childhood-onset case is more likely to result when the father is affected than when the mother has the condition
E. Presymptomatic testing in families affected by HD is possible

6. In HD, genetic anticipation results from the instability of a trinucleotide repeat that lies in which region of the gene?
A. The 5′ untranslated region of the gene, altering the level of transcriptional activity of the gene
B. Within an exon in the protein-coding sequence
C. Deep within an intron
D. In an intron, at a splice site close to an exon
E. In the 3′ untranslated region

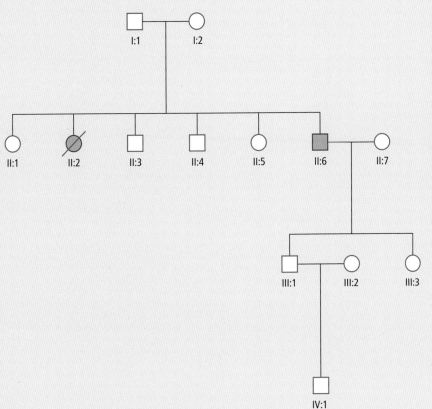

Fig. 14.6 Billy, individual IV:1 in this family, aged 28, mentions to his family doctor that he is worried that he may develop dementia at an early age. Billy met his grandfather (II:6) recently in a nursing home and was dismayed to discover that his grandfather had forgotten his name and that he had, in fact, developed Alzheimer disease, like Billy's grandfather's late elder sister (II:2). These two individuals had been diagnosed with the condition at the ages of 78 and 74. Billy was sufficiently concerned about the possible implications for himself that the family doctor decided to refer him to see a geneticist for advice. See Question 4 in Self-assessment.

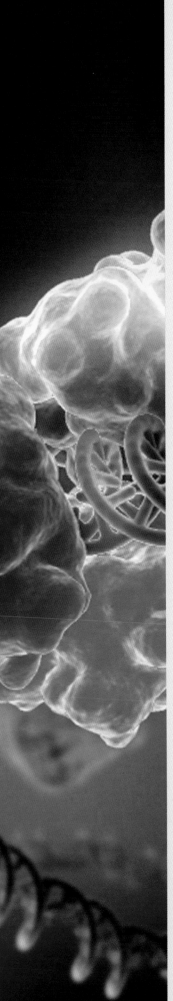

CHAPTER 15
Strong family history – typical Mendelian disease

Key Topics

Introduction

Many single-gene disorders that are inherited in a typical Mendelian manner are known. In this chapter, common well-recognised examples of the three most common Mendelian inheritance mechanisms are described in order to illustrate how individuals at risk can be identified and how, for such typical situations, approximate risks can be calculated. The clinical and molecular details of most of the other well-known examples of such conditions are now available from online sources such as GeneReviews and Online Mendelian Inheritance in Man (OMIM) (see Further reading and Chapter 19).

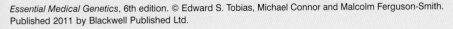

Cystic fibrosis

Cystic fibrosis (CF) is an autosomal recessive condition affecting, in the UK, 1 in 2500 newborns, with a carrier frequency of approximately 1 in 20–25. In Caucasians, it is, in fact, the commonest life-limiting autosomal recessive condition, although survival beyond the age of 30 is, fortunately, now increasingly observed. Carriers are less frequent in African–American and Asian populations (1 in 65 and 1 in 90, respectively). The main clinical manifestations of the disease are, in the classical form, recurrent lung infections with bronchiectasis and obstructive lung disease, exocrine pancreatic insufficiency (85–90% of cases) and male infertility (97%) due to congenital bilateral absence of the vas deferens (CBAVD). Neonatal screening for elevated serum immunoreactive trypsin levels can be undertaken in the general population with confirmation of the affected status of an individual by DNA mutation analysis and/or by the detection in a sweat sample (of at least 75 mg) of an increased concentration of chloride (>60–70 mM) on two occasions. Depending on the genotype (see below), a milder phenotype may be observed: either non-classical CF (in which there may not be pancreatic insufficiency and/or male infertility) or just CBAVD (which accounts for 6% of all male infertility).

The underlying cellular abnormality is a defective chloride ion channel, which leads to an increased thickness of secretions, for instance in the respiratory tract and exocrine pancreas.

The gene and its mutations

The gene responsible, located at 7q31.2, encodes the cystic fibrosis transmembrane conductance regulator (CFTR), in which over 1000 different mutations have now been reported. The most common of these, named ΔF508, accounts for approximately 70% of the CF alleles in Northern Europeans but only 35–40% of CF alleles in African–Americans and just 30–35% of CF alleles in Ashkenazi Jews. The ΔF508 mutation consists of an in-frame deletion of 3 bp, corresponding to one full codon. Although resulting in the loss from the 1480 amino acid protein of just a single amino acid, phenylalanine at position 508, this prevents the CFTR protein from folding correctly and from inserting into the plasma membrane. Instead, the protein molecules are destroyed by one of the cell's protein degradation mechanisms. This involves the addition of molecular tags consisting of ubiquitin protein molecules and subsequent protein breakdown in cellular compartments called proteasomes.

The other CFTR mutations (which are mostly missense, frameshift, nonsense or splicing mutations) are individually much rarer in the UK, each accounting for <3% of the CF alleles except in certain ethnic groups such as the Ashkenazi Jewish population (in which the W1282X mutation is particularly common, accounting for approximately 45% of mutant alleles). Different mutations can affect the function of the CFTR protein in five recognised ways: defective protein production (e.g. due to W1282X), protein processing (as with ΔF508), protein regulation and two similar mechanisms, defective conductance and reduced CFTR functioning, which are associated with a milder phenotype such as non-classical CF or even just CBAVD.

Genetic counselling

As with other autosomal recessive conditions, the parents of an affected child are expected to be carriers (i.e. heterozygotes), each possessing one mutant allele in addition to one normal copy of the gene. The risk of recurrence to such parents will be 1 in 4, or 25% (see Fig. 8.8). A healthy adult sibling of an affected individual will possess either a normal (N/N) or heterozygous mutant (N/M or M/N) genotype, but not a homozygous mutant (M/M) genotype, with the consequent chance of being a carrier of 2 in 3. The calculation of risk to offspring is described in detail below.

Testing

Laboratory testing for the commonest CFTR mutations can currently detect around 90% of mutations in Northern Europeans. The identification of the two causative mutations in an affected individual allows the subsequent search for and identification of carriers in the family by cascade screening. Testing children for carrier status is, however, not usually carried out until they are old enough to discuss and understand the test's implications. Analysis for specific known mutations can be undertaken when requested in prenatal diagnosis (e.g. by chorionic villus sampling at 10 or 11 weeks of gestation) or even in preimplantation genetic diagnosis (PGD) (see Chapter 12). If the causative mutation cannot be identified in the proband, prenatal diagnosis may still be possible by linkage analysis provided that paternity is certain and that the diagnosis of CF is not in doubt.

In Fig. 15.1, a typical affected family is illustrated, in which the sister (III:2) of an affected individual seeks genetic counselling. Providing there is no consanguinity between her and her partner and that her partner has no family history of the condition himself, then their chance of having an affected child, assuming a population CF carrier frequency of around 1 in 20, is: (her chance of being a carrier, i.e. 2 in 3) × (her partner's chance of being a carrier, i.e. 1 in 20) × (the chance of the child of two carriers being affected, i.e. 1 in 4). Thus, the chance of having an affected child is 2/3 × 1/20 × 1/4 = 2/240 or 1/120. If her brother possesses two identified mutations detectable on the standard screening test, then it would be appropriate for her to undergo the standard screening test. If she is found not to have any detectable mutation, then she can be reassured that she does not possess either of her affected brother's two CFTR mutations. In addition, her chance of being a carrier is now actually much less than the population frequency (if she has also undergone screening for the other relatively common mutations that are contained within the standard screen). If she is found to be a carrier, however, it would be appropriate for her partner to also undergo a CFTR mutation screen by sending his blood sample to a diagnostic molecular genetics laboratory. If he is found to be a carrier, then the couple's chance of having an affected child would become: her carrier risk × his carrier risk × 1/4, i.e. 1 × 1 × 1/4 = 1/4 (or 1 in 4), and prenatal diagnosis (and perhaps even PGD) could be discussed. If, as is more likely, no

mutation is detected in his blood, then assuming a mutation detection rate of 90%, his chance of being a mutation carrier drops markedly to only 1/191, as calculated using Bayes' theorem (see Table 15.1 and Appendix 1). With the couple's chance of having an affected child now only 1/191 × 1 × 1/4 = 1/764, they can be reassured that their chance is very low indeed. Figure 15.2 shows the general carrier risks for relatives of an individual affected by an autosomal recessive condition.

Other general points

There are many other autosomal recessive conditions. In most of them, there is a wide range of reported mutations in the underlying gene, but there is often a subset of relatively frequent specific mutant alleles in a particular population. For instance, in the more common form of congenital adrenal hyperplasia, testing for a panel of around ten specific mutations can detect at least 80% of mutant alleles, and in haemochromatosis, just two *HFE* gene mutations (resulting in the C282Y and H63D amino acid substitutions) account for nearly all the mutant alleles (see Chapter 17). CF is atypical in being associated with a single predominant mutation (i.e. the ΔF508 CFTR mutation in Northern Europeans) that accounts for such a high proportion of mutant alleles.

CF is also atypical in having a relatively high carrier frequency, although the frequency is by no means the highest (as the carrier frequency for Gilbert syndrome is approximately 1 in 2, as mentioned below).

It should also be remembered that a single clinical phenotype may result from mutations in different genes. In this situation, termed 'locus heterogeneity' (see Chapter 8), two affected parents could have an unaffected child (if one affected parent possesses mutations in one gene but the other parent has mutations in a different gene).

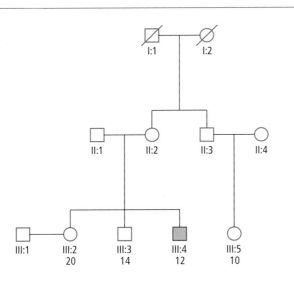

Fig. 15.1 Linda (III:2 in the pedigree), the 20-year-old apparently healthy elder sister of a boy affected by cystic fibrosis, comes to the genetics clinic. She hopes to have a child and seeks advice regarding the risks to her future child. Her partner (III:1) is healthy, not related to her and has no family history of genetic conditions himself. See text and Self-assessment questions 1–3 for a discussion of the risks.

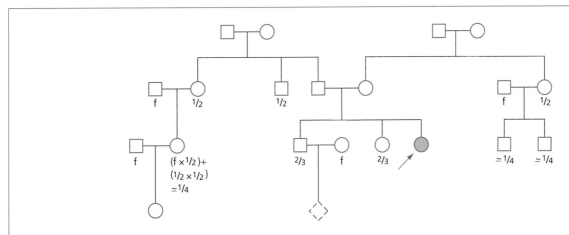

Fig. 15.2 Autosomal recessive trait in a family, with carrier risks indicated for each individual. f, General population carrier frequency.

Table 15.1 Calculation of CF carrier risk using Bayes' theorem in an individual with a prior carrier risk of 1 in 20, who then tests negative on a CF mutation screening test that detects 90% of *CFTR* mutant alleles

	Carrier	Not a carrier
Prior risk	1/20	19/20
Conditional information (negative mutation screen, i.e. the chance of him having a negative mutation screen if he *is* a carrier (1/10) or if he *is not* a carrier (1))	1/10	1
Joint odds (product of first two entries)	1/200	19/20 = 190/200
Final carrier risk (carrier joint odds, divided by the sum of the carrier and non-carrier joint odds)	(1/200)/((1/200) + (190/200)) = (1/200)/(191/200) = 1/191	

With autosomal recessive conditions, affected children sometimes have consanguineous parents. Similarly, parental consanguinity suggests (although does not prove) that an undiagnosed condition affecting their child is autosomal recessively inherited.

While a vertical pattern of inheritance is only rarely observed in families affected by autosomal recessive conditions, it can occur when there is a high degree of consanguinity or when the population carrier frequency is relatively high. This 'pseudodominant inheritance' has been observed, for instance, with Gilbert syndrome for which the carrier frequency of the *UGT1A1* gene promoter region mutation is as high as 50% in North America and Europe (see Chapter 9).

Finally, compared with autosomal dominant disorders, autosomal recessive conditions usually show much less phenotypic variability and lack of penetrance is much less common.

Duchenne and Becker muscular dystrophies

Duchenne muscular dystrophy (DMD) is an X-linked recessive genetic disorder. It is the most severe form of childhood muscular dystrophy and is also the most common type, affecting approximately 1 in 3000–3500 male births.

Males with the condition are usually affected under the age of 5 years, with delayed walking and a progressive proximal muscle weakness. They become unable to walk, due to weakness and contractures, at the age of 7–13 (with a mean age of 9). Calf hypertrophy (or 'pseudohypertrophy') due to fatty infiltration is often present and there is typically marked elevation of serum creatine kinase. In addition, respiratory failure, requiring nocturnal ventilation, is common in the late teens, and cardiomyopathy is almost always present with an increased risk of arrhythmia. Other problems include scoliosis in over 90% of boys with DMD (often requiring major surgery) and a non-progressive learning disability in over 90%. With appropriate specialist care, including nocturnal ventilation, the mean age of death is now around 25 years.

Typically, an electromyogram is abnormal and muscle biopsy shows characteristic histology with an absence of dys-trophin protein. The condition results from the absence of this large rod-like protein from the muscle fibre membrane (the sarcolemma). There, it normally plays a crucial role in linking the muscle fibre inner structural cytoskeleton (composed of F-actin) to the extracellular matrix proteins (via binding to dystroglycan proteins).

The gene and its mutations

The 3685 amino acid dystrophin protein is encoded by the *DMD* gene at Xp21.2, an enormous gene consisting of 79 exons distributed over 2.2 Mb of genomic DNA (Fig. 15.3). In fact, on account of its size, it takes over 16 hours for the gene to be transcribed and spliced. The commonest type of *DMD* mutation, accounting for 60–65% of cases, is a large intragenic deletion (often affecting either exons 3–8 or exons 44–60) that causes a frameshift during protein translation. Exon duplications account for around a further 5%. Protein-truncating frameshift or nonsense mutations account for the majority of the remainder. Generally, the severely shortened proteins are degraded. Around 10–20% of female *DMD* mutation carriers have mild to moderate muscle weakness (with an average age of onset of 33 years) as a result of a skewed pattern of X chromosome inactivation (see Chapter 6).

On account of the high proportion of frameshift mutations among the gene alterations responsible for DMD, an exciting area of research at present is the development of antisense oligonucleotides that may, in the future, be administered to a DMD patient with a frameshift mutation. Such oligonucleotides can cause skipping of an exon, resulting in restoration of the reading frame and the generation of a functional (albeit shortened) form of dystrophin. The disorder could therefore, in theory, be converted from the lethal Duchenne form to the milder Becker type, described below (see Aartsma-Rus *et al.*, 2009, in Further reading). The antisense oligonucleotides required for an individual patient would be selected in order to target the specific exon affected. The long-term effects of repeated administration and the 'off-target effects' (i.e. those resulting from non-specific binding of the oligonucleotides to other genes) in humans are, however, not yet known.

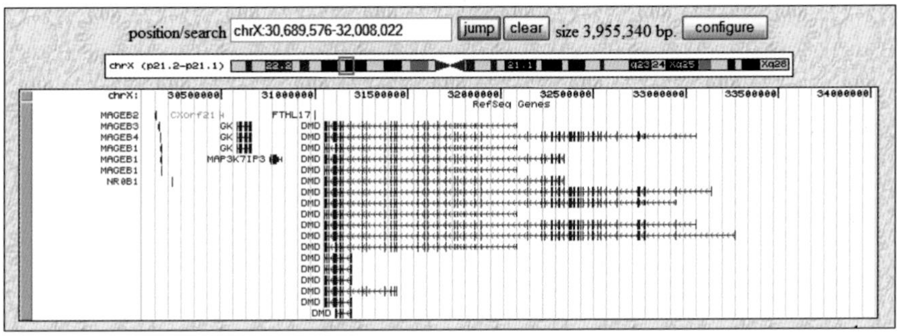

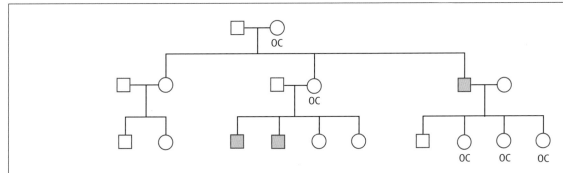

Fig. 15.3 The *DMD* gene, the largest gene found in nature to date, spanning approximately 2.2 Mb of genomic DNA on the short arm of the X chromosome. In this University of California, Santa Cruz (UCSC) genome browser window (see Chapter 19 for further details; Kent et al. (2002) The human genome browser at UCSC. Genome Res.12(6):996–1006. http://genome.ucsc.edu/), the complexity of the *DMD* gene can be seen. It contains at least eight independent tissue-specific promoters and two polyadenylation sites. In addition, the RNA is differentially spliced. The gene thus generates a large set of protein isoforms. The nearby glycerol kinase (*GK*) gene can occasionally be lost together with *DMD* in a contiguous gene deletion. Interestingly, although *DMD* is the largest gene identified to date at the genomic level, its encoded protein, dystrophin (3685 amino acids) is not the largest protein, which is actually another muscle cell protein named titin (composed of 34,350 amino acids). Titin is encoded by a considerably more compact gene (approximately 281 kb in size at the genomic level).

Fig. 15.4 X-linked recessive trait in a family, with obligate carriers (OC) indicated (in a condition which, unlike DMD, does not preclude reproduction).

Genetic counselling

Females may be identified as being obligate (i.e. certain) DMD carriers (e.g. those who have both an affected brother and son; see Fig. 15.4) and carrier detection is also possible by combined biochemical and DNA analyses. An assay for elevated serum creatine kinase (median of three separate measurements) may be combined with pedigree risk information and the results of DNA analyses (using Bayes' theorem; see Appendix 1). Although the biochemical creatine kinase tests may be available for carrier detection, the results do not always correlate with carrier status, as a consequence, for instance, of skewed X inactivation. Combining the biochemical and other data, therefore, is often valuable when counselling non-obligate carrier females. In the absence of a family history, two-thirds of mothers of affected boys will be carriers, with a high risk of recurrence for their own pregnancies and those of other female relatives.

As the inheritance pattern is X-linked recessive, in each pregnancy a carrier will have a 1 in 4 (25%) chance of having an affected male child (see Fig. 8.11). She will, of course, also have a 25% chance of having a carrier female child, a 25% chance of a normal male child and a 25% chance of having a female child with a normal DMD genotype.

Prenatal diagnosis by DNA analysis can be carried out if in that family the pathogenic mutation has been identified or if informative linked markers can be used to identify the mutant allele. If prenatal diagnosis is carried out, fetal sexing is generally performed first, with subsequent DMD genetic analysis when the fetus is identified as being male. PGD may be offered, for instance to select female embryos in families in which no pathogenic DMD mutation can be identified.

It should be noted that, in the absence of a family history of the condition, the mother of an affected boy may not appear on blood testing to be a DMD carrier. A significant possibility remains, however, that she may possess the causative mutation in some of her egg cells as a result of the mutation having arisen very early in her development. This situation, known as 'gonadal mosaicism' is described in more detail in Chapter 9 and also applies to autosomal dominant conditions (see Other general points under Neurofibromatosis type 1, below).

Becker muscular dystrophy

Becker muscular dystrophy (BMD) is similar to DMD but is a milder condition, with a frequency of approximately 1 in 20,000 male births, and is caused by mutations in the same gene as for DMD. The age of onset of progressive muscular weakness is later, with a mean of 11 years. Affected males may remain ambulant until their 60s, learning disability is less common and severe than in DMD and lifespan can be normal. Again, calf pseudohypertrophy and markedly elevated serum creatine kinase are typically present with an abnormal electromyogram and muscle biopsy. In contrast to the absence of dystrophin in DMD muscle, on immunohistochemistry the protein may appear to be normal or to be present in reduced quantity with patchy staining. This results from the mutations being in frame rather than a frameshift, with the consequence that dystrophin is produced, albeit shorter and less functional than in its normal form.

Other general points

DMD is inherited in a manner that is typical of X-linked recessive conditions, with unaffected or mildly (and variably) affected female carriers (due to X inactivation), more severely affected males and a lack of male-to-male transmission. At the molecular genetic level, an atypical aspect of the condition, perhaps on account of the unusually large associated gene, is the high frequency of underlying large intragenic deletions.

Not all X-linked conditions are recessive, of course. As discussed in Chapter 8, a relatively small number are inherited as dominant traits and, as mentioned in Chapter 9, some of those cause male lethality *in utero*. An X-linked condition can even be inherited in a way that appears in a pedigree similar to an autosomal dominant condition. This 'pseudo-autosomal' inheritance is a well-recognised feature of the condition known as Léri–Weill dyschondrosteosis. The underlying gene, *SHOX*, is located within the small part of the short arm of the X chromosome that is known as the pairing or pseudoautosomal region and within which recombination can take place with a homologous region on the Y chromosome (see Chapters 6 and 9).

Mutations that are associated with DMD are typically stable, remaining unchanged when transmitted to successive generations within a family. In contrast, those associated with another X-linked recessive condition, fragile X syndrome, are unstable, with a tendency to mutation expansion upon transmission (as discussed in more detail in Chapters 9 and 16).

Neurofibromatosis type 1

Neurofibromatosis type 1 (NF1), previously known as von Recklinghausen disease, is an autosomal dominantly inherited syndrome whose principal manifestations involve tissues derived from the neural crest. It has an incidence in the UK of approximately 1 in 3500 live births. The condition generally causes multiple café au lait patches, mostly on the trunk (Fig. 15.5), with skin neurofibromas (Fig. 15.6) from adolescence onwards. In addition, affected individuals tend to have short stature and macrocephaly.

For an individual to be regarded as affected by NF1, he or she should strictly have been found to satisfy two or more of the diagnostic criteria (see Table 15.2). These include: having an affected first degree affected relative with NF1, the presence of at least six café au lait patches, a minimum of two skin neurofibromas (or one plexiform neurofibroma), and two or more iris Lisch nodules (Fig. 15.7) which may not appear until adulthood. Learning difficulties are common, present in 30%, but are severe in 3% or less.

In addition to the above manifestations, however, patients affected by NF1 are at increased risk of developing malignant change in a plexiform neurofibroma, phaeochromocytomas, optic gliomas and other central nervous system tumors, hypertension, scoliosis and spinal cord or root compression (hence the operation scar in Fig. 15.6). Annual examination is recommended to detect such potential complications (absent in around 65%) and includes a check of peripheral vision (to detect optic gliomas, which occur most often in the first 6 years

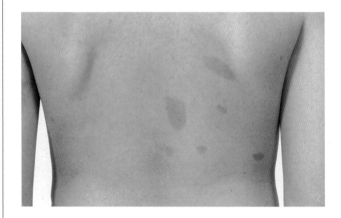

Fig. 15.5 Café au lait patches (coffee-coloured macules) on the skin of Stewart, an 18-year-old catering assistant, who visits a dermatologist. He has eight of these pigmented skin patches (measuring 2–5 cm in diameter) on his abdomen and limbs, as well as three small (1 cm diameter) soft lumps just beneath his skin. He is otherwise apparently healthy. His mother had considerable difficulties with arithmetic, reading and writing at school and has several similar pigmented cutaneous patches, although she was unaware of their possible significance. There is no other family history of note. Stewart's dermatologist suspects that he may have NF1 and refers him to the genetics clinic for further advice. See question 7 in Self-assessment. Image kindly provided Dr Margo Whiteford, Ferguson-Smith Centre for Clinical Genetics, UK.

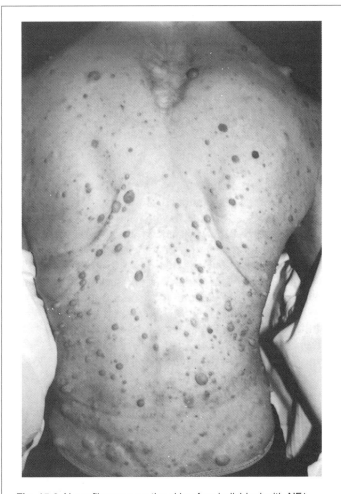

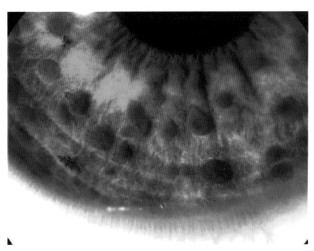

Fig. 15.7 Lisch nodules visible on the iris of a patient affected by NF1. Image from http://www.nature.com/eye/journal/v19/n3/ fig_tab/6701478f1.html. Reprinted with permission from Nature Publishing Group: P Cackett, J Vallance and H Bennett; Neurofibromatosis type 1 presenting with Horner's syndrome, Eye 19:351–3; copyright 2005.

Fig. 15.6 Neurofibromas on the skin of an individual with NF1. The scar from previous spinal cord decompression surgery is visible at the top of the image.

of life), the spine (as scoliosis requiring surgery occurs in 5%), the legs (as pathological fracture of the tibia occurs in 1–2%) and blood pressure (as hypertension occurs in 2%). NF1 accounts for one-third of patients with optic gliomas and about 5% of cases of phaeochromocytoma, although the frequencies of optic glioma and phaeochromocytoma in individuals affected by NF1 are only around 5% (mostly asymptomatic) and 1–2%, respectively (see Huson *et al.*, 1989; Ferner *et al.*, 2007; in Further reading).

The gene and its mutations

The *NF1* gene at 17q11.2 is large, comprising 60 exons spanning over 350 kb, and encodes a very large protein of 2818 amino acids. Around half of affected individuals possess a *de novo NF1* mutation. The estimated new mutation rate of 1 in 10,000 is, in fact, one of the highest for a human disorder. Most mutations are paternal in origin, but there is no signifi-

Table 15.2 Diagnostic criteria for NF1 based on the findings of the NIH Consensus Development Conference, 1988 (see review on NF1 in the GeneReviews website for further information)

Diagnosis requires that two or more of the following criteria be met:
An affected first-degree affected relative with NF1
At least six café au lait macules (at least 15 mm in size in a postpubertal individual; 5 mm if prepubertal)
A minimum of two skin neurofibromas or one plexiform neurofibroma
Axillary, groin or neck freckling
Two or more iris Lisch nodules (visible on slit-lamp examination)
Associated bony dysplasia (dysplasia of the sphenoid bone or dysplasia or thinning of the long bone cortex)
An optic pathway glioma

cant observed paternal age effect. Full mutation analysis of the gene is currently laborious (and not routinely performed in the UK) on account of the gene's size and large number of exons, the presence of several *NF1* pseudogenes and the wide spectrum of genetic alterations. Many mutations have been described, of which around 80% are predicted to cause truncation of the encoded protein. There is no clear genotype–phenotype correlation at present, other than the association of *NF1* gene deletions (of 1.2–1.4 Mb) with dysmorphic features, increased numbers of neurofibromas and significant developmental delay (in addition to the typical NF1 manifestations). In addition, the relatively few NF1 patients with these large *NF1* gene deletions (which encompass the entire *NF1* gene) appear to be more predisposed to malignant peripheral nerve sheath tumours (MPNSTs).

In accordance with the Knudson model of tumor suppressor gene function (see Chapter 13), in benign neurofibromas and in NF1-associated MPNSTs, phaeochromocytomas and astrocytomas, the normal copy of the *NF1* gene often undergoes loss of heterozygosity or point mutation. The protein encoded by the *NF1* gene, neurofibromin, is normally localised in the cytoplasm of the cell and bears considerable similarity to the catalytic domains of GTPase-activating proteins. By stimulating the GTPase activity of the signal-transducing ras proteins, neurofibromin helps to prevent overactivity of the ras signalling proteins in the cellular signalling pathway, which promotes cell proliferation. Thus, loss of neurofibromin results in the abnormal persistence of the GTP-bound (i.e. active) form of ras.

Careful clinical evaluation (including ophthalmology examination) of the parents is necessary to determine whether one of them is clinically affected, with the phenotype often being mild and occasionally segmental, i.e. mosaic (arising from a post-zygotic mutation).

Genetic counselling

Each child of an individual affected by NF1 will have a 50% chance of being affected, with the penetrance being almost 100% but the clinical severity being very variable. Following the birth of an affected child to parents who are not clinically affected, there is a small possibility of recurrence of the condition in the next pregnancy on account of the chance of gonadal mosaicism (see Chapter 9), although the risk is less than 1%. Where a parent has segmental NF1, the risk is intermediate and difficult to quantify.

Prenatal diagnosis is theoretically possible by DNA analysis, e.g. in families in which the causative mutation has been identified. In practice, however, in the UK, prenatal diagnosis for the condition is usually not requested.

Identification of affected individuals and predictive testing may be carried out by genetic analysis if the familial mutation has been identified. In the UK, however, identification of affected children is generally carried out by careful clinical examination, and those at risk of having inherited NF1 are monitored during childhood.

Other general points

NF1 is typical of autosomal dominant conditions in its high degree of phenotypic variability between and within families (i.e. 'variable expression'). As mentioned in Chapter 9, the additional factors that may contribute to the variability in the phenotypic expression of such conditions include environmental factors and modifier genes (many of which remain to be identified). Like many autosomal dominant conditions such as achondroplasia (but unlike many others, such as the acute porphyrias), NF1 has a high penetrance.

As mentioned above, a high proportion of NF1 cases are the result of a *de novo* mutation in the associated gene. Some autosomal dominant conditions, such as Apert syndrome or Cornelia de Lange syndrome, result from new mutations in almost all cases, whereas in others, such as Huntington disease, the proportion of new mutations is very low.

The gene that is responsible for NF1 is unusual in that it is one of the approximately 90 recognised tumour suppressor genes. Mutations in these genes, discussed in much more detail in Chapter 13, generally cause loss of function of the encoded protein. In addition, the DNA contained in the tumour cells of an affected individual typically possesses an abnormality in both copies of such genes, rather than just in the copy bearing the inherited mutation.

There are a few autosomal dominant conditions whose inheritance patterns display particularly unusual features. These features include imprinting, for example in Prader–Willi, Angelman and Beckwith–Wiedemann syndromes (see Chapters 6 and 9) and, as more recently discovered, in hereditary paraganglioma caused by *SDHD* mutations. In addition, genetic anticipation due to unstable length mutations is a feature of several conditions, such as myotonic dystrophy, Huntington disease and several spinocerebellar ataxias (as described in Chapter 9).

Finally, as mentioned above and in Chapter 9, where a child is affected by a condition that can be autosomal dominantly inherited but has apparently unaffected parents, there is a small chance that the mutation may be present in the gonadal cells of one of the parents. In this situation, known as 'gonadal mosaicism', there is a small recurrence risk for future siblings of the affected child. Although small, this risk can represent an important potential hazard in counselling such families. Gonadal mosaicism should be especially considered as an alternative to autosomal (or X-linked) recessive inheritance in families in which unaffected parents have had two children who have been affected by the same condition, particularly if the disorder is normally autosomal dominantly inherited.

SUMMARY

- CF is the commonest life-limiting autosomal recessive disorder. It results from a defective chloride ion channel encoded by the *CFTR* gene on chromosome 7, leading to an increased thickness of secretions.
- Parents of an individual with an autosomal recessive disorder are expected to be carriers and the unaffected siblings of the affected individual will each have a 2/3 chance of being a carrier. The parents' recurrence risk of having an affected child will be 1 in 4.
- Typically, autosomal recessive conditions show greater penetrance and less intrafamilial phenotypic variation than autosomal dominant conditions.
- Identification of the causative mutations in autosomal recessive conditions in a family permit cascade screening, identifying carrier relatives. There are often a few relatively common specific mutations, with frequencies depending on which population is studied.
- DMD, the commonest and most severe childhood muscular dystrophy, is an X-linked recessive disorder.

- Mutations in the responsible gene on chromosome Xp result in the absence of dystrophin from the muscle fibre membrane, the sarcolemma. As in other X-linked recessive disorders, there is a 1 in 4 (25%) risk to a female carrier of having an affected son and also a 25% chance of having a carrier daughter.
- Approximately 10–20% of female carriers of *DMD* mutations have muscular weakness as a result of skewed X chromosome inactivation.
- BMD is a similar condition to DMD but with a milder phenotype. It results from mutations in the *DMD* gene. However, as these are not frameshift mutations, they permit the formation of dystrophin protein, albeit in a less functional form than normal.
- Like many other autosomal dominant conditions, NF1 has very variable expression. New mutations are particularly frequent in this condition, accounting for around 50% of cases.
- Gonadal mosaicism occurs in both X-linked recessive and autosomal dominant conditions.

FURTHER READING

Aartsma-Rus A, Fokkema I, Verschuuren J, Ginjaar I, van Deutekom J, van Ommen GJ, den Dunnen JT (2009) Theoretic applicability of antisense-mediated exon skipping for Duchenne muscular dystrophy mutations. *Hum Mutat* **30**:293–9.

Ferner RE, Huson SM, Thomas N, Moss C, Willshaw H, Evans DG, Upadhyaya M, Towers R, Gleeson M, Steiger C, Kirby A (2007) Guidelines for the diagnosis and management of individuals with neurofibromatosis 1. *J Med Genet* **44**:81–8.

Firth HV, Hurst JA (eds) (2005) *Oxford Desk Reference: Clinical Genetics*. Oxford University Press:Oxford.

Harper PS (2010) *Practical Genetic Counselling*, 7th edn. Hodder Arnold:London .

Huson SM, Compston DAS and Harper PS (1989) A genetic study of von Recklinghausen neurofibromatosis in south east Wales. II. Guidelines for genetic counselling. *J Med Genet* **26**:712–21.

Young I (2007) *Introduction to Risk Calculation in Genetic Counselling*, 3rd edn. Oxford University Press: Oxford.

WEBSITES

GeneReviews at the GeneTests website:

http://www.geneclinics.org/

Human Gene Mutation Database at the Institute of Medical Genetics in Cardiff:

http://www.hgmd.cf.ac.uk/ac/index.php

Online Mendelian Inheritance in Man (OMIM):

http://www.ncbi.nlm.nih.gov/sites/entrez?db=OMIM

Self-assessment

1. With regard to the situation outlined in Fig. 15.1, the chance of Linda being a carrier is:

A. 100%
B. 67%
C. 50%
D. 25%
E. 12%

2. If Linda's partner has a brother who has a daughter affected by cystic fibrosis (CF), then (prior to performing mutation analysis) the chance for the couple (III:1 and III:2) of having an affected child is:

A. 1 in 120
B. 1 in 16
C. 1 in 12
D. 1 in 8
E. 1 in 6

3. Again with regard to Fig. 15.1, the chance of III:5, the daughter of the affected boy's maternal uncle, being a carrier is closest to:

A. 100%
B. 67%
C. 50%
D. 25%
E. 12%

4. With regard to the family shown in Fig. 15.8, which are the obligate carrier females in the pedigree?

5. Using just the information in the pedigree in Fig. 15.8, if Helen (III:2) has a child, what is the chance of the child being an affected male?

A. 1 in 16
B. 1 in 8
C. 1 in 4
D. 1 in 2
E. 2 in 3

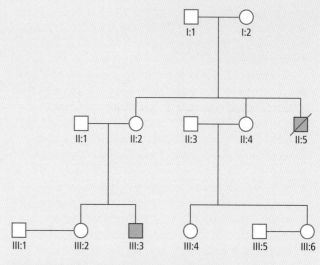

Fig. 15.8 In this family, two individuals have been diagnosed with DMD, Jason (II:5), who died at the age of 25, and Mark (III:3), who is just 15. Mark's sister, Helen (III:2), hopes to have a child soon and seeks genetic counselling first. See questions 4–6 in Self-assessment.

6. Helen's cousin, Lucille (III:6 in Fig. 15.8), also wishes to have a child. Again, using the pedigree information alone, what is the chance that Lucille's child would be an affected male?

A. 1 in 16
B. 1 in 8
C. 1 in 4
D. 1 in 2
E. 2 in 3

7. Which of the following is not a common clinical feature of NF1?

A. Café au lait patches
B. Axillary freckling
C. Phaeochromocytoma
D. Inguinal freckling
E. Lisch nodules

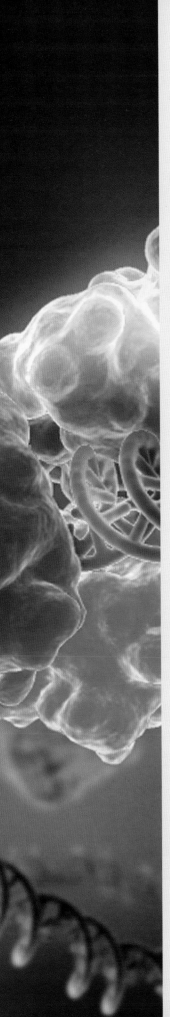

CHAPTER 16

Strong family history – other inheritance mechanisms

Key Topics

Introduction

Although a great many genetic conditions are single-gene disorders that follow autosomal dominant, autosomal recessive or X-linked recessive mechanisms of inheritance, there are several conditions whose inheritance patterns reflect the atypical Mendelian or non-Mendelian mechanisms described in earlier chapters. These mechanisms include genetic anticipation (as occurs, for example, in myotonic dystrophy and fragile X syndrome), mitochondrial inheritance, imprinting and chromosome translocations, which are all discussed further below as well as in Chapters 7, 9 and 10.

Essential Medical Genetics, 6th edition. © Edward S. Tobias, Michael Connor and Malcolm Ferguson-Smith.
Published 2011 by Blackwell Published Ltd.

Myotonic dystrophy

Myotonic dystrophy (dystrophia myotonica or DM), a condition with a frequency of around 1 in 7500, is autosomal dominantly inherited with genetic anticipation. It typically involves progressive muscle weakness in early adult life, especially of the face, sternomastoids and distal limb muscles. In addition, there is typically myotonia, which can be observed as difficulty in relaxing clenched hands (particularly in cold weather) and cataracts, especially in the posterior part of the lens (85%). There is also a tendency to cardiac conduction defects, a susceptibility to diabetes mellitus and risks associated with general anaesthesia. Additional clinical features include frontal baldness and gonadal atrophy in males, fatigue, daytime sleepiness, gastrointestinal symptoms and pigmentary retinopathy. Affected individuals are advised to undergo regular (e.g. annual) ECGs (to detect conduction defects), blood sugar tests (for diabetes mellitus) and assessment of their vision (for ocular cataract).

As mentioned in Chapter 9, the genetic basis of DM is an unstable length mutation of a CTG repeat tract within the 3′ untranslated region (UTR) of the *DMPK* gene and it is therefore one of the conditions in which genetic anticipation is observed. Normal individuals show stable minor length variations of this region (with 4–37 CTG repeats) whereas in DM expansion into the clinically affected range (from 50 to over 2000 repeats) is seen, with these larger repeat tracts being unstable. The phenotypic expression is very variable and there is a general (but incomplete) correlation between the size of the repeat sequence and the clinical severity (50–99 CTG repeats: mild; 100–1000: classic affected and 1000–2000: congenital). Carriers of small amplifications may have no symptoms, normal electromyograms and normal slit-lamp examinations. Further repeat tract expansion, however, can result in more severely affected offspring, with the chance of a large increase in repeat tract size at transmission being more likely from female carriers. Those female carriers who have DM symptoms or signs may have a congenitally affected floppy infant at risk of neonatal death or severe respiratory problems and subsequent physical and mental disability. Conversely, the length of the mutation may occasionally decrease at transmission and this is more common for paternal (10%) than maternal (3%) transmission. For the offspring of an affected female, on average 50% are unaffected, 29% are affected in later life, 12% die neonatally and 9% have severe neonatal hypotonia and significant learning disability (Fig. 16.1). For an affected male, half of his offspring are affected and half are unaffected, with neonatal cases being rare.

Presymptomatic carrier detection and prenatal diagnosis are possible by DNA analysis by PCR and, occasionally, Southern blotting. In the UK, laboratories generally now use a 'triplet repeat-primed' polymerase chain reaction (TP-PCR) to permit the identification of the large pathogenic repeat tracts that could otherwise not be amplified using standard flanking PCR primers (see Fig. 16.2). Standard PCR with primers that

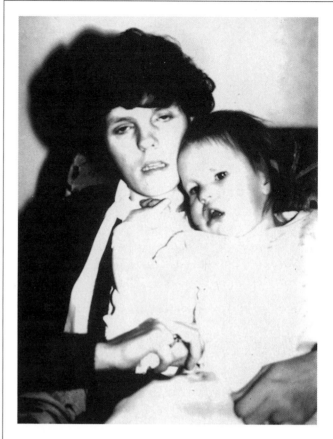

Fig. 16.1 Mother and child with myotonic dytrophy.

flank the (CTG)$_n$ repeat region is carried out separately at the same time as the TP-PCR. The TP-PCR result is particularly valuable when only one product is detected on the standard PCR analysis. In this situation, the TP-PCR will help to determine whether the patient is homozygous for a normal allele or whether the patient possesses one normal allele and a mutant allele that is too large (e.g. containing over 100 CTG repeats) to be amplified successfully by the standard PCR. Although the TP-PCR will (unlike standard PCR) detect the presence of a large *DMPK* mutation, it will not permit the determination of the precise size of the repeat tract. For this purpose, a Southern blot would be required, although, in practice, the measurement of the precise size of a TP-PCR-detected large *DMPK* mutation is often not necessary.

The mechanism of pathogenicity of the repeat expansion is complex but is currently believed to result from the abnormal *DMPK* mRNA, which indirectly exerts a toxic intracellular effect on the splicing of other genes such as the chloride channel 1 (*CLCN1*) gene that appears to be responsible for the myotonia. In addition, the expression of genes adjacent to *DMPK*, such as *SIX5* and *DMWD*, appear to be reduced, possibly due to condensation effects on the chromatin by the expanded repeat tract. The molecular pathogenesis has been reviewed by Lee and Cooper, 2009 (see Further reading).

(a)

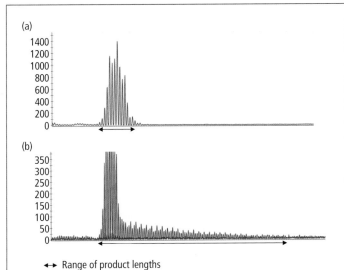

(b)

↔ Range of product lengths

Fig. 16.2 Electropherograms showing the results of TP-PCR from (a) a patient with two small normal-range *DMPK* alleles and (b) a patient affected by DM. For TP-PCR, one of the PCR primers used consists of *DMPK*-specific sequence but the other is designed to bind to the CTG triplet repeat itself. In (a), a small range of product lengths is generated, reflecting the slightly differing binding positions of the $(CTG)_n$-binding primer. In (b), however, there is a much greater range of PCR product lengths (along the *x*-axis) as a result of the presence of a large mutant allele. As a fluorescent dye is attached to one of the TP-PCR primers, the products can be detected by an automated DNA sequencer. The green trace visible in (b) should be ignored for this analysis. Figures adapted from images kindly provided by Dr Alexander Cooke, Institute of Medical Genetics, Glasgow, UK.

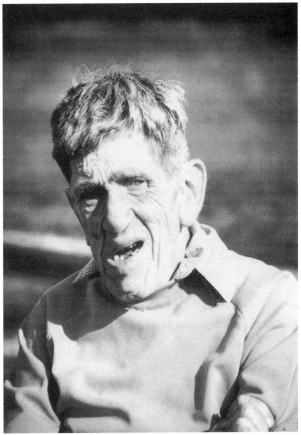

Fig. 16.3 Typical facies of an individual affected by fragile X syndrome.

Fragile X syndrome

Like DM, fragile X syndrome exhibits genetic anticipation. The inheritance pattern of this condition, however, unlike that of most others that involve genetic anticipation, is X-linked recessive rather than autosomal dominant.

Fragile X syndrome is the most common inherited cause of significant learning disability. Down syndrome, in contrast, although commoner, usually occurs as the result of a *de novo* genetic abnormality (trisomy 21) without being inherited. The frequency of fragile X syndrome is around 1 in 5000 males. In affected males, the phenotype can be severe, but it can also affect up to 50% of carrier females, albeit with milder learning disability. Males with the full mutation have significant learning disability and 50% have enlarged testes after puberty. Less consistent features include large ears, a long face and prognathism (Fig. 16.3).

The underlying genetic abnormality is located in the *FMR1* gene on the long arm of the X chromosome. The inheritance is consequently X-linked, although there are unusual features. The precise genetic basis of the condition is an unstable length mutation in the CGG trinucleotide repeat (normally 6–54

repeats with a median of 30 repeats) in the 5' UTR of the *FMR1* gene (see Chapter 9). Individuals affected by fragile X-associated learning disability will almost always possess a full mutation, with over 200 trinucleotide repeats. This results in hypermethylation of *FMR1* and thus suppression of its transcription. This, in turn, results in loss of production of the *FMR1*-encoded protein, FMRP. This protein regulates translation by binding to mRNA molecules (see Pfeiffer and Huber, 2009; in Further reading). Its presence is believed to be necessary for the normal development of the neuronal dendritic spines and synapses that are required for normal learning and memory. In contrast, male and female carriers of the premutation (smaller length mutations consisting of approximately 55–200 repeats) do not have learning disability. Approximately 40% of males with a premutation, however, become affected by fragile X-associated tremor/ataxia syndrome (FXTAS) consisting of a late onset (generally over 50 years), progressive intention tremor and subsequent cerebellar ataxia. Female premutation carriers may also develop FXTAS (albeit with a lower risk than males). In addition, approximately 20% of females possessing a *FMR1* premutation develop premature ovarian failure (with cessation of menstruation prior to the age of 40).

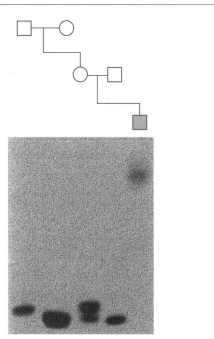

Fig. 16.4 DNA analysis of a family with fragile X syndrome. Note instability of the larger (mutant) allele. Direction of DNA migration was from top to bottom.

It is also now recognised that at the upper end of the 'normal' range is an intermediate range with alleles containing 41–54 repeats. For alleles in this range, it appears at present that female carriers have no significant risk of having affected offspring but the number of repeat units may increase slightly by one or two repeats when transmitted to a child.

The diagnosis of the condition can be confirmed in the molecular genetics laboratory. The length of the *FMR1*-associated CGG repeat tract can be determined by PCR or (particularly where a large repeat length is present) by Southern blotting. On Southern blotting, in males with the premutation, the size of the DNA fragment containing the CGG repeat is usually increased by 150–500 bp. A similar increase in size is seen in females possessing the premutation and their second band (migrating faster on an electrophoretic gel) represents the normal X chromosome (Fig. 16.4). In affected males the normal band is replaced by a single larger band (of approximately 1–4 kb, containing 230 to over 1000 repeats plus surrounding DNA), multiple discrete larger bands or a smear of fragments (representing somatic instability of the mutation). Female carriers of the full mutation (whether normal or having learning disability) have a normal-sized band, in addition to the mutant band or bands seen in the affected males (Fig. 16.4).

With regard to the transmission of the condition, atypical X-linked inheritance is observed on account of the instability of the length mutation. All daughters of clinically normal males with the premutation (normal transmitting males) inherit the premutation, which may then be passed on to the next generation either intact or with expansion to the full mutation. Further expansion of the full mutation can occur in somatic tissues or at female meiosis. Thus, affected relatives usually each possess different length mutations and show phenotypic variability. In practice, all mothers of affected males possess either the premutation or the full mutation. On average, 50% of the sons of a female who possesses a full mutation will have learning disability. Similarly, on average, half of the daughters of a full mutation carrier mother will receive the full mutation (and, as mentioned above, about half of these individuals will have learning disability to some extent). For mothers with the premutation, the risk of expansion to the full mutation at meiosis is related to the size of the mother's premutation. In a study of the children of around 1500 premutation carrier females, the risk was calculated to range from 5% (for 60–69 CGG repeats), 31% (for 70–79 CGG repeats) and 58% (for 80–89 CGG repeats) to 94–100% (for over 100 CGG repeats).

Prenatal diagnosis by DNA analysis is possible in the first trimester, but prediction of which females with the full mutation will be affected is not yet possible.

Mitochondrial disorder

Mitochondrial disorders represent a large group of largely overlapping conditions primarily affecting muscle and nerve cells but which can affect multiple tissue types. Examples (see Table 10.11) include mitochondrial myopathy, encephalopathy, lactic acidosis and stroke-like episodes (MELAS) and myoclonic epilepsy with ragged-red fibres (MERRF). Some mitochondrial disorders affect just a single organ, such as the eye in Leber hereditary optic neuropathy (LHON or Leber optic atrophy). This condition results in painless, midlife loss of central vision. Generally, however, the organs that are affected in mitochondrial conditions include the brain (encephalopathy, seizures, dementia, migraine and stroke-like episodes), skeletal muscle (proximal myopathy), heart (cardiomyopathy) and eyes (optic atrophy, pigmentary retinopathy, external ophthalmoplegia and ptosis).

Investigations that are carried out when a mitochondrial disorder is suspected from the clinical features generally include blood DNA testing (if the clinical features suggest a particular disorder), blood (and cerebrospinal fluid) lactate and fasting glucose (because of the association between mitochondrial dysfunction and diabetes mellitus). The investigations may also include neuroimaging (CT or MRI), neurophysiology (EEG or EMG), cardiac investigations (ECG and echocardiography) and a muscle biopsy for respiratory chain complex studies.

Mitochondrial diseases result from defective function of the mitochondrial respiratory chain and this can result from one of many different mutations in the mitochondrial DNA itself. For example, one of three specific mutations in the respiratory complex I (NADH dehydrogenase) genes is present in around 95% of affected individuals with LHON. Such mutations are inherited from the mother but not from the father and all the children of an affected mother are at risk. The severity of the phenotype, however, may vary not only according to which specific mutation is present but also depending on the level of heteroplasmy, i.e. the proportion of mitochondrial DNA molecules that are abnormal (see Chapters 5 and 10).

It is now recognised that mitochondrial disorders can also result from nuclear gene mutations and thus be inherited in an autosomal dominant, recessive or X-linked manner. For instance (as mentioned in Chapter 10), mutations in one of the nuclear genes (particularly *SCO2*) encoding one of the polypeptides within the last enzyme complex (complex IV or cytochrome *c* oxidase) of the mitochondrial respiratory chain can result in severe autosomal recessive mitochondrial disease. In addition, a mutation of the DNA polymerase γ (*POLG*) gene located on nuclear chromosome 15 results in an autosomal dominantly inherited tendency to mitochondrial DNA deletions and progressive external ophthalmoplegia, i.e. eye muscle weakness (see Hudson and Chinnery, 2006, in Further reading). Generally, those mitochondrial conditions that result directly from nuclear gene mutations have an earlier onset (typically in childhood) than those that are caused by mitochondrial DNA abnormalities.

Imprinting-related disorder

As mentioned in Chapter 9, there are a few genetic conditions in which the phenotypic effect of a gene alteration is dependent upon which parent has passed on the abnormal allele. The reason for this is that, in contrast to most autosomal loci, in which both alleles are together either transcriptionally active or inactive, these specific genes are only expressed (in at least the relevant tissues) from either the maternal or the paternal copy. The non-expressed copy is transcriptionally repressed by a process known as imprinting in which one gene copy is silenced by DNA methylation. The establishment of the imprint, involving DNA methylation of specific alleles, is believed to occur as they pass through the male or female germline. Examples of this effect underlie Angelman and Prader–Willi syndrome (the clinical features of which are discussed in Chapter 6) and the fetal overgrowth syndrome Beckwith–Wiedemann syndrome. In Angelman and Prader–Willi syndromes, the copy of the associated gene (or genes) that is normally transcriptionally active is the one that has been transmitted from the mother or the father, respectively (Fig. 16.5). It is the occasional loss of this active copy of the gene (or genes) that results in the

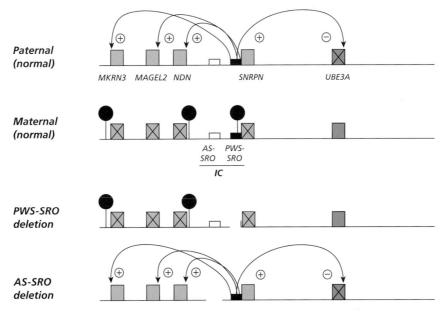

Fig. 16.5 Model of normal and abnormal gene expression control by the Prader–Willi syndrome (PWS)/Angelman syndrome (AS) imprinting centre (IC). Black circles represent sites of CpG methylation. Arrows indicate transcriptional control. The PWS/AS IC contains two functional regions: the 'PWS shortest region of overlap' (PWS-SRO) and the AS-SRO. Normally, on the paternally inherited chromosome 15, the PWS-SRO is unmethylated and active. It activates transcription of the *SNRPN*, *MKRN3*, *MAGEL2* and *NDN* genes (shaded blue), while in the brain it suppresses expression of the *UBE3A* gene (shaded red) possibly via antisense transcription of it. On the normal maternal chromosome 15, PWS-SRO is methylated and inactivated by a mechanism that depends on the presence of AS-SRO on the same chromosome. Consequently, the pattern of gene expression is reversed. In PWS patients with IC PWS-SRO microdeletions, a maternal gene expression pattern results, with loss of *SNRPN*, *MKRN3*, *MAGEL2* and *NDN* transcription. In AS patients with IC microdeletions that remove the AS-SRO, on maternal transmission the PWS-SRO fails to undergo methylation and inactivation, leading to the paternal regulatory pattern with loss of *UBE3A* expression. Modified from Horsthemke and Wagstaff, 2008 (see Further reading).

condition. Therefore, a deletion or inactivating mutation affecting the maternal copy of this region, at 15q11–13, can result in Angelman syndrome, while similar alterations affecting the paternal copy can cause Prader–Willi syndrome.

In Angelman syndrome, the disorder results in 70–75% of cases from a deletion, in approximately 5% of cases from paternal uniparental disomy (in which both copies of chromosome 15 are contributed by the father) and in 3% from an imprinting defect. These abnormalities will all show an abnormal methylation pattern upon standard genetic analysis at the neighbouring *SNRPN* gene. In an additional 10–20% of cases, however, the underlying defect is a mutation in the *UBE3A* gene at this locus, which will not be detected upon methylation analysis. As mentioned previously in Chapter 6, the *UBE3A* gene encodes a ubiquitin protein ligase enzyme. As the normal function of UBE3A is to chemically mark specific proteins (with ubiquitin tags) for subsequent degradation, in Angelman syndrome it may be the abnormal accumulation of these target proteins (resulting from the absence of UBE3A) that leads to the characteristic neurological abnormalities.

Genetic investigations of individuals affected by Angelman syndrome include cytogenetic analyses (karyotype and fluorescence *in situ* hybridisation (FISH) for deletion of the Angelman syndrome/Prader–Willi syndrome critical region) and *SNPRN* methylation studies. If there is no cytogenetic abnormality, then, if the methylation is abnormal, additional analyses may include uniparental disomy (UPD) testing (which requires the parents' DNA samples). If there is no cytogenetic or methylation abnormality, then *UBE3A* mutation analysis would be considered, particularly if a family history is present.

The clinically distinct Prader–Willi syndrome, in contrast, results from loss of expression of the paternal allele at the same 15q locus. At the critical region within this locus, it is the paternally inherited copies of the *MKRN3*, *MAGEL2*, *NDN* and *SNRPN* genes (which are normally expressed in the tissues involved, e.g. in the brain) that are believed to be most important in causing the phenotype. As for Angelman syndrome, investigations of a case of Prader–Willi syndrome would normally include cytogenetic analysis, methylation studies and possibly UPD testing. As in Angelman syndrome, there is a deletion present in around 75% of cases (detectable on karyotyping or by FISH), although it is of course on the paternal chromosome. Of the remaining 25% of cases, almost all show UPD (maternal in Prader–Willi syndrome), and only around 1% of overall cases possess an imprinting defect.

In genetic counselling of such families, where the parental karyotypes are normal, the recurrence risk is very low where the proband's phenotype is the result of a *de novo* deletion or of paternal UPD. If however, a parent possesses a chromosomal translocation or if the proband possesses an inherited *UBE3A* mutation (or an inherited imprinting centre defect), the recurrence risk could be much higher. The possibility of offering prenatal diagnosis would then need to be considered. The imprinting centre is a small region of 35 kb of genomic DNA located just upstream of the *SNRPN* gene (Fig. 16.5). It contains two imprint control elements that are responsible for establishing and maintaining the paternal and maternal imprints. Inherited microdeletions that affect the imprinting centre region account for only 10–20% of imprinting defects but are associated with a 50% recurrence risk. The remainder of the imprinting defects are the result of incompletely explained abnormalities of methylation and are associated with a very small risk (<1%) of recurrence in siblings. These non-deletion, epigenetic (i.e. not affecting the DNA sequence itself) imprinting defects may result from errors occurring in imprint erasure in primordial germ cells, in imprint establishment in the gametes or in its maintenance in postzygotic cells (see Horsthemke and Wagstaff, 2008; in Further reading).

Individuals with Prader–Willi syndrome or Angelman syndrome almost never reproduce. There is a theoretical possibility, however, that if a proband who had Prader–Willi syndrome as the result of an inherited deletion at 15q11–13 were to have a child, then there would be a 50% chance of the child having Prader–Willi syndrome if the proband was male or Angelman syndrome if the proband was female. For an example of a reported family illustrating this, see Fig. 9.6.

Chromosomal translocation

A translocation is the transfer of chromosomal material between chromosomes. Three main types are identified: reciprocal, Robertsonian (centric fusion) and insertional (see Chapter 7). Robertsonian translocations only involve the acrocentric chromosomes (i.e. chromosomes 13–15, 21 and 22), whereas reciprocal translocations may involve any of the chromosomes, including the sex chromosomes. If the transfer results in no overall loss or gain of chromosomal material, then the person will usually be healthy and is said to have a balanced translocation. The birth frequency for balanced translocations is 1 in 500, with approximately equal numbers of the centric fusion and reciprocal types but relatively few insertional translocations. Most of the Robertsonian translocations are inherited, with only around 10% being *de novo*, whereas, of the reciprocal translocations, approximately half are inherited and half are *de novo*.

The carrier of a balanced translocation can be reassured that their health and lifespan would be expected to be unaffected. Problems may arise, however, during meiosis with the possible production of chromosomally unbalanced offspring. Some of these fetuses will spontaneously abort, but, if liveborn, the children often exhibit multiple dysmorphic features and usually have learning difficulties. On theoretical grounds, the majority of offspring should be chromosomally unbalanced, but the actual risk is much lower because of embryonic inviability and gametic selection. The risk of unbalanced offspring depends upon the type of translocation and which parent is the carrier (Table 16.1).

The risks for reciprocal translocations vary somewhat in different families, reflecting the wide variety of possible breakpoints and rearrangements. Exchanges of whole arms of

Table 16.1 Risks of chromosomally unbalanced offspring, at birth, for carriers of balanced structural rearrangements. See Gardner and Sutherland (2004) in Further reading for further details

The risks of chromosomally unbalanced offspring for the carriers of pericentric inversions, reciprocal translocations and insertions vary significantly, depending upon such factors as the size and site of the abnormal segment, the family history and whether there have been published reports of liveborn individuals with related chromosomal imbalances. See Table 18.9 for risks at amniocentesis (rather than at birth).

Rearrangement	Carrier	Risk of unbalanced offspring at birth (%)
Robertsonian translocation 13;14	Father	<1
Robertsonian translocation 13;14	Mother	1
Robertsonian translocation 14;21	Father	<1
Robertsonian translocation 14;21	Mother	10–15
Robertsonian translocation 21;22	Father	<1
Robertsonian translocation 21;22	Mother	10–15
Robertsonian translocation 21;21	Either parent	100
Paracentric inversion	Either parent	<1
Pericentric inversion*	Either parent	1–10% (see table legend)

*excluding the common pericentric inversion of chromosome 9, which is a normal variant.

non-acrocentric chromosomes rarely produce viable offspring and, if ascertainment is via recurrent miscarriages only, the risk of chromosomally abnormal viable offspring is often said to be 5% or less. The assessment of the risk of viability of chromosomally unbalanced fetuses, however, is likely also to involve: (i) determination of the length of the potentially unbalanced chromosomal segments (the haploid autosomal length or HAL) with higher risks being associated with shorter HALs; (ii) consultation of empiric (i.e. observed outcome) reference data; (iii) study of published phenotypes of affected cases that possessed similar chromosomal imbalances; and (iv) consideration as to whether a 3:1 segregation (mentioned in Chapter 7) is a likely outcome. The latter, which has a greater associated risk of trisomic segments, is more likely, for instance, for some female carriers of a reciprocal translocation between chromosomes 11 and 22. If ascertainment of a parental balanced reciprocal translocation is via a family history of a liveborn affected child or a termination of pregnancy with multiple congenital anomalies, the risk will generally be said to be high, for example 20% or greater. Fetal karyotyping after amniocentesis or chorionic villus sampling (CVS) may provide reassurance in a pregnancy at risk. About half of unbalanced fetuses detected at the time of CVS will generally have spontaneously aborted before the time of amniocentesis. A family study should always be undertaken to detect other relatives who are outwardly healthy translocation carriers, who will be at similar reproductive risk.

A *de novo* apparently balanced translocation where both parents have normal chromosomes is usually not associated with clinical abnormality. Occasionally (<10%), however, in reciprocal but not in Robertsonian translocations, genes may be damaged at the break points and produce imbalance and an abnormal phenotype. This is a cause for concern when a *de novo* reciprocal translocation is an incidental finding at amniocentesis, even when the ultrasound scan is apparently normal.

When the parent is a carrier of an inversion, the risk to the offspring depends on the location on the chromosome of the inverted segment. Thus, if the inversion is paracentric (i.e. does not encompass the centromere), then the risk is very low. If, however, the inversion is pericentric (i.e. the inverted segment includes the centromere), then the risk may be high, particularly if the inverted region is large with small distal normal chromosomal segments (see Chapter 7).

Further details regarding the calculation of risks resulting from parental chromosomal aberrations are given in Gardner and Sutherland (2004) and Young (2007), in Further reading.

SUMMARY

- DM and fragile X syndrome are examples of autosomal dominant and X-linked inheritance, respectively, that is atypical as a result of genetic anticipation.

- In DM, the genetic anticipation is due to expansion of a repeat tract within the 3′ UTR of the *DMPK* gene. This indirectly interferes with the splicing of several genes.

- Females affected by DM are at particular risk of having severely affected children.

- Fragile X syndrome, the commonest inherited cause of mental retardation, affects all males and up to 50% of females, who inherit the full mutation (an expanded trinucleotide repeat in the 5′ UTR of the *FMR1* gene).

- The mother of a male affected by fragile X syndrome will possess either the premutation or the full mutation.

- Angelman syndrome and Prader–Willi syndrome are both imprinting disorders. Deletions affecting the maternal chromosome at the region at 15q11–13 can cause Angelman syndrome, while those affecting the paternal chromosome can cause Prader–Willi syndrome. High recurrence risks may apply if a parent possesses a predisposing chromosome abnormality, or if the condition has been caused by an inherited microdeletion or point mutation.

- Chromosome translocations may be reciprocal, Robertsonian or, more rarely, insertional. Carriers of apparently balanced reciprocal translocations are usually healthy but are at risk of having abnormal offspring, particularly if there is a family history of a liveborn affected child or a termination of pregnancy with multiple congenital anomalies.

FURTHER READING

Gardner RJM, Sutherland GR (2004) *Chromosome Abnormalities and Genetic Counseling*, 3rd edn. Oxford University Press: Oxford.

Harper PS (2010). *Practical Genetic Counselling*, 7th edn. Hodder Arnold: London.

Horsthemke B, Wagstaff J (2008) Mechanisms of imprinting of the Prader–Willi/Angelman region. *Am J Med Genet A* **146A**:2041–52.

Hudson G, Chinnery PF (2006) Mitochondrial DNA polymerase-γ and human disease. *Hum Mol Genet* **15** (review issue no. 2):R244–52.

Lee JE, Cooper TA (2009) Pathogenic mechanisms of myotonic dystrophy. *Biochem Soc Trans* **37**: 1281–6.

Pfeiffer BE, Huber KM (2009) The State of Synapses in Fragile X Syndrome. *Neuroscientist* **15**:549–67.

Young ID (2007) *Introduction to Risk Calculation in Genetic Counseling*. Oxford University Press: Oxford.

WEBSITES

GeneReviews:
http://www.genetests.org

Online Mendelian Inheritance in Man (OMIM):
http://www.ncbi.nlm.nih.gov/sites/entrez?db=omim

Self-assessment

1. Which of the following are correct regarding the pregnant 19-year-old in Fig. 16.6 who may be clinically affected by myotonic dystrophy (DM)?
A. Identification of the pathogenic gene alteration would normally be undertaken by DNA sequencing of the gene
B. If the repeat expansion has been detected in her DNA, prenatal diagnosis will be possible
C. Prediction of the degree of severity of the phenotype in her future child would be reliable using prenatal DNA analysis
D. Her child, if congenitally affected, is likely to have a 'tented mouth' appearance with an inability to smile
E. Genetic testing should be offered to her close relatives, in case they too have DM

2. In relation to the information given in the scenario described in Fig. 16.7, which of the following statements are correct?
A. Carol is a carrier of a full fragile X mutation
B. As Carol is healthy and does not have learning difficulties, the chances of her having children affected by fragile X are very low
C. If she were to have a son, the chance of him being affected would be approximately 50%

D. Prenatal diagnosis would be available if she wished, in order to determine the sex and fragile X mutation status of the fetus
E. If, following chorionic villus sampling testing, the fetus were found to be female with a full fragile X mutation, examination of the number of repeats present in the full mutation would predict the severity of the learning difficulties in the future child

3. With regard to the family shown in Fig. 16.8, which of the following are correct?
A. Arthur's father's children from his second marriage (II:1 and II:2) are now at significant risk of developing Leber hereditary optic neuropathy (LHON)
B. Arthur himself is not at risk of transmitting the condition to his offspring
C. Prenatal diagnosis would be a straightforward way of determining which of Arthur's sister's children are likely to be severely affected in the future
D. Arthur's sister (II:4), being only mildly affected, can be reassured that she is unlikely to pass the disorder on to her children
E. The mutation rate in mitochondrial DNA is lower than in nuclear DNA

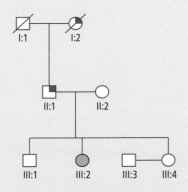

Fig. 16.6 A 19-year-old woman (individual III:4), at 7 weeks' gestation in her first pregnancy, mentions to her general practitioner in the UK that she had heard that her sister (III:2) was recently diagnosed in New York State with DM. On questioning, it transpires that their father (II:1) and his mother (I:2) were both affected by cataracts in their adult life. On further discussion, the 19-year-old herself mentions a difficulty she has noticed in letting go of shopping bag handles, particularly in cold weather. She asks whether she might be affected by the same condition as her sister and whether there are any tests that could help determine this. She also asks whether, if she is affected, her unborn child may be affected (see Self-assessment question 1).

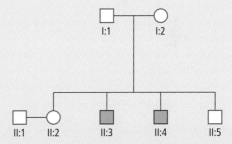

Fig. 16.7 Carol (II:2), a 26-year-old teacher, seeks genetic advice prior to marrying her partner, to whom she is not related. She is healthy and studied mathematics at university, but is aware that two of her three brothers (II:3 and II:4) have required special schooling on account of their significant learning difficulties. She is concerned that there might be a familial tendency that could have implications for her future children. It has transpired that one of Carol's affected brothers (II:3) was recently tested and was found to possess a fragile X gene alteration with a product size corresponding to approximately 220 CGG repeats. Carol herself has now undergone genetic testing and has been found to possess 104 repeats. She asks about her risk of having affected children and whether prenatal testing can be relied upon to detect which children are going to be affected (see question 2 in Self-assessment).

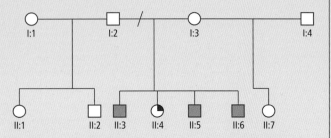

Fig. 16.8 A 25-year-old man, Arthur (II:6), is investigated on account of progressive central visual loss. He is aware that his two elder brothers (II:3 and II:5) became progressively affected by a similar condition from around the age of 30 and are now legally blind. In addition, his sister (II:4) has been affected but to a much milder extent. Arthur has a central scotoma and undergoes blood DNA testing for Leber hereditary optic neuropathy. He is found to possess the m.11778G>A mutation in his mitochondrial DNA. Arthur's parents, now divorced, have each married new partners and had further children (see question 3 in Self-assessment).

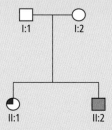

Fig. 16.9 A male neonate (II:2) is investigated on account of difficult feeding with a poor suck, severe floppiness, hypogonadism and small hands. His saliva is noted by a junior doctor as being unusually 'stringy' and thick. His elder sister (II:1) has moderate learning difficulty but has never been fully investigated. The baby boy is suspected to have Prader–Willi syndrome and undergoes genetic testing. His karyotype and FISH studies are found to be normal with no detectable deletion at 15q11–13. Methylation analysis does, however, reveal an abnormality with, very unusually, the paternal chromosome carrying a maternal imprint. Following analysis of his DNA, he is subsequently found to possess an imprinting centre microdeletion at the 5′ end of the *SNRPN* locus on chromosome 15. His mother (I:2), and subsequently his older sister, are both found to possess the same microdeletion. His parents are concerned that their next child might be similarly affected (see question 4 in Self-assessment).

4. Which of the following are true statements with regard to the information given in the scenario shown in Fig. 16.9?
   A. Although not found in this neonate, cytogenetically detectable deletions at the 15q11–13 region are more common than uniparental disomy (UPD)
   B. In Prader–Willi syndrome, UPD is likely to be paternal in origin
   C. The recurrence risk following the birth of a child with Prader–Willi syndrome on account of an inherited imprinting centre microdeletion may be up to 50%
   D. Mutations in the imprinting centre are frequently the cause of the syndrome
   E. In Angelman syndrome, UPD is again a possible cause, but will be paternal in origin

5. Which of the following is correct, in relation to the family shown in Fig. 16.10?
   A. The health of Ann herself would not be expected to be significantly adversely affected as a result of the translocation
   B. This translocation is the least common of the constitutional non-Robertsonian translocation in humans
   C. There is a significant risk to Ann's offspring, but she could still have a healthy child
   D. Prenatal diagnosis would be available
   E. Ann's parents should be tested for the translocation if possible, so that the appropriate relatives can subsequently be offered a chromosome test in order that carriers can be identified

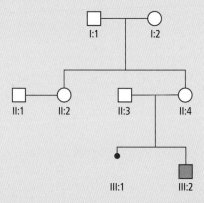

Fig. 16.10 Colin and his wife, Ann (II:2), attend the genetics clinic after being referred by Ann's family doctor. The doctor was concerned after hearing that Ann's sister, Paula (II:4), had recently (following a previous miscarriage) given birth to an infant with multiple congenital anomalies. This, it emerged, had led to Paula having a chromosome test. The karyotype had, in fact, revealed that Paula was a carrier of an apparently balanced translocation between chromosomes 11 and 22, known as t(11;22)(q23;q11). Ann is tested at the genetics clinic and unfortunately is found to possess the same translocation. She is concerned that she may never be able to have a healthy child and seeks advice (see question 5 in Self-assessment).

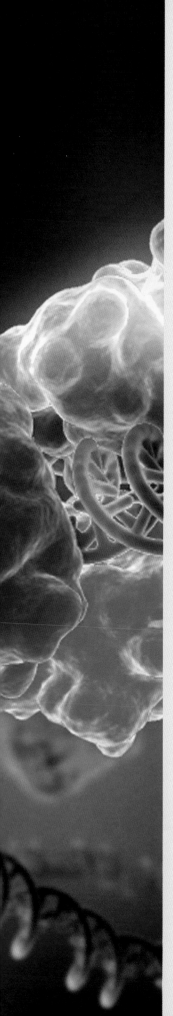

CHAPTER 17

Screening for disease and for carriers

Key Topics

Introduction

In this chapter, commonly used forms of prenatal and neonatal screening for specific conditions are described, in addition to examples of situations in which carrier detection is carried out in adults. Population screening entails the testing of a whole population in order to detect those at risk of a genetic disease either for themselves or for their offspring. This approach is not appropriate for all genetic diseases as certain principles need to be observed (Table 17.1). Thus, although many genetic diseases are well defined, they are too rare to merit a whole population screening programme. There must also be an advantage to early detection. For example, prenatal diagnosis (e.g. of neural tube defects or Down syndrome) provides the option of selective termination, neonatal diagnosis (e.g. of cystic fibrosis) permits presymptomatic therapy, and carrier detection (e.g. for β-thalassaemia or Tay–Sachs disease, as described below) permits genetic counselling and possibly prenatal diagnosis in a future pregnancy. Any test used for population screening must be sensitive or cases will be missed and yet it must be sufficiently specific to prevent the need for re-testing large numbers of false-positive cases. The sensitivity of a screening test is measured by determining the proportion of affected persons detected, and its specificity from the proportion of unaffected persons testing as normal (see Table 17.2).

Essential Medical Genetics, 6th edition. © Edward S. Tobias, Michael Connor and Malcolm Ferguson-Smith.
Published 2011 by Blackwell Published Ltd.

Table 17.1 Principles of a screening programme

Clearly defined disorder

Appreciable frequency

Advantage to early diagnosis

Few false positives (specificity)

Few false negatives (sensitivity)

Benefits outweigh the costs

See the National Screening Committee website in Further reading for full details of the selection criteria used to determine whether or not screening should be recommended.

Table 17.2 Screening test sensitivity, specificity and predictive values

Screening test result	Clinical status	
	Affected	**Unaffected**
Positive	True positive (TP)	False positive (FP)
Negative	False negative (FN)	True negative (TN)

The *sensitivity* can be calculated from TP/(TP + FN), whereas the *specificity* is TN/(FP + TN). The *positive predictive value* is the proportion of those testing positive who are actually affected. This is calculated from TP/(TP + FP). Similarly, the *negative predictive value* is the proportion of those who have a negative test result who do not have the condition: TN/(FN + TN).

Prenatal screening

Two major prenatal screening programmes that have become widely available are (i) fetal ultrasound scanning in the second trimester for structural malformations such as neural tube defects (NTDs) and, more recently, (ii) screening for Down syndrome by combined ultrasound and biochemical screening (CUBS) in the first trimester.

Neural tube defect

As over 95% of all children with NTDs are born to couples with no relevant family history, it is clear that only by screening all of the pregnant population can most pregnancies at risk be identified. In the first trimester, most women have a 'dating scan' to confirm the stage of gestation. The ultrasound scan at this early stage can detect almost all cases of anencephaly but visualisation of spina bifida is difficult at this stage of gestation.

In addition, detailed ultrasound screening for fetal malformations in the second trimester is now widely available in many countries. Previously, in many geographical regions, detailed ultrasound scanning was confined to pregnancies at increased risk of a specific condition. Performed at 18–22 weeks of gestation, it can detect many serious structural abnor-

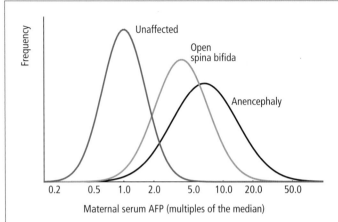

Fig. 17.1 MSAFP in normal pregnancies and pregnancies affected by neural tube defects. (The distribution is log Gaussian and hence medians rather than means are used). Figure kindly provided by Jenny Crossley and David Aitken, Yorkhill Hospitals, Glasgow.

malities affecting the fetus, such as malformations of the central nervous system, heart, kidneys, limbs and intestines (see Table 12.14). The ability to detect NTDs (including spina bifida) with a higher sensitivity and specificity (although published data show large variations in these figures) than maternal serum α-fetoprotein (MSAFP) screening (see below) has led to ultrasound scanning now being the recommended method of screening for NTDs in the UK. There are, however, limitations to the range of abnormalities that can be detected by ultrasound scanning, and this is particularly true of some cardiac and brain abnormalities.

Prior to the introduction of detailed ultrasound scanning, MSAFP was widely used to detect neural tube defects. α-Fetoprotein (AFP) is the major fetal plasma protein and has a similar structure and function to albumin in the adult. AFP is made initially by the yolk sac and later by the liver. It peaks in the fetal bloodstream at around 12–14 weeks of gestation and falls thereafter. It is found in the amniotic fluid at approximately 0.01% of the concentration found in fetal serum. Most of this is derived from fetal urine and the maximum concentration is attained at 14–15 weeks of gestation. Fetal AFP reaches the maternal bloodstream and is detectable at levels 1000 times less than those found in amniotic fluid. The MSAFP rises from 13 weeks of gestation to a peak at around 32 weeks of 250 ng/ml before falling towards term (Fig. 17.1). Correct interpretation of MSAFP results depends critically on the accurate estimation of gestation. In pregnancies where the fetus has a NTD or certain other malformations, MSAFP is elevated by leakage into the amniotic fluid from exposed fetal capillaries (Table 17.3).

Where a second-trimester ultrasound is not routinely available, measurement of MSAFP may instead be undertaken at 15–20 (optimum 17) completed weeks of gestation. If the level is above the 95th centile (equivalent to two multiples of the

Table 17.3 Causes of elevated maternal serum and amniotic fluid AFP

Cause	MSAFP	Amniotic fluid AFP
Underestimated gestation	+	–
Overestimated gestation	–	+
Fetal blood in amniotic fluid	+/–	+
Multiple pregnancy	+	–
Threatened abortion	+*	–
Missed abortion	+	+
Anencephaly	++	++
Open spina bifida	+	+
Closed spina bifida	–	–
Isolated hydrocephalus	–	–
Anterior abdominal wall defect	+/–	+
Fetal teratoma	+/–	+/–
Maternal hereditary persistence of AFP	++	–
Congenital nephrotic syndrome	+	+
Skin defects	+	+
Placental haemangioma	+	+

++, Very elevated; +, elevated; –, not elevated.
*MSAFP returns to normal within a week after symptoms subside.

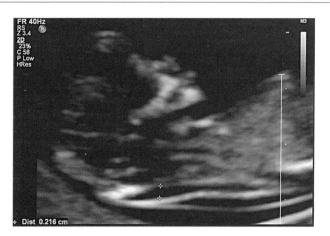

Fig. 17.2 Fetal ultrasound scan. The NT measurement between the points indicated by '+' was 2.16 mm.

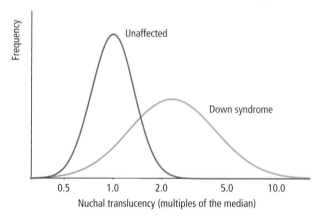

Fig. 17.3 NT measurements in normal pregnancies and in those affected by Down syndrome. Figure kindly provided by Jenny Crossley and David Aitken, Yorkhill Hospitals, Glasgow.

median), then a detailed fetal ultrasound is generally indicated in order to detect a possible NTD or other defect (Table 17.3).

The causes of elevated AFP in maternal serum (and amniotic fluid) are listed in Table 17.3. Amniocentesis was historically occasionally undertaken (to permit analysis of the amniotic fluid AFP level and acetycholinesterase electrophoresis pattern) in order to reduce the rate of false-positive NTD detection. In practice, on account of the efficacy of detailed ultrasound scanning, amniocentesis is now rarely used in the UK for the diagnosis of NTDs alone.

Unexplained elevations of MSAFP are associated with an increased risk of spontaneous miscarriage, premature labour, stillbirth, low birth weight and perinatal death.

Down syndrome

The recommended method of screening for Down syndrome in the UK is now CUBS in the first trimester (at 11 + 0 to 13 + 6 weeks' gestation). This method is regarded as superior to current biochemical second-trimester screening protocols, in terms of improved sensitivity and specificity, in addition to the consequent earlier diagnosis of an affected pregnancy. It includes a measurement of the fetal nuchal translucency (NT)

and also the measurement of biochemical markers. The NT represents the ultrasound-translucent area of fluid between the skin and the soft tissue that overlies the cervical spine in the fetal neck (Fig. 17.2). Its average normal thickness (at its widest point) is 1.4–1.5 mm at 13 weeks of gestation (when measured in the sagittal plane). The NT thickness is often increased in Down syndrome (Fig. 17.3) and also in trisomy 18 and trisomy 13. For instance, 84% of Down syndrome pregnancies, but only 4.5% of those that are unaffected, have a NT measurement of 2.5 mm or greater. The biochemical markers used in the first trimester currently include free β human chorionic gonadotrophin (β-hCG, which is increased in Down syndrome-affected pregnancies) and pregnancy-associated plasma protein A (PAPP-A), which is reduced in such pregnancies (Fig. 17.4). This combination, depending on the institution, is said to give a Down syndrome detection rate of approximately 85–90%, with a false-positive rate of around 3.5% (see Table 17.4). To meet the new UK National Screening Committee recommendations (>90% detection rate for a false-positive rate of <2%),

Table 17.4 Examples of methods used to screen for Down syndrome

Test	Characteristics	Detection rate	False-positive rate
Age alone	Chorionic villus sampling or amniocentesis offered to all pregnant mothers aged 35 or older	55%*	20%*
Triple marker	Classic 'triple test' using three serum markers in second trimester (14–20 weeks) (AFP and total hCG, or AFP and free β-hCG)	65–70%	5–6%
Quadruple marker	Four maternal serum markers in second trimester (AFP, hCG, UE3 and inhibin A)	75%	5%
Combined (CUBS)	First trimester (10–13 weeks) ultrasound NT and serum (free β-hCG and PAPP-A)	85–90%	3.5%
Contingent	CUBS plus standard second-trimester tests	>90%	2%

Data obtained predominantly from Aitken *et al.*(2007) with addition of updated results for CUBS.
*Calculated figures for this method in 2008, when the median age at delivery in the UK was 30 years. Previously, these figures were lower on account of the younger maternal age distribution. For instance, in 1992, when the median age at delivery was 26 years, the detection rate using age alone was 32% with a false-positive rate of 7%.

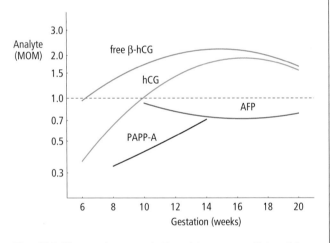

Fig. 17.4 Changes in concentrations (shown as multiples of the median or MOM) of four analytes in maternal serum with increasing gestation in pregnancies affected by Down syndrome. Figure kindly provided by Jenny Crossley and David Aitken, Yorkhill Hospitals, Glasgow.

Table 17.5 Variations in protein levels in maternal serum in chromosomally abnormal pregnancies

Protein level in maternal serum (trimester)	Trisomy 21	Trisomy 18	Trisomy 13
AFP (second trimester)	L	L	N/H
hCG (second trimester)	H	L	N
Free β-hCG (first trimester)	H	L	L
PAPP-A (first trimester)	L	L	L
UE3 (second trimester)	L	L	L*
Inhibin A (second trimester)	H	N	H*

L, low; H, high; N, normal. Measurements of both UE3 and inhibin A are increasingly becoming incorporated into second-trimester screening protocols. Data from Aitken *et al.* (2007); see Further reading.
*Based on small numbers.

however, new protocols will be required. These will involve some or all women having more than one sample taken at different stages of pregnancy. For example, the contingent protocol incorporates maternal age, NT, free β-hCG and PAPP-A in the first trimester and uses a high cut-off to achieve a Down syndrome detection rate of 60% at a low false-positive rate of 1.2%; 75% of the pregnancies are identified as very low risk and can be reassured without further tests. The remaining pregnancies are retested in the second trimester using the standard biochemical markers. The outcome is an overall detection rate of >90% for a false-positive rate of 2%, and the need for chorionic villus sampling (CVS) and amniocentesis is reduced to a minimum. The first-trimester screening

does not include AFP as it is not discriminatory for either NTDs or Down syndrome at that stage (see Fig 17.4, which shows the distributions of maternal serum AFP, hCG, free β-hCG and PAPP-A in Down syndrome and unaffected pregnancies).

For those women who are unable to undergo CUBS (for instance because of booking after 14 weeks of gestation), quadruple biochemical screening may be offered. This consists of the measurement of MSAFP, hCG or free β-hCG, unconjugated estriol 3 (UE3) and inhibin A. For instance, MSAFP levels are generally reduced in the second trimester to an average of 0.7 multiples of the median in pregnancies affected by trisomy 21 or other autosomal trisomies (see Fig. 17.4).

Although the normal ranges of these measurements are known in addition to the observed increases or decreases in such measurements with trisomic pregnancies (Table 17.5), the molecular mechanisms of these changes are not understood. In addition, it should be noted that appropriate population control values are required, as levels of MSAFP are, for instance, generally lower (by 6%) in Asian women and higher (by 15%) in black people.

For those pregnancies that are assessed by such first- or second-trimester screening as being at significant risk of being affected by Down syndrome (or trisomy 18 or 13), invasive testing by CVS or amniocentesis, respectively, can be offered, with subsequent testing by quantitative fluorescent polymerase chain reaction (QF-PCR; see Chapter 7).

Historically, screening for fetal chromosomal abnormalities, of which trisomy 21 is numerically the most important, was confined to the offer of CVS or amniocentesis to mothers of 35 years and older, in view of the rising incidence with maternal age (see Table 18.8). This was later followed by the offer of second-trimester biochemical screening to all pregnant women, combining information from maternal serum biochemistry (MSAFP and hCG measurement) with maternal age risk, and so extending screening to identify those younger mothers who were also at increased risk. This gave a greater sensitivity of 65–70% for a false-positive rate of 5–6%, compared with a sensitivity of just 32% for a false-positive rate of 7% using maternal age alone (Table 17.4).

A recent study concluded that, from 1989 to 2008 in England and Wales, the number of live births affected by Down syndrome would have been expected to increase by 48% (from rising maternal age), but this appears to have been fully offset by improvements in available antenatal screening with more subsequent terminations, such that the birth frequency has remained almost unchanged (see Morris and Alberman, 2009, in Further reading).

While NT is probably the most effective marker of fetal chromosomal abnormalities that is widely available at present, in order to benefit from the information that it provides, women must attend the screening clinic within the fairly narrow gestational window mentioned above, at 11 + 0 to 13 + 6 weeks' gestation. As mentioned above, for those attending too late, second-trimester screening may be offered. It should also be noted that fetal abnormalities other than aneuploidy, such as cardiac defects, may be associated with an abnormally high first-trimester NT measurement. Therefore, when the NT is significantly increased (e.g. over 2.5 multiples of the median or over 3.0 mm) but the fetus is found to be chromosomally normal, a second-trimester ultrasound or fetal echocardiogram is advisable.

Future methods of trisomy detection may involve the detection of abnormalities of the fetal DNA or RNA in maternal blood. There is, in fact, growing evidence that the detection of trisomic pregnancies from fetal nucleic acid in the maternal circulation is possible, although it is currently very costly (see Fan *et al.*, 2008, in Further reading). If reliable, it could provide a non-invasive means of detection that is even more sensitive than CUBS.

Neonatal screening

Neonatal screening was first introduced in 1961 (for phenylketonuria) and its success has encouraged the development of other neonatal screening tests. These tests are generally performed on a dried blood spot, which is collected from a heel prick within the first 5–7 days of life (e.g. on a blood spot card). In many Western countries, virtually all newborns are tested in this way.

Depending on geographical location, different neonatal screening tests are performed for a number of childhood conditions, which may include phenylketonuria (PKU), congenital hypothyrodism, cystic fibrosis (CF) and haemoglobinopathies (Table 17.6). With the availability of advanced methods of detection such as tandem mass spectrometry, the range of screening tests that are possible has increased greatly. In Scotland, for instance, the neonatal screening tests currently performed routinely are those that detect PKU, congenital hypothyroidism and CF (see below). Testing for medium chain acyl co-A dehydrogenase deficiency (MCADD) and sickle-cell disorder are being added in 2010. Other countries have more expansive screening programmes.

PKU is a treatable autosomal recessive condition with learning disability that is caused by a deficiency of phenylalanine hydroxylase, resulting from mutations in the *PAH* gene on chromosome 12. For children with PKU, early diagnosis and therapy are mandatory if normal development is to occur. However, few if any physical signs are present in the neonate. The presence of an increased level of blood phenylalanine in the dried blood spot is now detected by tandem mass spectrometry (but was previously identified by the Guthrie bacterial inhibition assay). Mild elevations of phenylalanine due to prematurity or delayed enzyme maturation are not uncommon and these can be excluded by repeat testing. False negatives are rare.

Similarly, with congenital hypothyrodism, early diagnosis and therapy will permit normal development, yet few physical

---

Table 17.6 Examples of conditions that are included in neonatal screening programmes

Phenylketonuria

Congenital hypothyroidism

Cystic fibrosis

Galactosaemia (no longer recommended in the UK)

Congenital adrenal hyperplasia (not in the UK)

Haemoglobinopathies (e.g. sickle-cell disease)

Medium chain acyl coA dehydrogenase deficiency (MCADD; introduced in England in March 2009; being introduced in Scotland in 2010)

See the National Screening Committee website in Further reading for a complete table of conditions for which screening is recommended in the UK.

Table 17.7 Signs in infants with congenital hypothyroidism at the time of diagnosis by newborn screening

Prolonged jaundice	80%
Open fontanelles	60%
Poor feeding	60%
Large tongue	47%
Hypothermia	40%
Umbilical hernia	35%
Hoarse cry	18%
Increased TSH	100%

signs are present in the newborn (Table 17.7). Thyroid-stimulating hormone (TSH) is measured on the dried blood spot. Neonates with primary hypothyroidism have elevated levels of TSH. The recall rate is 0.05% and false negatives appear to be rare. The incidence of congenital hypothyroidism is 1 in 3000–4000 in the UK compared with 1 in 900 in Asians and 1 in 20,000–30,000 in African-Americans. Although occasional cases are due to recessive enzyme defects (in which case there is usually a goitre), the majority are sporadic failures of normal thyroid development with a low recurrence risk.

Cystic fibrosis

CF is the most common serious autosomal recessive disorder in northern Europe and the USA. As described in Chapter 15 in detail, CF is inherited as an autosomal recessive trait and is caused by a variety of mutations (over 1000) in the CF transmembrane conductance regulator (*CFTR*) gene. The incidence of the condition in the UK is 1 in 2500 newborns and it is much less common in native Africans and Asians than in European Caucasians. A 3 bp deletion, resulting in loss of a single amino acid at position 508 (ΔF508) is the single commonest mutation. This mutation accounts for 70% of mutant alleles in Caucasians. The protein in patients with ΔF508 is abnormally processed after translation and is degraded before it reaches its site of function. Most of the other mutations are individually uncommon, although a few are associated with particular ethnic groups, such as the W1282X mutation, which accounts for approximately half of the mutant alleles in Ashkenazi Jews.

Those individuals affected by the condition commonly go on to develop chronic lung disease secondary to recurrent infection, pancreatic insufficiency and, in males, infertility due to congenital bilateral absence of the vas deferens (CBAVD). The clinical severity is very variable, depending to some extent on the genotype. Individuals homozygous for the ΔF508 *CFTR* mutation generally all have pancreatic insufficiency but the severity of the lung disease varies considerably. Survival of

individuals affected by CF is into early adulthood, increasingly beyond the age of 30.

Neonatal testing is being made available in an increasing number of regions as it is believed that early prophylactic intervention with antibiotics improves the clinical outcome. The initial screening test, performed on a blood spot, measures serum immunoreactive trypsinogen levels in the newborn period. This trypsinogen is produced by the pancreas and its release into the circulation is elevated in CF, probably on account of abnormal pancreatic duct secretions. This test has a high sensitivity but not specificity, and additional testing is appropriate for those neonates that have elevated initial immunoreactive trypsinogen (IRT) results (Fig. 17.5). Further testing involves a repeat IRT assay, and, if this is again elevated, a molecular genetic screen of the *CFTR* gene for the commonest mutations is undertaken. If two pathogenic mutations are detected, CF is diagnosed and sweat testing is usually carried out for diagnostic confirmation. If only one *CFTR* mutation is detected, then a further IRT assay is carried out at 27 days of life. If this is now below the pre-defined cut-off value (e.g. 60 ng/ml), then the child is regarded as being a CF carrier. If, however, it is instead again found to be greater than the threshold value, then a sweat test (and possibly a more complete *CFTR* mutation analysis) is generally undertaken, in case the child is actually affected, possessing a second mutation that was not detected by the initial *CFTR* mutation screen. With this strategy, currently used to test approximately 60,000 neonates annually in Scotland, CF mutation screening is required for approximately 360 of these babies. Of these, around 30 (1 in 12) are found to be affected (and approximately 30 to be carriers). The positive predictive value of the IRT test for detecting CF is therefore around 1 in 12, or 8.3%.

A randomised controlled trial has shown that neonatal CF screening reduces the frequency of severe malnutrition among affected children who were screen-detected (see Southern *et al.*, 2009, in Further reading). In addition to the clinical benefits for the children detected early, the parents can be counselled regarding the possibility of recurrence, they can be offered prenatal diagnosis and cascade screening of relatives can be initiated.

Carrier detection in the adult population

The purpose of adult carrier screening is to allow reproductive choices to be made at an early stage, ideally prior to conception. At the present time, population genetic screening for carrier detection in the UK is mainly focused on ethnic groups who are at high risk for particular single-gene disorders such as thalassaemia and Tay–Sachs disease (Table 17.8). Such testing is offered on a voluntary participation basis. Participation in population carrier screening programmes worldwide, which are mainly for β-thalassaemia, is, however, mandatory in some countries (see Zlotogora, 2009, in Further reading, for a detailed review). Carrier screening for many other genetic

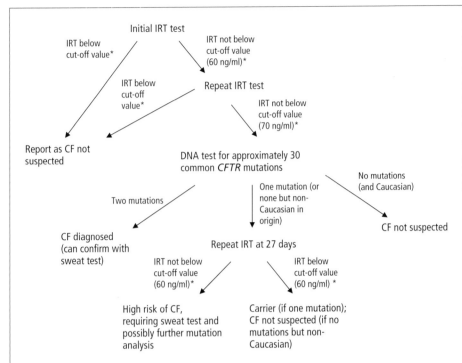

Fig. 17.5 Neonatal screening strategy in Scotland for the detection of CF by immunoreactive trypsinogen (IRT) and mutation analysis. The cut-off values used (indicated by *) are currently 60 ng/ml and 70 ng/ml, depending on the stage of the test in the protocol. The strategy has been simplified slightly for illustrative purposes. Figure adapted from details provided by Joan Mackenzie and Arlene Brown, Yorkhill Hospitals, Glasgow.

Table 17.8 Examples of population groups for which carrier screening is most appropriate

Condition(s)	Ancestral/population group(s)
β-Thalassaemia and glucose-6-phosphate dehydrogenase deficiency	Mediterraneans, Indians, Middle East populations, Thais, people of Middle Eastern, South-east Asian, Mediterranean or African descent
Sickle-cell disease	African-Americans, black Africans, West Indians, Asian Indians, Mediterraneans (especially Greeks and Middle East populations)
Tay–Sachs disease	Ashkenazi Jews

conditions such as haemochromatosis or CF is available in the UK to those individuals who attend genetics clinics on account of a family history of the condition.

β-Thalassaemia

β-Thalassaemia is an autosomal recessive condition in which there is reduced or absent synthesis of the β-subunit (or chain) of haemoglobin. In contrast, in sickle-cell anaemia, the β-haemoglobin is synthesised at the normal level but is structurally abnormal. The diagnosis in β-thalassaemia homozygotes can be made by the finding of severe hypochromia,

microcytosis with target cells in the blood film and an increased proportion of haemoglobin F (HbF, consisting of two α-chains and two γ-chains ($\alpha_2\gamma_2$). The proportion of haemoglobin A_2 (HbA_2: $\alpha_2\delta_2$) is usually also increased. Homozygotes (or compound heterozygotes) have severe chronic anaemia due to ineffective erythropoiesis and haemolysis, and generally die before the age of 20 unless they receive repeated blood transfusions. Lifespan is often reduced despite such supportive measures, particularly as a result of myocardial disease. The latter results from transfusion-related siderosis, even with regular iron chelation therapy.

As in sickle-cell anaemia (see below), the β-chain abnormalities become clinically significant once the synthesis of haemoglobin switches physiologically from HbF to haemoglobin A (HbA: $\alpha_2\beta_2$) perinatally. There is a range of clinical severity depending upon the particular molecular lesion, i.e. reduced synthesis (in the presence of a 'β+' thalassaemia allele) or absent synthesis (when there is a 'β0' thalassaemia allele) of the β-globin chain and the coexistence of other haemoglobinopathies (for example those known as Hb S, C, E, O$_{Arab}$ and Lepore). Bone marrow transplantation, when available, from an HLA-identical sibling can be curative.

The heterozygote frequency of β-thalassaemia varies widely in different populations but is especially high in Mediterranean countries and south-east Asia. Thus, persons from these ethnic groups merit carrier screening. The carrier state ('β-thalassaemia minor') is detected by the finding of microcytosis (mean cell volume <80 fl), a low mean cell haemoglobin level (less than 27 pg) and an increased HbA$_2$ concentration (more than 3.5%; normal upper limit 2.5%) upon electrophoresis of haemoglobin. Carrier detection permits genetic counselling and prenatal diagnosis (by DNA analysis on chorionic villus samples or, less commonly, by fetal blood sampling and haematological analysis) for couples who are both heterozygotes. In such couples, therefore, following the detection of carrier status, molecular genetic analysis is usually carried out to identify the pathogenic mutations in the β-haemoglobin locus, *HBB*. The condition is caused by over 200 different mutations in the β-globin gene cluster (*HBB*) on 11p15.5. Large gene deletions are rare, with the majority of mutations being single-nucleotide substitutions, deletions or insertions. Selection has resulted in a higher carrier frequency for β-thalassaemia in Mediterranean (e.g. 1 in 6 Cypriots and 1 in 14 Greeks), Asiatic Indian (1 in 6 to 1 in 50) and Chinese (1 in 50) populations. In each population, a few (between four and ten) specific mutations tend to be particularly prevalent, such as a β-globin splice site mutation at nucleotide 5 of intron 1 (c.92 + 5G>C) in the Indian and Thai populations and a specific nonsense mutation (p.Gln39X) in Sardinians. The introduction of couple screening, particularly in Cyprus and Sardinia, has substantially reduced the birth frequency of β-thalassaemia homozygotes

Sickle-cell disease is another autosomal recessive haemoglobinopathy that occurs in individuals from the Mediterranean and India, but is especially prevalent in black Africans. Heterozygotes for this condition can be detected by the demonstration of sickle cells on exposure of red cells *in vitro* to a (chemically-induced) very low oxygen concentration (the Sickledex test), HPLC, isoelectric focusing or DNA analysis. The detection of heterozygotes permits genetic counselling and alerts the anaesthetist prior to general anaesthesia. As for β-thalassaemia, most of the many globin chain structural variants are single amino acid substitutions resulting from point mutations. The commonest sickle-cell disease allele, named HbS, contains a single nucleotide substitution in codon 6 of the β-globin gene on chromosome 11. This results in the replacement of the polar glutamic acid by the non-polar amino acid valine. As a consequence, it permits HbS to polymerise on deoxygenation, leading to red blood cell distortion into the sickle shape. Individuals affected by sickle-cell disease are most commonly homozygous for HbS. Some patients, however, are compound heterozygotes, possessing a single HbS allele in combination with, for example, an HbC or a β-thalassaemia allele. The precise proportions vary according to the geographic region. The clinical phenotypes that result from the SS and Sβ⁰ genotypes are generally more severe than those due to SC and Sβ⁺ disease. However, carrier screening for sickle-cell disease has not been utilised to the same extent as for β-thalassemia.

Tay–Sachs disease

Tay–Sachs disease (TSD) is an autosomal recessive neurodegenerative condition that results from mutations in the α-chain of β-*N*-acetylhexosaminidase A (HexA). Typically, progressive neurological abnormalities are evident from late infancy, leading to death, usually by the age of 4 years. Deficiency of HexA activity leads to accumulation of the enzyme's substrate, GM_2 ganglioside, in the lysosomes and consequent neuronal toxicity. The diagnosis is facilitated by the finding of a 'cherry-red' macular spot (present in 90%) and confirmed by the detection of reduced serum HexA activity.

The heterozygote frequency for this autosomal recessive trait is 1 in 30 for Ashkenazi Jews but only 1 in 300 for Sephardic Jews and other ethnic groups. Carriers are detected by the measurement of serum HexA (leucocyte HexA is more reliable during pregnancy) or by DNA analysis. In Ashkenazi Jews, there are two particularly common mutations: a 4 bp insertion in exon 11 and a splice-site mutation in intron 12. Carrier detection permits genetic counselling and prenatal diagnosis for couples at risk. Prenatal diagnosis is possible by DNA analysis or by assay of HexA in chorionic villi (or amniocytes). The incidence of TSD in the Ashkenazi Jewish population of North America was previously 1 in 3600 births. Following extensive education, population carrier screening and genetic counselling, however, the incidence has been reduced by over 90% (see Kaback, 2000, in Further reading).

In addition to Ashkenazi Jews, other population groups have been identified in which carriers are relatively frequent. These include those of Louisiana Cajun and Eastern Quebec French Canadian descent (see Roe and Shur, 2007, in Further reading).

Haemochromatosis

Haemochromatosis is an autosomal recessive condition in which there is progressive iron accumulation. Untreated, the complications can include diabetes mellitus, hepatic cirrhosis, cardiomyopathy, arthropathy, impotence and hepatocellular carcinoma (usually in cirrhotic livers).

Among Caucasians, the disorder almost always results from mutations in the *HFE* gene at chromosome 6p21. There are only two common mutations, C282Y and H63D. The pathogenicity of H63D is lower than that of C282Y. Therefore, the condition may develop clinically in C282Y homozygotes and in C282Y/H63D compound heterozygotes (albeit much less commonly), but it does not occur in H63D homozygotes. The carrier frequency in Caucasians is approximately 1 in 10. Carrier detection within an affected family is usually possible by direct DNA analysis. The clinical penetrance in homozygotes has been found to be age dependent and appears to be low (probably less than 5%, although the precise figure is unclear). The penetrance is believed to be higher in those C282Y homozygotes who are first-degree relatives of an affected individual than in homozygotes detected in the general population, presumably because the former are more likely to carry (unidentified) disease-modifying gene variants. In addition, risks to C282Y homozygote females are approximately ten times lower than in males. It is common practice to offer genetic testing to the parents and adult siblings of an affected person. If an affected individual has children, his partner can be offered genetic testing to determine the risk to the children. If she is a carrier (or declines testing), the offspring can be offered testing from their teenage years.

Those individuals who are found to be C282Y homozygotes (or C282Y/H63D compound heterozygotes) can be offered regular iron testing and, if this becomes significantly abnormal, they can undergo regular venesection as required to prevent clinical complications. Iron tests in those affected typically show an increased serum iron, transferrin saturation (the preferred screening test to detect affected individuals), serum ferritin and iron content in a liver biopsy (which may be performed to detect cirrhosis if the serum ferritin concentration is found to be greater than 1000 ng/ml). Repeated venesection to reduce the iron overload improves the prognosis and, if commenced prior to development of the above complications, life expectancy is normal. Heterozygotes usually remain clinically unaffected.

Presymptomatic screening of adults

Presymptomatic clinical screening of adults may be offered to clinically unaffected relatives of individuals affected by inherited conditions in which there is a delayed onset of symptoms. In families in which the causative mutation or mutations has been identified in an affected individual, the relatives can be offered genetic counselling and mutation testing. The aim is to identify those family members who, although not yet affected, are at significant risk of developing the condition and who thus may benefit from clinical screening. This screening includes, for example: surveillance for tumours and/or prophylactic surgery in carriers of genes for inherited forms of cancer (see Chapter 13); the cardiac monitoring of carriers of a familial hypertrophic cardiomyopathy mutation; and therapy with β-blockers or an implantable cardioverter defibrillator (ICD) in relatives possessing a familial long QT syndrome mutation.

In the future, identification of the 'at-risk' genotype for the common chronic diseases of adulthood may be possible, and screening to identify these individuals might, for instance, permit avoidance of the environmental trigger(s) and so help to prevent disease. Many studies have, in fact, already identified several common gene variants (mostly single-nucleotide polymorphisms or SNPs) that each confer a slightly higher or lower likelihood of developing the condition. The analysis of several such variants in combination could contribute to the estimation of the chance of developing a condition. In practice, at present, such tests are costly, the non-genetic triggers are often unknown and knowledge regarding the many genetic factors is incomplete. The clinical value of testing for such gene variants is therefore, at present, controversial and this type of test is not currently available in genetic clinics in the UK.

SUMMARY

- A population screening programme should satisfy certain criteria. Such criteria include: an appreciable frequency of the disorder, an advantage to early detection, a sufficiently low false-positive test rate (i.e. high specificity) and a sufficiently low false-negative test rate (i.e. high sensitivity). In addition, the costs must be outweighed by the benefits.
- Widely available screening for *prenatal screening* includes screening for Down syndrome by first-trimester CUBS and also screening for structural malformations (such as NTDs) by fetal ultrasound scanning in the second trimester.
- *Neonatal screening* may include tests for childhood conditions such as PKU, congenital hypothyroidism, CF, haemoglobinopathies, MCADD and sickle-cell disorder.

- Screening of *adults* by DNA testing may be offered, to detect mutation carriers, in order to permit informed reproductive choices to be made at an early stage. Such testing is often offered to members of ethnic groups that have high carrier frequencies for specific single-gene disorders (such as β-thalassaemia or Tay–Sachs disease).
- Adults who themselves are at significant risk of developing particular adult-onset diseases may be offered appropriate clinical screening. For instance, clinical screening may be offered with the aim of detecting tumours at an early stage in those individuals who have inherited a cancer predisposition gene mutation. Where such a mutation has been identified in an affected relative, it may be possible to offer a presymptomatic DNA test, with appropriate counselling and follow-up.

FURTHER READING

Aitken DA, Crossley JA, Spencer K (2007) Prenatal screening for neural tube defects and aneuploidy. In *Emery & Rimoin's Principles & Practice of Medical Genetics*, 5th edn. Edited by Rimoin DL, Connor JM, Pyeritz RE & Korf BR. Churchill Livingstone: Edinburgh.

Fan HC, Blumenfeld YJ, Chitkara U, Hudgins L, Quake SR (2008) Noninvasive diagnosis of fetal aneuploidy by shotgun sequencing DNA from maternal blood. *Proc Natl Acad Sci* **105**:16266–71.

Kaback MM (2000) Population-based genetic screening for reproductive counseling: the Tay–Sachs disease model. *Eur J Pediatr* **159**:S192–5.

Morris JK, Alberman E (2009) Trends in Down's syndrome live births and antenatal diagnoses in England and Wales from 1989 to 2008: analysis of data from the National Down Syndrome Cytogenetic Register. *BMJ* **339**:1188.

Roe AM, Shur N (2007) From new screens to discovered genes: the successful past and promising present of single gene disorders. *Am J Med Genet C Semin Med Genet* **145C**:77–86.

Southern KW, Mérelle MM, Dankert-Roelse JE, Nagelkerke AD (2009) Newborn screening for cystic fibrosis. *Cochrane Database Syst Rev* CD001402.

Stenhouse EJ, Crossley JA, Aitken DA, Brogan K, Cameron AD, Connor JM (2004) First-trimester combined ultrasound and biochemical screening for Down syndrome in routine clinical practice. *Prenat Diagn* **24**:774–80.

Vadiveloo T, Crossley JA, Aitken DA (2009) First-trimester contingent screening for Down syndrome can reduce the number of nuchal translucency measurements required. *Prenat Diagn* **29**:79–82.

Zlotogora J (2009) Population programs for the detection of couples at risk for severe monogenic genetic diseases. *Hum Genet* **126**:247–53.

WEBSITES

UK National Screening Committee:

- **http://www.screening.nhs.uk** (for information and a policy summary regarding screening for various conditions in the antenatal, newborn, childhood and adult periods)
- **http://www.screening.nhs.uk/criteria** (for the detailed criteria used in deciding whether screening should be undertaken for a particular condition)

Self-assessment

1. A 35-year-old woman in her first pregnancy undergoes, in the first trimester, biochemical serum screening (for free β-hCG and PAPP-A) and ultrasound fetal nuchal translucency measurement. She is found to be at elevated risk of having a child with Down syndrome and is offered an invasive test (by chorionic villus sampling (CVS) or later amniocentesis, followed by DNA and karyotype analysis). Which of the following are true?

A. The nuchal translucency measurement detects the fluid beneath the skin of the neck of the fetus and the amount of this fluid is often increased in Down syndrome
B. The biochemical measurements vary with the gestation
C. Smoking does not affect the biochemical measurements
D. Following CVS or amniocentesis, detection of trisomy 21 can be performed rapidly by quantitative fluorescent polymerase chain reaction (QF-PCR) with subsequent confirmation by full karyotyping
E. There is no possibility of an unrelated chromosome abnormality being detected, e.g. a sex chromosome anomaly, in this situation

2. With regard to the situation illustrated in Fig. 17.6, which of the following are true statements?

A. A single raised immunoreactive trypsinogen (IRT) result from a neonate is a reliable indicator that the child is affected by cystic fibrosis (CF)
B. Testing of parents should be offered following the detection in a child of even just one *CFTR* mutation, in order to permit the detection of CF mutation carriers in the family by cascade screening and genetic counselling of relatives who may be at risk of having an affected child
C. The ΔF508 *CFTR* mutation is a frameshift mutation

D. The ΔF508 mutation is pathogenic on account of reduced translation and thus impaired CFTR protein synthesis
E. In the absence of any other family history of CF, the healthy aunts and uncles of the affected neonate will now each have a chance of approximately 50% of being carriers

3. A healthy 27-year-old Greek Cypriot woman is found on screening to have an abnormally small red blood cell volume with a mean cell volume of 76 fl and mean cell haemoglobin content of just 22 pg. Which of the following are correct?

A. There is a strong possibility that she is a carrier of β-thalassaemia
B. Haemoglobin electrophoresis in a β-thalassaemia carrier would be expected to show a reduced proportion of HbA₂
C. If she is found to be a carrier, then her partner should be offered screening for β-thalassaemia carrier status
D. Mutation analysis is generally too difficult to carry out, because of the wide variety of mutations
E. Most mutations are deletions

4. Mr and Mrs Miller, an Ashkenazi Jewish couple in New York, undergo carrier testing for Tay–Sachs disease shortly after marrying each other. Both are found to be carriers. Which of the following are true?

A. Prenatal diagnosis is possible
B. The condition typically results in death in the early teenage years
C. The carrier frequency is particularly high in Sephardic Jews

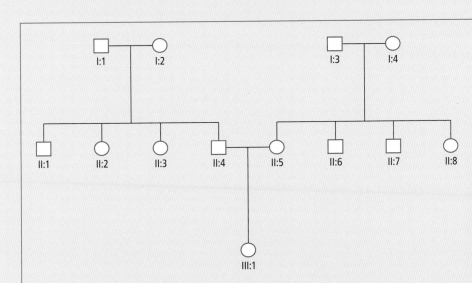

Fig. 17.6 A healthy couple are referred to the genetics clinic after their daughter, Fiona (individual III:1), is found on genetic testing to be homozygous for the ΔF508 *CFTR* mutation. She was tested after elevated serum immunoreactive trypsinogen (IRT) levels were detected on routine neonatal screening. See question 2 in Self-assessment.

D. Enzyme replacement therapy for the condition is widely available

E. GM$_2$ ganglioside accumulation in the mitochondria is responsible for neuronal death

5. Robert, a 25-year-old man seeks advice. His brother, William, was recently diagnosed with haemochromatosis at the age of 44 after developing liver cirrhosis and diabetes mellitus and was found to possess two C282Y mutant alleles in the HFE gene. Robert himself is well but has not yet undergone any investigations. Which of the following are correct?

A. The risk that Robert is a heterozygote is 2/3

B. The chance that he will develop haemochromatosis is approximately 25%

C. If Robert is found, in due course, to have an early form of haemochromatosis, treatment by regular venesection should give him a normal life expectancy

D. If Robert's wife is not a carrier, he need not be concerned that their children will develop the condition

E. If William's wife has a chance of being a carrier of 10%, then William's son, Greig, will at present have a chance of 1 in 20 of having inherited two *HFE* mutations

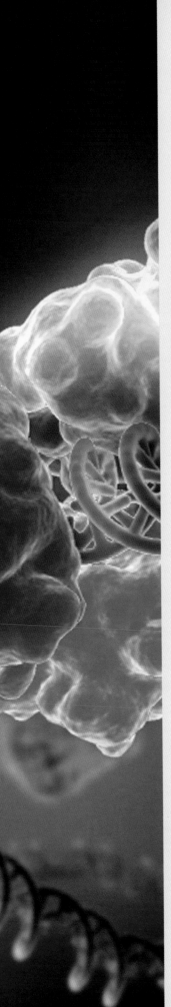

CHAPTER 18

Family history of one or more congenital malformations

Key Topics

Introduction

A *malformation* is a primary error of normal development or morphogenesis of an organ or tissue. All malformations are thus congenital (i.e. present at birth), although they may not be diagnosed until later, especially if they are microscopic or if internal organs are involved. Malformations may be single or multiple and may be of minor or major clinical significance. About 14% of newborns have a single minor malformation, 3% of newborns have a single major malformation and 0.7% of newborns have multiple major malformations (Table 18.1). The frequency of major malformations is even higher in early pregnancy (10–15%), but the majority of these fetuses abort spontaneously (Fig. 18.1). Table 18.2 lists some common minor congenital malformations. These are of no functional significance individually but should alert the clinician to the possibility of an associated major malformation, which coexists in about 20% of infants with multiple minor malformations.

A *disruption* (or secondary malformation) is a morphological defect due to breakdown of a previously normal organ or tissue. Disruptions can arise at any stage of gestation after initial morphogenesis. Similarly, *deformations* arise after the embryonic period and are alterations in shape caused by unusual mechanical forces. About 2% of newborns are affected, with multiple deformations in one-third of these. Malformations and deformations may coexist, and there is an increased risk of deformation (8%) in the presence of a major congenital malformation, especially if the latter involves the central nervous system (CNS) or urinary tract.

Essential Medical Genetics, 6th edition. © Edward S. Tobias, Michael Connor and Malcolm Ferguson-Smith.
Published 2011 by Blackwell Published Ltd.

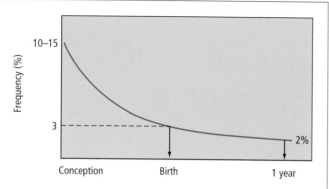

Fig. 18.1 Frequency of major congenital malformations.

Table 18.1 Classification and birth frequency of congenital malformations and deformations

Classification		Frequency
Minor malformation	Single	140 in 1000
	Multiple	5 in 1000
Major malformation	Single	30 in 1000
	Multiple	7 in 1000
Deformation	Single	14 in 1000
	Multiple	6 in 1000

Table 18.2 Examples of minor congenital malformations

Epicanthic folds

Upslanting or downslanting palpebral fisssures

Coloboma

Ear tag or pit

Bifid uvula

Single transverse palmar crease

Fifth-finger clinodactyly

Soft-tissue syndactyly

Mongolian spot

Haemangioma

Umbilical hernia

Minor hypospadias

Single umbilical artery

Aetiology

Table 18.3 indicates the identifiable causes of congenital malformations. Multifactorially inherited disorders constitute the commonest identifiable cause, followed by monogenic and

Table 18.3 Aetiology of major congenital malformations

Idiopathic	50%
Multifactorial	30%
Monogenic	7.5%
Chromosomal	6%
Maternal illness	3%
Congenital infection	2%
Drugs, X-ray, alcohol	1.5%

Table 18.4 Causes of congenital deformation

Intrinsic	Neuromuscular disease, connective tissue defects, CNS malformations
Extrinsic	Primigravidae, small maternal stature, oligohydramnios, breech presentation, uterine malformation, multiple pregnancy

chromosomal disorders. Thus, genetic conditions account for at least one-third of all congenital malformations of known aetiology.

Visible duplication or deficiency of any of the autosomes is almost invariably associated with learning disability, postnatal growth deficiency and dysmorphic features. Multiple malformations and intrauterine growth retardation are also commonly seen and correlate roughly in severity with the extent of the chromosomal imbalance. The phenotypes of over 250 single-gene disorders include major congenital malformations (including tissue dysplasias) as a consistent or frequent feature. Recognition of these single-gene disorders and of inherited structural chromosome rearrangements is of clinical importance in view of their high recurrence risks.

Maternal conditions that are associated with an increased risk of fetal malformation include diabetes mellitus, epilepsy, alcohol abuse and phenylketonuria. The risk is also increased (to about 6%, especially for cleft lip and congenital heart disease) for a mother with epilepsy, although here it is difficult to separate the risk due to the disease and that due to her medications (e.g. fetal valproate syndrome, described below). Untreated maternal phenylketonuria carries a high risk to the fetus for mental retardation, microcephaly (Fig. 18.2) and congenital heart disease (25%).

Deformations, such as congenital dislocation of the hip or talipes equinovarus (club foot), are caused by any factor that restricts the mobility of the fetus and so causes prolonged compression in an abnormal posture. Causes may be primarily intrinsic or extrinsic (Table 18.4). Deformations are correctible by pressure, and complete resolution is usual in the newborn period (Table 18.5).

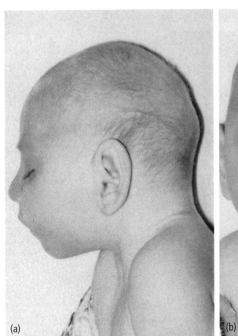
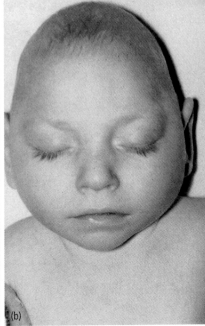

Fig. 18.2 (a, b) A child with microcephaly. The ears look relatively large as the head is so small.

Table 18.5 Examples of congenital deformation
Talipes (club foot)
Congenital dislocation of the hip
Congenital postural scoliosis
Plagiocephaly
Torticollis
Mandibular asymmetry

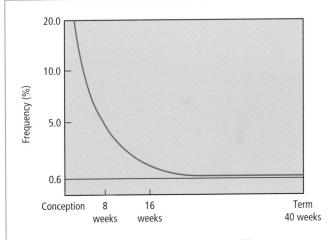

Fig. 18.3 Frequency of chromosomal abnormalities.

Chromosomal disorders

Chromosomal disorders are traditionally regarded as those conditions that are associated with cytogenetically visible changes in the chromosomes. Approximately 20% of all conceptions have a chromosomal disorder, but most of these fail to implant or are spontaneously aborted, with the result that the birth frequency is only 0.6% (Fig. 18.3). Among early spontaneous abortions, the frequency of chromosomal disorders is 60%, whereas in late spontaneous abortions and stillbirths, the frequency is 5%. The types of chromosomal abnormality differ within these different groups. Table 18.6 shows the types of chromosomal abnormality seen in early spontaneous abortions. With the exception of chromosome 1, each type of autosomal trisomy has been seen, and trisomy 16 is especially frequent. In contrast, trisomy 16 is never seen in the newborn because no recognisable embryo is formed. Triploid fetuses may survive to term, but the majority abort. Thus, in general, the chromosomal abnormalities that cause early spontaneous

Table 18.6 Chromosomal findings in early spontaneous abortions	
Apparently normal	40%
Abnormal:	60%
Trisomy	30%
45,X	10%
Triploid	10%
Tetraploid	5%
Other	5%

Table 18.7 Chromosomal disorders in newborns

Disorder	Birth frequency
Balanced translocation	1 in 500
Unbalanced translocation	1 in 2000
Pericentric inversion	1 in 100
Trisomy 21	1 in 700
Trisomy 18	1 in 3000
Trisomy 13	1 in 5000
47,XXY	1 in 1000 males
47,XYY	1 in 1000 males
47,XXX	1 in 1000 females
45,X	1 in 5000 females

Table 18.8 Frequency of trisomy 21 at birth and at prenatal diagnosis in relation to maternal age

Maternal age (years)	At birth	At amniocentesis	At chorionic villus sampling
20	1 in 1500	1 in 1200 (E)	1 in 750 (E)
25	1 in 1350	1 in 1000 (E)	1 in 675 (E)
30	1 in 900	1 in 700 (E)	1 in 450 (E)
35	1 in 380	1 in 300	1 in 240
37	1 in 240	1 in 190	1 in 130
39	1 in 150	1 in 120	1 in 75
41	1 in 85	1 in 70	1 in 40
43	1 in 50	1 in 40	1 in 25
45	1 in 28	1 in 22	1 in 13

E, estimated frequency.

abortion tend to be those with the most severe effects on the fetus. Sex chromosome abnormalities are rare among early abortuses, with the notable exception of 45,X (Turner syndrome), which is discussed in Chapter 6.

Table 18.7 indicates the commonest chromosomal disorders seen in newborns. Not all of these chromosomal changes are associated with disease, but, in general, autosomal abnormalities tend to be more severe than sex chromosomal abnormalities, and deletions tend to be more severe than duplications. In those with autosomal abnormalities, learning disability, multiple congenital malformations, dysmorphic features and growth retardation (pre- and postnatal) are common, as mentioned above. Although the pattern of features may suggest which chromosomal disorder is present, no individual clinical feature is pathognomonic for a given chromosomal abnormality.

The exact recurrence risk varies with the type of chromosome abnormality, but, for couples at high risk, prenatal diagnosis is always an option. Parental karyotypes need not be performed if the affected child has regular aneuploidy, but must be examined if the child has a partial duplication or deletion. Extended family studies will be required if a parent has a balanced structural rearrangement. Chromosomal structural aberrations such as translocations, deletions and inversions are discussed in detail in Chapter 7.

Trisomy 21 (Down syndrome)

The overall birth incidence of trisomy 21 is 1 in 700 live births. The incidence at conception is much greater, but more than 60% are spontaneously aborted, and at least 20% are stillborn. The incidence increases with increasing maternal age (Table 18.8). Thus, the incidence at the 16th week of pregnancy (a common time for amniocentesis) is 1 in 300 for a 35-year-old mother, rising to 1 in 22 at 45 years.

The facial appearance, which is a combination of dysmorphisms, often permits a clinical diagnosis. The palpebral fissures are upslanting, with speckling of the iris (Brushfield spots), the nose is small and the facial profile is flat (Fig. 18.4a). Antenatally, ultrasound examinations at 10–13 weeks of gestation may reveal increased fetal nuchal translucency if this is measured (see Chapter 17). In the neonate, hypotonia may be marked and redundant folds of skin around the neck are a feature of this and several other chromosomal disorders. The skull is brachycephalic with misshapen, low-set ears. A single palmar crease (Fig 12.4 and 18.4b) is often present (50%) and the little fingers may be short and incurved (clinodactyly; 50%). In addition, a wide gap between the first and second toes may be present.

Learning disability is a significant feature. The IQ is usually less than 50 and, if not, mosaicism should be suspected. Congenital heart malformations, especially endocardial cushion defects, are present in just over 40%, and duodenal atresia may occur. Other complications include cataracts (2%), epilepsy (10%), hypothyroidism (20–40%), acute leukaemia (1–2%) and atlantoaxial instability (symptomatic in 2–3% but radiologically evident in 18%).

When serious cardiac malformations are present, death during infancy is common, but otherwise survival well into adult life is usual. Trisomy 21 accounts for about one-quarter of all moderate and severe learning disability in children of school age. Most will walk and develop simple language. Puberty is often delayed and incomplete, with adult heights about 150 cm. Presenile dementia commonly supervenes after 40 years of age. The neuropathological appearance is very similar to that in Alzheimer disease (see Chapter 14).

Aetiology

Most cases (95%) of Down syndrome result from regular trisomy 21 (Fig. 18.5). This arises from non-disjunction, usually at the first (75%) but sometimes at the second meiotic

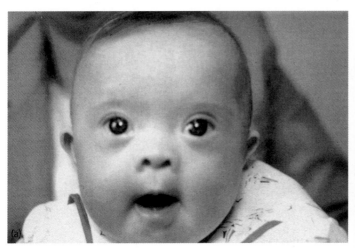

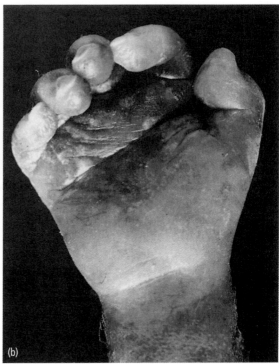

Fig. 18.4 Trisomy 21 phenotype. (a) Facies. (b) Single palmar crease in affected fetus.

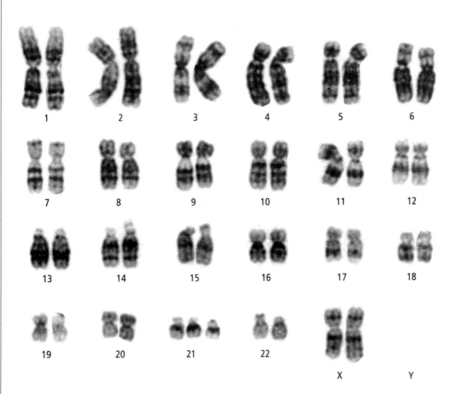

Fig. 18.5 Trisomy 21 karyotype. A 34-year-old woman seeks genetic advice following the birth of a girl with Down syndrome. Chromosome analysis performed neonatally has revealed this karyotype. There is no other family history suggestive of chromosome abnormalities. See question 2 in Self-assessment.

Table 18.9 Risks of chromosomally unbalanced offspring (at amniocentesis) for carriers of balanced structural rearrangements. See Table 16.1 for risks at birth.

Rearrangement	Carrier	Risk of unbalanced offspring at amniocentesis (%)
Robertsonian translocation 13;14	Either parent	1
Robertsonian translocation 14;21	Father	1
Robertsonian translocation 14;21	Mother	15
Robertsonian translocation 21;22	Father	5
Robertsonian translocation 21;22	Mother	10–15
Robertsonian translocation 21;21	Either parent	100
Reciprocal (on average)	Either parent	12
Insertional (on average)	Either parent	50
Pericentric inversion*	Father	4–15
Pericentric inversion*	Mother	8–15

*Excluding the common pericentric inversion of chromosome 9, which is a normal variant.

division. Overall, the mother contributes the extra chromosome in 90% of cases and the father in 10% (see Gardner and Sutherland, 2004, in Further reading). At least 1% of patients have mosaicism with normal and trisomy 21 cell lines. This may arise from mitotic non-disjunction in a normal zygote or loss of a chromosome 21 from a trisomic zygote (mitotic rescue). The clinical features in these chromosomally mosaic individuals tend to be milder than in the full syndrome. In 3–4% of cases, the child will have received the extra copy of chromosome 21 from a parent who is a carrier of a balanced translocation involving chromosome 21 (particularly a 14;21 Robertsonian translocation, see Fig. 7.8) or the child has a *de novo* translocation (see Chapters 7 and 16). The region of chromosome 21 that is most important in contributing to the phenotype is believed to be the so-called Down syndrome critical region (DSCR) at 21q22. Within the DSCR, two genes in particular, *DYRK1A* and *RCAN1*, may be responsible for the neuropathology in the condition (see Park *et al.*, 2009, in Further reading).

Recurrence risk

For young parents who have produced a child with trisomy 21 (or mosaic trisomy 21), the risk of recurrence of trisomy 21 or other major chromosomal abnormality at amniocentesis is around 1.5% (risk at birth 1%). This is a low risk, but many couples still seek reassurance by fetal karyotyping in future pregnancies. When the mother is 40 years of age or older, the age-specific risk should be used (Table 18.8) and the couple offered the choice of having prenatal screening before considering invasive tests. The recurrence risks (at amniocentesis) for carriers of a balanced translocation are given in Table 18.9.

Affected persons rarely reproduce. Men with trisomy 21 are generally infertile, but offspring of females with trisomy 21 are recorded, and rather less than one-half are affected.

Prenatal diagnosis and screening

Table 18.8 indicates that the risk of Down syndrome increases with maternal age. In the past, increased maternal age was used as an indication for fetal karyotype analysis by amniocentesis or chorion villus sampling (CVS). This is no longer advocated, as two-thirds of cases occur in women under 35 years and, in most, the risk of fetal loss is higher than the detection rate. Instead, women, irrespective of their age, may be offered screening tests in the first trimester based on a combination of maternal age, ultrasound measurement of nuchal translucency and the levels of maternal serum pregnancy-associated plasma protein A (PAPP-A) and free β human chorionic gonadotrophin (β-hCG). In one new protocol under consideration, women at high risk in the first trimester may choose CVS; those with a very low risk may be reassured, and those 25% with an intermediate risk may proceed to further maternal serum tests in the second trimester. In this 'contingent' protocol, the overall Down syndrome detection rate has been estimated as >90% for a false-positive rate of 2%. Improved biochemical screening has led also to a major reduction in invasive prenatal diagnostic tests and the consequent reduction in the loss of normal fetuses. Maternal age alone is no longer advised for the assessment of fetal Down syndrome risk in pregnancy (see Chapter 17 for further details).

Trisomy 18 (Edwards syndrome)

The incidence of trisomy 18 is 1 in 3000 live births with a maternal age effect. The incidence at conception is much higher, as is the case in trisomy 21, and 95% of affected fetuses abort spontaneously. At birth, there is a preponderance of females, which may reflect an excess of spontaneous abortion in affected males.

The birth weight is low, and multiple dysmorphic features are apparent in the newborn. These include: a characteristic

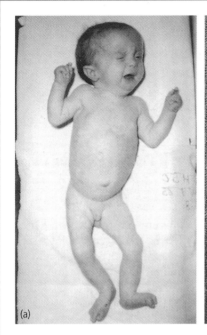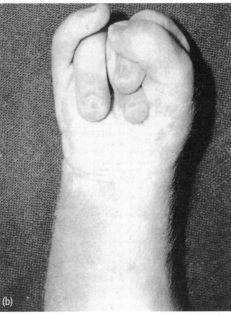

Fig. 18.6 Trisomy 18 phenotype. (a) General view. (b) Close-up of hand showing characteristic posture.

skull shape with a small chin and prominent occiput, low-set, malformed ears, clenched hands with overlapping index and fifth fingers, single palmar creases, rockerbottom feet and a short sternum (Fig. 18.6). In males cryptorchidism is usual.

Malformations of the heart, kidneys and other organs are frequent, and 30% die within a month. Only 10% survive beyond the first year, and these children show profound learning disability. Trisomy 18 usually results from maternal non-disjunction (95%, especially at the first meiotic division). Paternal non-disjunction is less common (5%) and rarely a parental translocation is responsible. Occasionally, mosaicism is seen, with a milder phenotype. For parents of a child with regular trisomy 18, the risk of recurrence or of other major chromosomal abnormality is 1.5% at amniocentesis.

Trisomy 13 (Patau syndrome)

The incidence of trisomy 13 is 1 in 5000 live births, with a maternal age effect. Multiple dysmorphic features are apparent at birth. These include: hypotelorism reflecting underlying holoprosencephaly, microphthalmia, cleft lip and palate, abnormal ears, scalp defects, redundant skin about the nape, clenched fists, single palmar creases (60%), postaxial (little finger side) polydactyly, prominent heels and cryptorchidism in the male (Fig. 18.7). Congenital heart disease is usual, and 50% die within a month. Only 10% survive beyond the first year, and these children show profound developmental delay. Trisomy 13 usually results from maternal non-disjunction (65%, especially the first meiotic division). Paternal non-disjunction is less common (10%). In about 20% of cases, one parent is a translocation carrier, and in about 5% of patients

mosaicism is present. The recurrence risk is less than 1% provided that neither parent is a carrier of a balanced translocation.

Triploidy

Triploidy occurs in 2% of all conceptions, but early spontaneous abortion is usual and survival to term is exceptional. The neonate with triploidy has marked low birth weight, disproportionately small trunk-to-head size, syndactyly, multiple congenital abnormalities and a large placenta with hydatidiform-like changes in many cases (Fig. 18.8). In most cases, the extra set of chromosomes is paternally derived, with 66% due to double fertilisation, 24% due to fertilisation with a diploid sperm and 10% due to fertilisation of a diploid egg. Sixty per cent are 69,XXY and most of the remainder are 69,XXX. Hydatidiform change is found only when there is a double paternal contribution. The recurrence risk is not known but is probably not increased above the general population risk.

Neural tube defects

In the development of the CNS, the neural groove appears at 20 days from conception and is mostly closed by 23 days. The anterior neuropore closes at 24 days and the posterior neuropore at 28 days. Defective closure of the neural tube may occur at any level. Failure at the cephalic end (anterior neuropore) produces anencephaly or an encephalocele, and failure lower down produces spina bifida. Overall, anencephaly (with or without spina bifida) accounts for 40% of neural tube defects

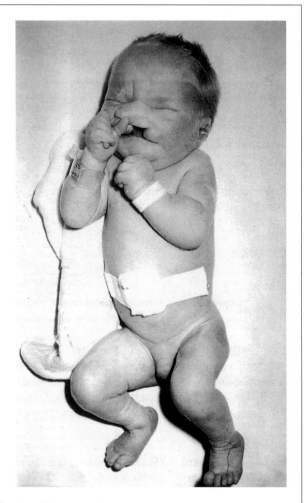

Fig. 18.7 Trisomy 13 phenotype.

Table 18.10 Classification of anterior abdominal wall defects

Type	Comments
Exomphalos	Umbilical cord attached to apex of sac; sac may contain liver and/or intestines; chromosomal abnormality in 30%; congenital heart disease (10%)
Gastroschisis	No sac and umbilical cord not involved in defect: may be associated areas of atretic intestine and congenital heart disease (20%)
Body stalk anomaly	Very short umbilical cord attached to apex of sac; severe spinal deformity; cloacal exstrophy; hypoplastic legs

or associated abnormalities have a particularly poor prognosis. In contrast, 60% of patients with closed lesions survive to 5 years and one-third are free of disability, with one-third moderately disabled and one-third severely disabled.

Encephaloceles are usually (95%) covered with intact skin (i.e. closed lesions). The degree of disability varies and depends upon the extent of nervous tissue involvement.

The frequency of NTDs shows geographical variation. In the USA, Africa and Mongolia, 1 in 1000 births are affected. In south-east England in the 1970s, 3 in 1000 births were affected and at that time the frequency was even higher in Ireland, Wales and the west of Scotland (5–8 in 1000). Subsequently, the frequency has fallen throughout the UK and the current frequency in the west of Scotland is 2 in 1000. The reasons for this fall in the UK are uncertain, as it began prior to the introduction of periconceptional folate supplementation (see below) and prenatal screening.

Epidemiological evidence and genetic analysis favour multifactorial inheritance with important environmental components. Genetic factors include polymorphisms in the *MTHFR* gene, which have been found to confer a relative risk of NTDs of around twofold. An environmental component, maternal levels of folic acid, has been identified, and supplementation with folic acid can reduce the recurrence risk in subsequent high-risk pregnancies. In the UK, the recurrence risk after an affected pregnancy is 3–4% and this risk is reduced to 1% by periconceptional folic acid supplementation begun *prior* to conception. In this situation, the recommended dose is 5 mg folic acid per day instead of the lower 400 μg dose that is recommended routinely in the UK to women planning a pregnancy (to be taken from at least 1 month before conception until the 12th week of pregnancy). The risk for offspring of an affected patient is also around 3–4% in the UK. For second-degree relatives, the risk is 1 in 70 and for third-degree relatives it is 1 in 150. After two or more affected children, the recurrence risk rises to 1 in 10. The recurrence risk is lower in countries with a lower incidence.

(NTDs), spina bifida alone for 50–55% and encephaloceles for 5–10%. Other malformations, particularly exomphalos (see Fig. 18.9 and Table 18.10) and renal malformations, coexist in 25%.

In anencephalic fetuses, the skin and cranial vault are missing (i.e. open lesions) and the exposed nervous tissue degenerates (Fig. 18.10). The hypothalamus is defective, and this leads to fetal adrenal atrophy with low maternal oestriols. Polyhydramnios may complicate the pregnancy. Stillbirth or neonatal death is invariable.

Spina bifida is most commonly lumbosacral with paralysis of the legs and sphincters. About 15–20% have a covering of intact skin (closed lesions) and these tend to cause less neurological disability than the open lesions. Hydrocephalus occurs in 80% (with aqueductal stenosis in about one-third). Without surgical therapy, only 20% of those with open lesions survive to 2 years. With surgery within 24 hours, 40% survive more than 7 years, but around 80% are severely disabled. Patients with gross paralysis of the legs, thoracolumbar or thoraco–lumbar–sacral lesions, kyphoscoliosis, hydrocephalus at birth

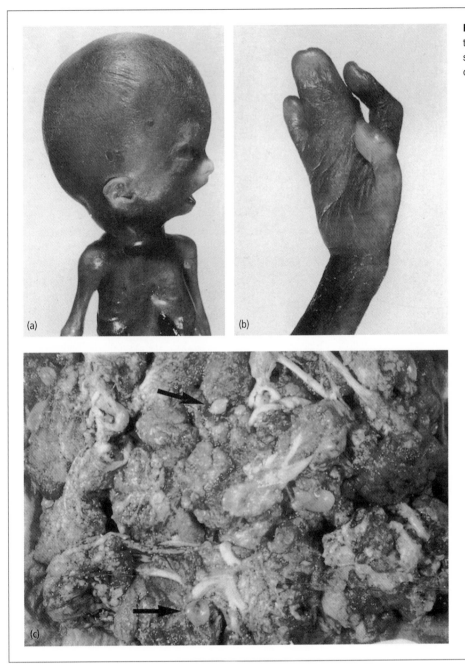

Fig. 18.8 Triploidy showing (a) trunk-to-head disproportion and (b) syndactyly. (c) Partial hydatidiform changes in the placenta.

Prenatal diagnosis is possible in pregnancies at risk by increasingly available second-trimester detailed ultrasound scanning or by assay of maternal serum α-fetoprotein (AFP). Although now rarely used for this purpose, if necessary, an amniocentesis can be performed to permit the analysis of amniotic fluid biochemistry (AFP assay and acetylcholinesterase pattern). In the general population, routine screening of pregnancies for spina bifida is now offered in the UK by detailed ultrasound scanning (or much less commonly by assay of maternal serum AFP), in the second trimester (see Chapter 17).

Isolated neural arch defects (spina bifida occulta) of one or two vertebrae (especially S1, S2 or L5) occur in about 23% of normal individuals. These localised defects are asymptomatic (but may be associated with an overlying hairy patch). They do not appear to increase the risk for siblings of a major NTD, but if three or more neural arches are involved, the lesion would be termed a closed spina bifida and would carry the usual recurrence risk.

Although most NTDs are multifactorial as outlined above, some are secondary to teratogenic influences (for example sodium valproate and maternal diabetes mellitus) and some are secondary to chromosomal or rare single-gene disorders. Trisomy 18 should be excluded if other congenital malformations coexist. Finally, encephalocele in combination with poly-

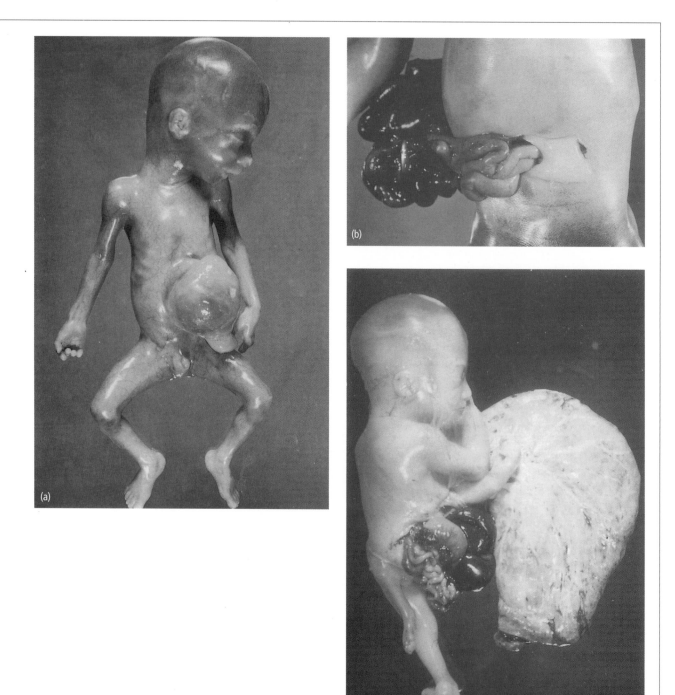

Fig. 18.9 Anterior abdominal wall defects. (a) Exomphalos. (b) Gastroschisis. (c) Body stalk anomaly.

dactyly and cystic kidneys is characteristic of an autosomal recessive disorder known as Meckel (or Meckel–Gruber) syndrome (Fig. 18.11), with which several genes are associated. These include *MKS1*, which encodes a flagellar protein, and *MKS3*, which encodes a transmembrane protein.

Teratogenic effects

Several environmental factors such as infectious agents or drugs, called teratogens, have been shown to cause malformations without acting as mutagens (Table 18.11). Numerous

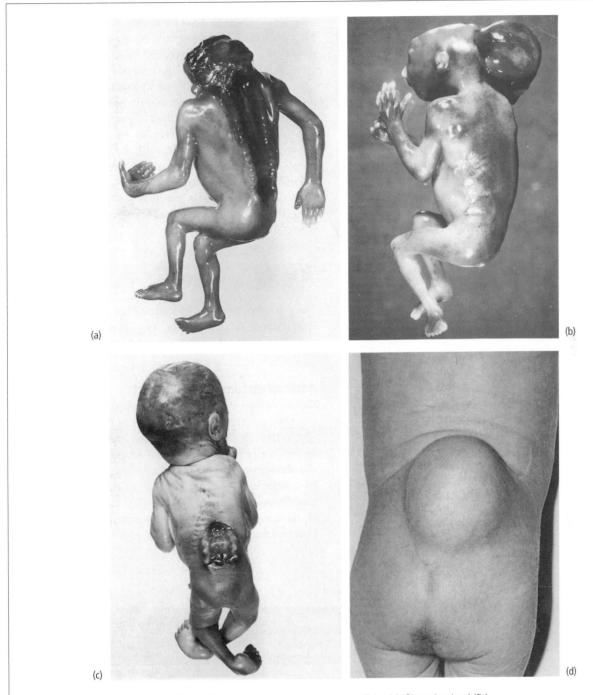

(a)

(b)

(c)

(d)

Fig. 18.10 NTDs. (a) Anencephaly. (b) Encephalocele. (c) Open spina bifida. (d) Closed spina bifida.

other agents are suspected to have teratogenic activity, but the difficulty lies in establishing the causal relationship, as animal experiments may not be directly informative (for example thalidomide is reported to be teratogenic in monkeys and rabbits, but not in rats or mice). Furthermore, retrospective studies are hampered by the facts that about 6% of all women experience a viral type of illness other than a cold during pregnancy and over 80% take one or more medications.

Malformations due to fetal infections with rubella, cytomegalovirus or toxoplasmosis are now uncommon in the UK. Each produces a distinctive pattern of malformations, often with evidence of active neonatal infection with jaundice, purpura and hepatosplenomegaly. The diagnosis is confirmed by the demonstration in the neonate of raised levels of specific antibodies, especially IgM. With the exception of cytomegalovirus infection where recurrent infection may involve the fetus,

Fig. 18.11 (a, b) Meckel syndrome showing polycystic kidneys, polydactyly and encephalocele.

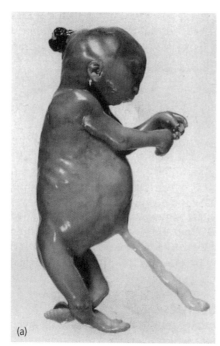
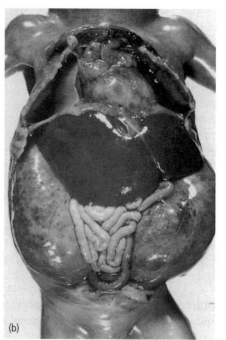

(a)

(b)

Table 18.11 Recognised human teratogens

Teratogen	Critical period	Malformations
Rubella	Most affected if infection in first 6 weeks; very low risk >16 weeks	Congenital heart disease (especially patent ductus arteriosus), cataracts, microcephaly, learning disability, sensorineural deafness, retinopathy, later insulin-dependent diabetes mellitus in 20%
Cytomegalovirus	Third or fourth month	Learning disability or microcephaly occurs in 5–10% with congenital infection
Toxoplasmosis	12% risk at 6–17 weeks, 60% risk at 17–28 weeks	Learning disability, microcephaly, chorioretinitis
Alcohol	First and second trimester, primarily.	Learning disability, microcephaly, congenital heart disease, renal anomaly, growth retardation, cleft palate, characteristic facies (see Fig. 18.12)
Phenytoin	First trimester; about 10% affected	Hypoplasia of distal phalanges, short nose, broad flat nasal bridge, ptosis, cleft lip and palate, learning disability, later increased risk of malignancy, particularly neuroblastoma
Thalidomide	34–50 days from last menstrual period	Phocomelia, congenital heart disease, anal stenosis, atresia of external auditory meatus
Warfarin	Exposure at 6–9 weeks results in structural abnormalities in 30%; after 16 weeks, learning disability alone may be seen	Hypoplastic nose, upper airway difficulties, optic atrophy, stippled epiphyses, short distal phalanges, learning disability
Lithium	First trimester	Congenital heart disease
Sodium valproate	First and third trimesters	NTD (1–2%), hypospadias, microstomia, small nose, long philtrum, long thin upper lip, developmental delay

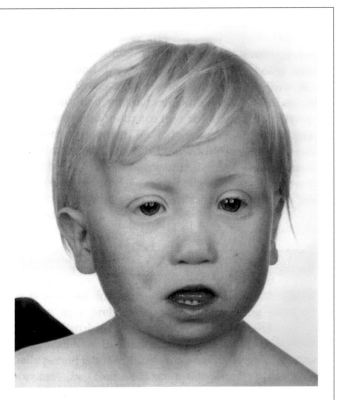

Fig. 18.12 Facies in the fetal alcohol syndrome.

maternal immunity generally prevents recurrence in a future pregnancy. If a pregnant woman has evidence of seroconversion during the critical period, then fetoscopic blood sampling to demonstrate evidence of fetal infection may be of value in deciding whether termination of pregnancy is indicated.

Treatment with spiramycin reduces the risk of fetal toxoplasmosis when the mother is infected, and if fetal seroconversion still occurs, then treatment, via the mother with additional antibiotics, is administered to reduce the incidence of sequelae.

Maternal alcohol ingestion of more than 150 g per day poses a substantial risk to the fetus, but lesser levels of intake may also be harmful. The facies in fetal alcohol syndrome exhibit short palpebral fissures and a smooth philtrum (Fig. 18.12).

In general, for these teratogenic agents, a critical period has been identified beyond which malformations appear much less likely. The early embryo is apparently relatively resistant to the action of teratogens, and for most organs the period of greatest vulnerability is from 4 to 8 weeks of gestation (from the last menstrual period). There also appear to be individual differences in susceptibility to these agents. For example, only 10–40% of offspring of mothers taking warfarin are affected by the drug. This susceptibility may reflect differences in, for example, fetal or maternal metabolism of the teratogen by the cytochrome P450 mono-oxygenases, probably on account of

person-to-person differences in combinations of genetic variants such as single-nucleotide polymorphisms (see Chapter 4). Although a few drugs including, for example, paracetamol, amoxicillin and cefuroxime, are generally considered non-teratogenic, for the majority of drugs their safety in pregnancy is unknown and, where possible, they should be avoided.

Multiple malformation syndromes

Multiple malformations, often a combination of minor and major, are present in 0.7% of newborns. In the majority, the combination is random, but in some neonates the pattern is non-random and one of over 2000 dysmorphic syndromes can be identified (see Jones, 2005, in Further reading, for many examples). In some cases, specific diagnosis can be verified by chromosomal analyses or, where a causative gene for the syndrome has been reported, DNA tests. Sequences and associations are subtypes of dysmorphic syndromes. In a sequence, the series of abnormalities can be causally related to a primary malformation. For instance in Potter sequence, there is pulmonary hypoplasia, amnion nodosum and flattened facies secondary to oligohydramnios, which itself may be caused by renal agenesis (or dysplasia) or by fetal obstructive uropathy (Fig. 18.13). Fetal abdominal distension and a consequent prune belly appearance is also a frequent result of the underlying renal or urological abnormality (Fig. 18.14). In an association, in contrast, there is a non-random combination of two or more structural defects that are not due to a single localised defect of embryogenesis. A well-known example is the VACTERL (or VATER) association, which includes vertebral defects, anal atresia, cardiac anomalies, tracheo-oesophageal fistula, renal abnormalities and limb defects. Recognition of these dysmorphic syndromes is important, as for many of them accurate recurrence risks and prenatal diagnosis can be provided. Searching the medical literature concerning rare syndromes is greatly facilitated by the computerised databases that are now available. These invaluable sources include the online GeneReviews, Online Mendelian Inheritance in Man (OMIM) and PubMed databases and the Winter–Baraitser Dysmorphology Database (see Further reading and Chapter 19).

Increasingly, previously unexplained dysmorphic syndromes (e.g. CHARGE association; see Johnson et al., 2006, in Further reading) and cases of multiple congenital malformations are being found to be due to abnormalities in single genes that were not previously recognised as being associated with human disease or to submicroscopic chromosomal lesions (see Other Microdeletion Disorders, below).

In addition, in particular syndromes such as Noonan syndrome (Fig. 18.15), the phenotype can result from mutations in one of several genes (e.g. *PTPN11/SHP2*, *SOS1* and *KRAS*) that encode proteins that lie on the same intracellular signalling pathway (Fig. 18.16). The phenotypic features in Noonan syndrome include short stature, learning disability, pulmonary stenosis, low-set ears and ptosis. For details of this

Fig. 18.13 Potter sequence due to bilateral renal agenesis. (a) Characteristic facies. (b) Amnion nodosum.

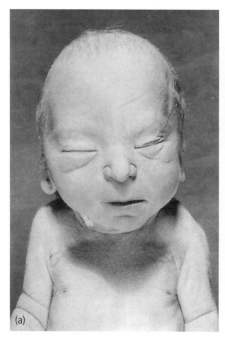
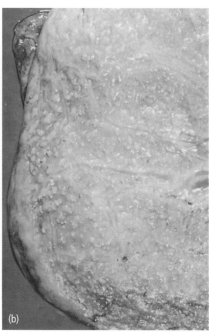

Fig. 18.14 Prune belly appearance secondary to fetal obstructive uropathy.

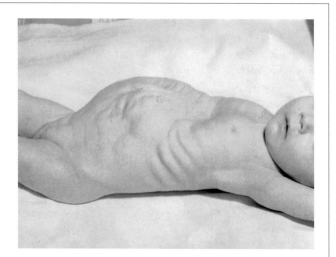

condition and the many other recognised dysmorphic syndromes the reader may wish to consult the comprehensive sources listed in Further reading, especially the books by Jones or by Baraitser and Winter, if available, or the electronic databases listed.

With regard to the CNS, although the most active period of CNS embryogenesis is from the 3rd to the 12th weeks, neuronal proliferation, migration, development of synapses and myelination continue throughout the whole pregnancy and up to 2–3 years of age. The brain thus has a longer period of developmental organisation than any other organ. This and its complexity account for its relatively high frequency of malformations. Often, those malformations contributing to idiopathic learning disability may be difficult to diagnose without detailed imaging or neuropathology, as only a small proportion of these malformations produce any external change. An example of a condition that involves significant CNS malformations but which *is* externally recognisable, however, is X-linked hydrocephalus. In addition to hydrocephalus, this syndrome is associated with corpus callosum hypoplasia, learning disability and hypoplastic and adducted thumbs (Fig. 18.17). It often arises as a result of mutations in *L1CAM*, a gene that encodes a neural cell–cell adhesion molecule.

In addition to a range of abnormalities affecting the facies, internal organs (e.g. the brain, heart and kidneys) and external genitalia, a variety of limb defects (e.g. those shown in Fig. 18.18) may be associated with malformation syndromes. For instance, severe upper limb reduction defects are a common finding in the well-recognised de Lange syndrome (Fig. 18.19). This syndrome also includes severe learning disability, growth retardation, congenital heart defects and characteristic facies with thin lips, synophrys and anteverted nostrils. It is now recognised that, in at least 50% of cases, de Lange syndrome results from mutations in the *NIPBL* gene, which encodes a protein that assists in sister chromatid cohesion and the long-range regulation of gene expression. Limb defects that affect the hands and feet are, however, in many syndromes often fairly subtle (e.g. Fig 18.20).

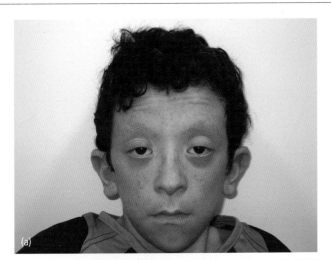

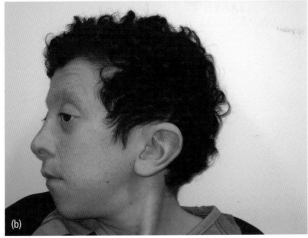

Fig. 18.15 (a, b) Noonan syndrome. A child possessing a mutation in the *SOS1* gene, which, in Noonan syndrome, is less commonly mutated than the *PTPN11* gene but which encodes a protein that participates in the same growth factor signalling pathway (see Fig. 18.16).

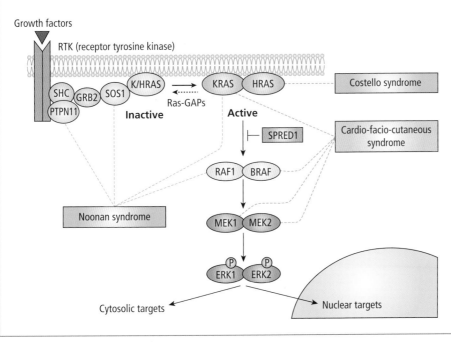

Fig. 18.16 The growth factor signalling pathway involved in the pathogenesis of Noonan syndrome. Redrawn with modifications from Tidyman and Rauen (2008), with permission from Cambridge Journals; see Further reading.

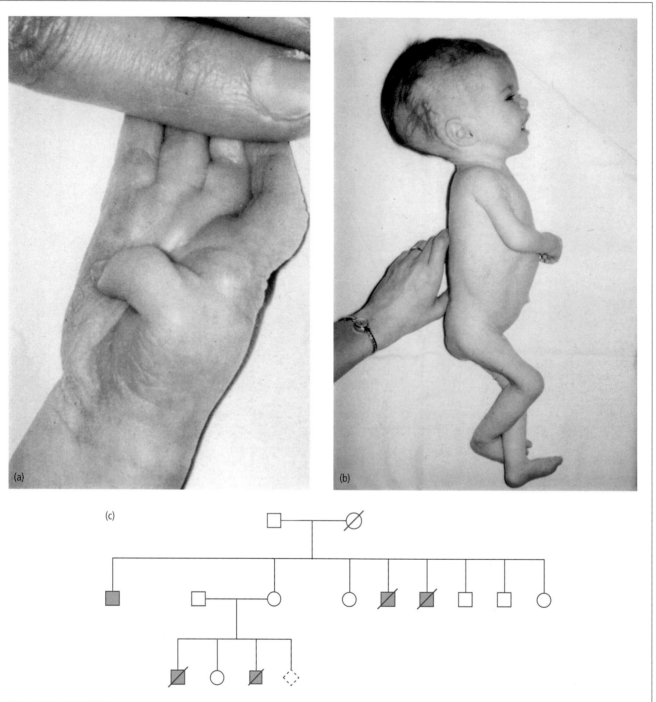

Fig. 18.17 (a, b) X-linked hydrocephalus. Note the characteristic adducted hypoplastic thumb in an affected male. (c) Example of a pedigree of a family with X-linked hydrocephalus.

In cases of perinatal death with multiple malformations, genetic counselling is facilitated by chromosome analysis, autopsy, whole-body radiography and clinical photographs (hence the mnemonic CARP). Chromosomal analysis may still be possible even 2–3 days after death by culturing and karyotyping fibroblasts from a post-mortem sample of the fascia lata. Recurrence risks depend upon the aetiology. However, if such investigations are all normal, if no syndrome is identified by an experienced clinical geneticist and if the parents are non-consanguineous, the recurrence risk on average is 2–5% (in addition to the general population risk). Reassurance by means of detailed ultrasound might be offered during subsequent pregnancies.

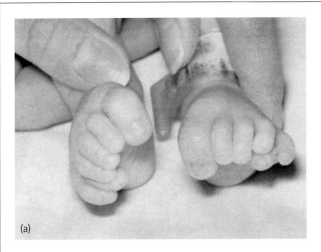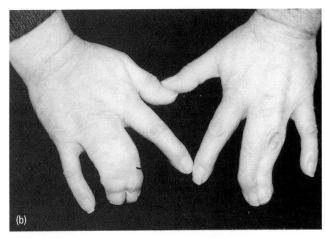

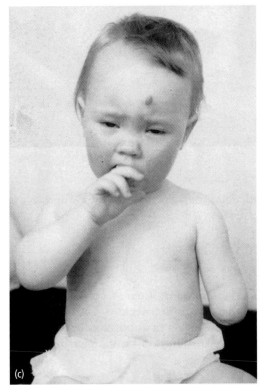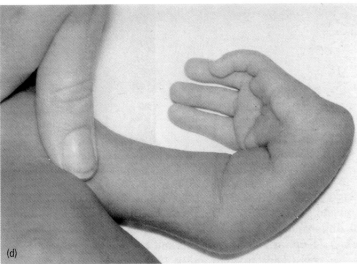

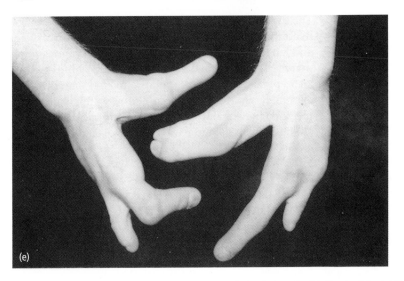

Fig. 18.18 Examples of limb defects. (a) Postaxial polydactyly. (b) Syndactyly. (c) Transverse limb amputation due to an amniotic band. (d) Radial aplasia. (e) Ectrodactyly. (f) Phocomelia. (g) Amelia.

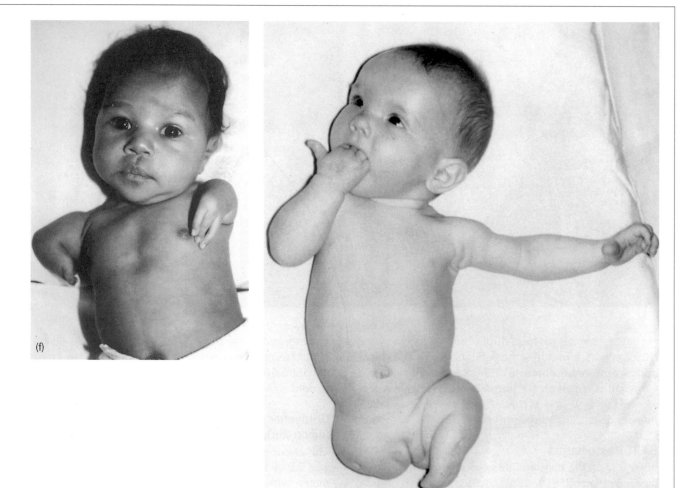

Fig. 18.18 (f, g *Continued*)

22q11 microdeletion syndrome

This syndrome manifests as a clinical phenotype involving several clinical features, with a spectrum ranging from velocardiofacial syndrome to the more severe DiGeorge syndrome. The clinical features include, particularly in more severe cases: failure to thrive, neonatal seizures secondary to hypoparathyroidism, and recurrent viral and fungal infections secondary to thymic aplasia. The hypocalcaemia and cell-mediated immunity defect both tend to improve during early childhood.

In approximately 75% of cases with a 22q11 microdeletion (i.e. a chromosome deletion that is close to the limit of light microscopy resolution), there is a congenital cardiac defect, a variety of which have been reported. These include: tetralogy of Fallot, ventricular septal defect, interrupted aortic arch, atrial septal defect, truncus arteriosus and transposition of the great arteries. There may be long thin fingers (Fig. 18.20) and

facial dysmorphisms are often present although subtle. These include a prominent nose (with 'squared-off' tip), hypertelorism, up- or down-slanting short palpebral fissures, ear abnormalities (e.g. with a flattened appearance superiorly) and a small mouth. A cleft palate (or submucous cleft palate) is common (10–15%) with velopharyngeal insufficiency present in around 30%. Growth retardation is common. Structural urinary tract abnormalities are present in around one-third of cases and learning difficulties are observed in approximately two-thirds. In addition, in adulthood, psychiatric disorders are described in around 20%. An accessible illustrated review of the condition has been published recently by Robert Shprintzen, who originally described the syndrome in 1978 (see Shprintzen, 2008, in Further reading).

A cytogenetically visible microdeletion at 22q11 is seen in 15–20% of patients. In the remainder, a deletion can be demonstrated using fluorescence *in situ* hybridisation (FISH) or

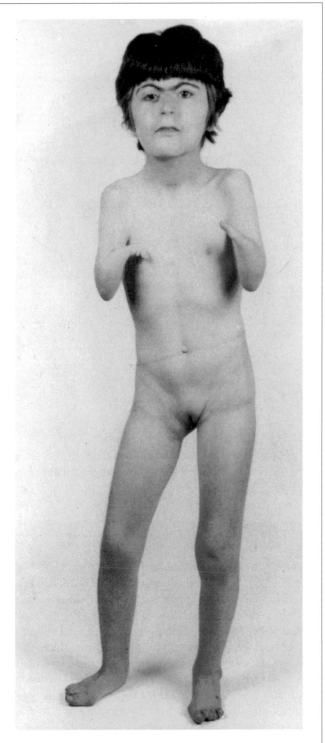

Fig. 18.19 De Lange syndrome.

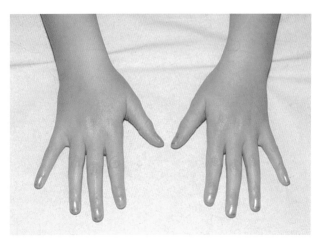

Fig. 18.20 Hands of a boy who was investigated on account of learning difficulties and a history of a ventricular septal defects and truncus arteriosus. Hypocalcaemia was detected neonatally. The presence of unusually long and tapering fingers was noted by a junior doctor. The karyotype analysis was normal but, on fluorescence *in situ* hybrisation, a microdeletion at 22q11 was detected. There was no notable family history. The parents sought genetic counselling. See question 6 in Self-assessment. Courtesy of Margo Whiteford, Yorkhill Hospitals, Glasgow.

more than 40 genes (Fig. 18.21). Haploinsufficiency for the *TBX1* gene probably contributes most to the phenotype, while the *CRKL* gene may play a more minor role. This deletion may be maternal or paternal in origin (i.e. there is no evidence for imprinting in this region), but the deletion occurs *de novo* in 94% of cases. The recurrence risk will be 50% when the deletion is present in a parent. In its absence in the parents, the risk is very small (approximately 1%) but not zero, on account of the small possibility of gonadal mosaicism. Prenatal diagnosis is possible by CVS or amniocentesis, and detection of the cardiac abnormalities, when present, may be possible on ultrasound examination of the fetus.

A growing number of cases of *duplication* of the same 3 Mb region are now being detected, although the clinical phenotype appears to be generally more variable and mild than is observed in individuals possessing deletions of this chromosomal region (see Portnoi, 2009, in Further reading). Interchromosomal homologous recombination at meiosis is believed to be the mechanism that generates both the microduplication and microdeletion at 22q11.2 (Fig. 18.22).

Other microdeletion disorders

In addition to the 22q11 microdeletion syndrome, several other conditions have been shown to be due to chromosomal microdeletions (Table 18.12). Such deletions have been shown to occur in many cases by recombination between low-copy-number DNA repeats that are present on either side of the region that becomes deleted. This is true for instance for the deletion associated with the velocardiofacial syndrome

alternatively by multiplex ligation-dependent probe amplification (MLPA) or array comparative genomic hybridisation (aCGH) (see Chapters 4 and 7). The deletion, which is flanked both proximally and distally by an identical long stretch of DNA sequence (the so-called 'low-copy repeat' sequences), typically spans approximately 3 Mb at 22q11.2 and includes

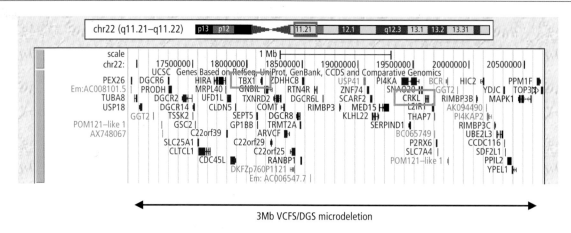

Fig. 18.21 Extent of the region of approximately 3 Mb on 22q that is most commonly deleted in patients with velocardiofacial syndrome (VCFS) and DiGeorge syndrome (DGS). The positions of the *TBX1* and *CRKL* genes are marked with orange-coloured boxes. It is believed that loss of one copy of *TBX1* is the major contributor to the clinical phenotype, with *CRKL* acting as a possible modifier. Modified from the UCSC genome browser (http://genome.ucsc.edu). Kent et al. (2002) 12(6):996–1006.

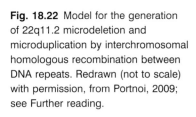

Fig. 18.22 Model for the generation of 22q11.2 microdeletion and microduplication by interchromosomal homologous recombination between DNA repeats. Redrawn (not to scale) with permission, from Portnoi, 2009; see Further reading.

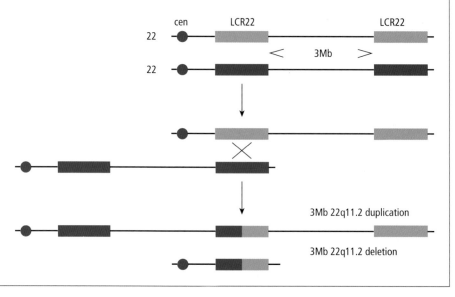

mentioned above and the 1.55 Mb deletion associated with Williams syndrome (Fig. 18.23).

Although smaller deletions can occasionally be detected, in most cases, as mentioned previously, the smallest cytogenetically visible deletion involves approximately 4–5 Mb. Thus, large numbers of genes can be lost or gained without producing cytogenetically visible changes. The clinical effects of such abnormalities are commonly learning disability, multiple congenital abnormalities and/or dysmorphic features. The detection of such deletions will often necessitate the use of more specialised testing such as FISH, MLPA or aCGH (see Chapters 4 and 7). With the growing use of such techniques, an increasing number of microdeletion syndromes are being described, such as those involving 1p36, 2q37, 9q34 and 16p11–12. The data regarding the genomic extents of the deletions detected by aCGH, together with (anonymised) details of the clinical phenotypes, are being catalogued (together with control data

from clinically unaffected individuals) in helpful databases such as the DECIPHER database (see Websites in Further reading).

Assessment of a child with multiple malformations

As discussed in detail in Chapter 12, a child with multiple malformations should be examined carefully with particular attention to the facies, head circumference, hands, feet and genitalia. This will normally be carried out initially by a paediatrician and the evaluation will include developmental assessment and noting the family history, in addition to details regarding the pregnancy (e.g. maternal illness and medications) and delivery. Chromosome analysis is useful and a rapid test for trisomy 21, 18 and 13 may initially be undertaken if such a diagnosis is suspected, followed by full karyotyping. Following

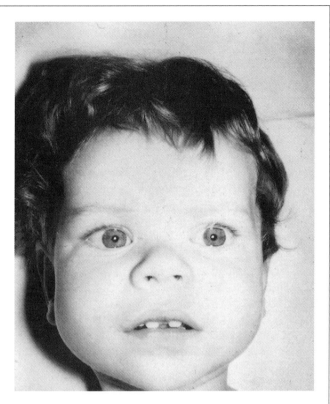

Fig. 18.23 Williams syndrome. In this syndrome, there is often short stature, learning disability, transient hypercalcaemia, supravalvular aortic stenosis and a characteristic facial appearance (with prominent lips and an anteverted small nose).

Table 18.12 Examples of conditions that may be caused by chromosomal microdeletions (e.g. 1–3 Mb in size)

Condition	Site of microdeletion
Alagille syndrome	20p12
Angelman syndrome	15q11–12
DiGeorge/velocardiofacial syndrome	22q11
Langer–Giedion syndrome	8q24
Miller–Dieker lissencephaly	17p13
Prader–Willi syndrome	15q11–12
Rubinstein–Taybi syndrome	16p13
Smith–Magenis syndrome	17p11
Sotos syndrome	5q35
Williams syndrome	7q11

karyotyping and testing as appropriate for suspected teratogens such as viral infections during pregnancy, a referral to the genetics service will then often be made for further advice or investigation (for instance where there is diagnostic uncertainty or where there may be implications for family members). The subsequent testing undertaken by geneticists may include specialised analyses for microdeletions (e.g. by FISH, MLPA or aCGH) or single-gene abnormalities (e.g. by DNA sequencing of specific genes).

Computer databases can now be searched as a means of identifying which rare syndrome or syndromes might be present. In practice, those clinical features that are best to use as search terms for this purpose are those that are most unusual in the general population and for which there is least ambiguity regarding their presence. The details of the various syndromes that result from such searches can then be studied to determine which syndrome most closely matches the patient being investigated. Further details regarding the use of such databases in medical genetics are provided in Chapter 19.

SUMMARY

- A *malformation* is present at birth and is a primary error of normal development of an organ or tissue. A *disruption*, in contrast, is a morphological defect that occurs by breakdown of a previously normally formed organ or tissue. A *deformation* (e.g. talipes) is an alteration in shape, caused by mechanical forces (such as compression), of a previously normally formed organ or tissue.
- A cytogenetically visible autosomal duplication or deletion generally causes learning disability, reduced growth and dysmorphic features.
- Autosomal abnormalities generally have more severe phenotypic consequences than those of sex chromosomes. The phenotypic effects of chromosomal deletions are usually greater than those of duplications.
- Trisomies 21, 18 and 13 are most often caused by maternal non-disjunction at the first meiotic division and the chance increases with increasing maternal age. In triploidy, in contrast, in which there is an extra set of all 23 chromosomes, the extra chromosomes are more often derived from the father than from the mother.
- A *sequence* (e.g. Potter syndrome) is a type of dysmorphic syndrome in which there is a series of abnormalities that are causally related to a primary malformation. An *association*, however, is a combination of different defects that are not due to a single anatomically localised abnormality of embryogenesis.

FURTHER READING

Baraitser M, Winter RM (1996) *Color Atlas of Congenital Malformation Syndromes.* Mosby-Wolfe: Philadelphia.

Gardner RJM, Sutherland GR (2004) *Chromosome Abnormalities and Genetic Counseling*, 3rd edn Oxford Monographs on Medical Genetics. Oxford University Press: Oxford.

Johnson D, Morrison N, Grant L, Turner T, Fantes J, Connor JM, Murday V (2006) Confirmation of CHD7 as a cause of CHARGE association identified by mapping a balanced chromosome translocation in affected monozygotic twins. *J Med Genet* **43**:280–4.

Jones KL (2006) *Smith's Recognisable Patterns of Human Malformation*, 6th edn. Saunders: Philadelphia.

Park J, Oh Y, Chung KC (2009) Two key genes closely implicated with the neuropathological characteristics in Down syndrome: *DYRK1A* and *RCAN1*. *BMB Rep* **42**:6–15.

Portnoi MF (2009) Microduplication 22q11.2: a new chromosomal syndrome. *Eur J Med Genet* **52**:88–93.

Reardon W (2008) *The Bedside Dysmorphologist*, 1st edn. Oxford University Press: Oxford.

Shprintzen RJ (2008) Velo-cardio-facial syndrome: 30 years of study. *Dev Disabil Res Rev* **14**:3–10

Tidyman WE, Rauen KA (2008) Noonan, Costello and cardio-facio-cutaneous syndromes: dysregulation of the Ras–MAPK pathway. *Expert Rev Mol Med* **10**:e37

Tolmie JL (2006) Down syndrome and other autosomal trisomies. In *Emery and Rimoins Principles and Practice of Medical Genetics*, 5th edn. Edited by Rimoin DL, Connor JM, Pyeritz RE, Korf BR. Churchill Livingstone: Edinburgh.

Winter–Baraitser Dysmorphology Database (proprietary software package). London Medical Databases Ltd.

WEBSITES

DECIPHER (DatabasE of Chromosomal Imbalance and Phenotype in Humans using Ensembl Resources):
https://decipher.sanger.ac.uk/application/

GeneReviews (expert-authored disease reviews; select 'GeneReviews' at this site):
http://www.geneclinics.org

Genetics Home Reference (of the US National Library of Medicine):
http://ghr.nlm.nih.gov/

OMIM (Online Mendelian Inheritance in Man):
http://www.ncbi.nlm.nih.gov/omim/

PubMed (database of journal publications with links to full text documents):
http://www.ncbi.nlm.nih.gov/sites/entrez/

Self-assessment

1. Which of the following are malformations?
A. Talipes equinovarus
B. Epicanthic folds
C. Bifid uvula
D. Umbilical hernia
E. Hypospadias

2. With regard to the woman whose daughter's karyotype is shown in Fig. 18.5, which of the following statements are correct?
A. The chance that either she or the girl's father has a chromosome abnormality that could predispose to Down syndrome is not significant
B. The additional chromosome 21 present in the girl is most likely to be maternal in origin
C. The aetiology is most likely to involve non-disjunction during mitosis
D. The chance that her next child will have Down syndrome is increased to 5%
E. If the additional chromosome 21 is detected in only some of the cells analysed (mosaicism), then the chance of recurrence will be increased

3. Which of the following conditions usually occurs as a result of the inheritance of additional chromosome(s) from the father?
A. Trisomy 13
B. Trisomy 18
C. Trisomy 21
D. Triploidy
E. Spina bifida

4. With reference to the family shown in Fig. 18.24, what is the approximate chance for the consultand's first child of being affected by a neural tube defect (NTD)?
A. 1 in 2
B. 1 in 10
C. 1 in 17
D. 1 in 25
E. 1 in 70

5. With reference to the affected boy in the family represented in Fig. 18.25, which of the following is the most likely cause of his problems?
A. An insertional mutation caused by sodium valproate
B. A frameshift deletion caused by sodium valproate
C. A nucleotide substitution caused by sodium valproate
D. Altered fetal gene expression caused by sodium valproate
E. A high-penetrance autosomal dominant condition

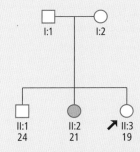

Fig. 18.24 Family from the West of Scotland in which the consultand (II:3), aged 19 (indicated with the arrow), seeks advice as she has recently married and wishes to start a family. Her elder sister (II:2) was born with spina bifida but no other medical problems. No other individual has been similarly affected in the family. See question 4 in Self-assessment.

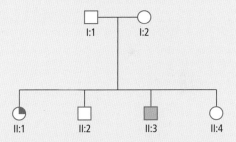

Fig. 18.25 Family in which a male child (II:3) is found neonatally to have the genital abnormality known as hypospadias. Subsequently, he is noted to be affected by developmental delay and to have an unusual facial appearance with a short nose, a smooth philtrum and a thin upper lip. The mother has epilepsy and was advised to continue taking her medication of sodium valproate during the pregnancy, as she had done during her previous pregnancies. It transpires that the boy's elder sister (II:1) has mild developmental delay and a similar facial appearance, but there is no other family history of such problems. See question 5 in Self-assessment.

6. In relation to the boy whose fingers are shown in Fig. 18.20, which of the following statements are correct?

A. It is most likely that one of the parents is a carrier of a similar deletion
B. Both parents should be offered testing for the deletion
C. If it is absent in the parents, recurrence of the same deletion in their future pregnancies cannot occur
D. If the child has offspring in the future, the risk for each of his children of being affected is 50%
E. The deletion may have arisen by homologous recombination between DNA repeats that flank a 3 Mb genomic region containing several genes

7. Which of the following most closely approximates the size of the smallest chromosome deletion that is visible using standard light microscopy?

A. 4 kb
B. 40 kb
C. 400 kb
D. 4 Mb
E. 40 Mb

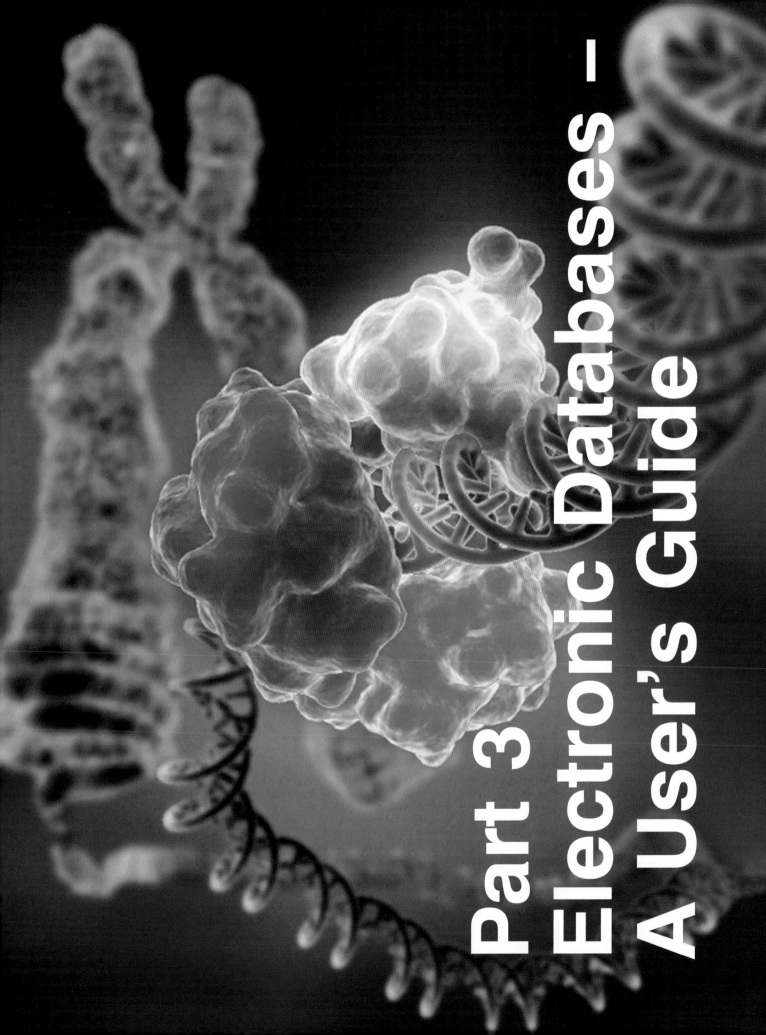

Part 3
Electronic Databases –
A User's Guide

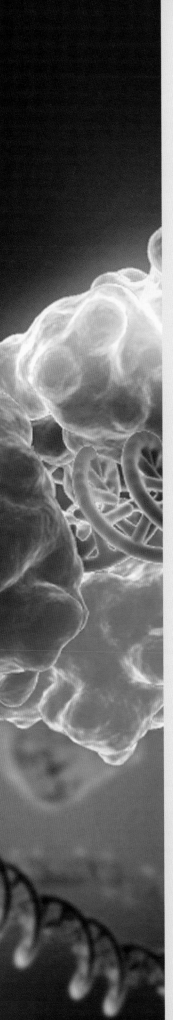

CHAPTER 19

Electronic databases – a user's guide

Key Topics

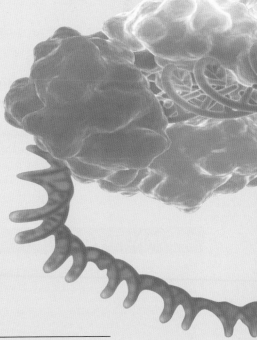

Essential Medical Genetics, 6th edition. © Edward S. Tobias, Michael Connor and Malcolm Ferguson-Smith.
Published 2011 by Blackwell Published Ltd.

Introduction

There are now many valuable online databases available, in most cases without cost, and it is essential for clinicians and scientists to be familiar not only with the range of resources available but also how to use them most efficiently. As in other areas, many of the available genetics-related databases are considerably more useful than others. Several different websites can provide very similar information, but differ markedly for instance in the presentation, ease of use and internal and external links. A great deal of time can be spent attempting to navigate through the various pages of a complicated database to find information that can be obtained more easily via a different route or even from a different website. There are often several different routes to obtaining the same data and many ways of reaching the same pages.

   In this chapter, a practical guide to the selection and use of many of the most useful genetics-related websites is provided in a question/answer format based on commonly encountered cases. The websites described here for specific purposes are those chosen for their mode of presentation and ease of use. The web addresses (URLs) for the websites mentioned are listed in the tables and are all provided as weblinks from this book's associated website (at **www.wiley.com/go/tobias**).

CASE I

You have just met a very large family known to be affected by a rare genetic condition called optic atrophy type 1. From the internet, how could you find the following:

1. Clinical information about the condition.
2. Its mode of inheritance.
3. The name and chromosomal location of the gene.
4. The names and contact details of laboratories undertaking mutation analysis for the condition.
5. Names and contact details of relevant patient support groups.

Answers are given in the following paragraphs.

Finding information regarding specific conditions and names of associated genes

The reference catalogue of human genetic conditions is the Online Mendelian Inheritance in Man (OMIM) database (Table 19.1), which began as a printed version compiled by the late Victor McKusick in the early 1960's. This database currently comprises around 20,300 entries including approximately 13,600 genes. For each condition, it provides the official name of the associated gene and its chromosomal location, followed by an enormous amount of information about the condition and its underlying genetics. This information, however, is incrementally compiled and can therefore be more difficult to read than the reviews mentioned below.

   In OMIM, to access the text description, the name of the condition of interest should be typed directly into the search box (Fig. 19.1). In the search results shown in Figs 19.2 and 19.3, the '1' after the '#' symbol in the catalogue number for this condition indicates that the inheritance of the condition is generally autosomal dominant. For autosomal recessive conditions, the first digit would be '2', for those that are X-linked recessive it would be '3' and for mitochondrially inherited conditions it would be '5'. It is necessary, however, to check the first paragraph of the detailed description as well as other related entries, as there is often genetic heterogeneity. The '#' symbol indicates that the condition has not been associated with a unique gene locus. In contrast, an asterisk ('*') would indicate that the condition is associated with a specific gene of known sequence. Full details of the nomenclature are available by clicking on 'Numbering System' beneath 'FAQ' at the left of the OMIM home page.

   More easily readable reviews of conditions are available at the linked GeneReviews directory (Table 19.1, Figs 19.4–19.6).

Table 19.1 Clinical information	
OMIM (Online Mendelian Inheritance in Man)	http://www.ncbi.nlm.nih.gov/omim/
GeneReviews (expert-authored disease reviews; select 'GeneReviews' at this site)	http://www.geneclinics.org
PubMed (online database of medical and biological journal publications with links to full text documents)	http://www.ncbi.nlm.nih.gov/sites/entrez/
Genetics Home Reference (Bethesda, MD, USA: National Library of Medicine)	http://ghr.nlm.nih.gov/

Type condition name in this box

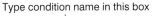
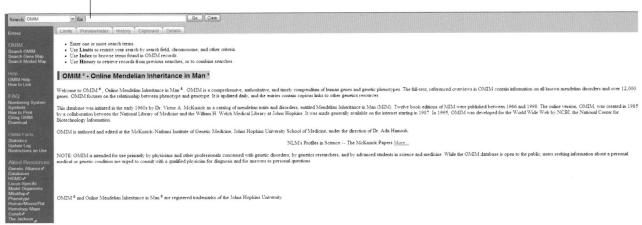

Fig. 19.1 OMIM home page. Searching by name of condition. Online Mendelian Inheritance in Man, OMIM™. McKusick-Nathans Institute of Genetic Medicine, Johns Hopkins University (Baltimore, MD) and National Center for Biotechnology Information, National Library of Medicine (Bethesda, MD) {9 June 2010}. Available from: http://www.ncbi.nlm.nih.gov/omim/.

Click here for further information

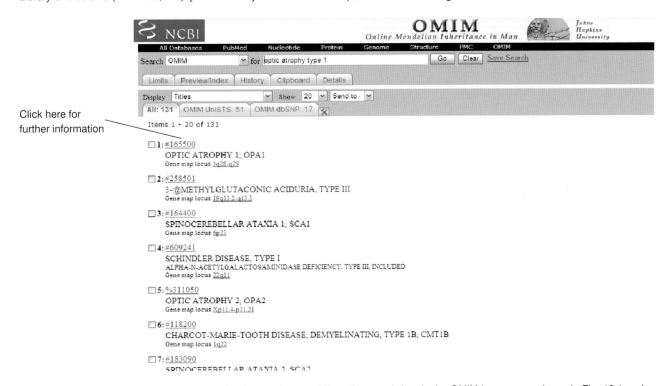

Fig. 19.2 OMIM search results, after typing 'optic atrophy type 1' into the search box in the OMIM home page shown in Fig. 19.1 and clicking on 'Go'.

These reviews are well written and generally expert authored. They contain reasonably comprehensive disease-orientated reviews summarising not only the clinical manifestations of each of a great many genetic conditions, but also the mode of inheritance, relevant publications and links to patient support groups (mainly in the USA). The databases can easily be searched using complete or incomplete search terms and each review has a hyperlinked table of contents. Clicking on the GeneTests link, in the top right of the page in OMIM, is another route to the relevant GeneReview.

As is the case for non-genetic medical conditions, PubMed is an invaluable, continually updated index of millions of clinical and scientific peer-reviewed articles that is provided as a service by the US National Library of Medicine (Table 19.1). This index allows searching for reviews separately and provides links to electronic PDF versions of the many articles.

For non-professionals, a useful website is the Genetics Home Reference, which is a service of the US National Library of Medicine and provides a 'consumer-friendly' guide to the genetics of more than 350 conditions (Table 19.1). This guide

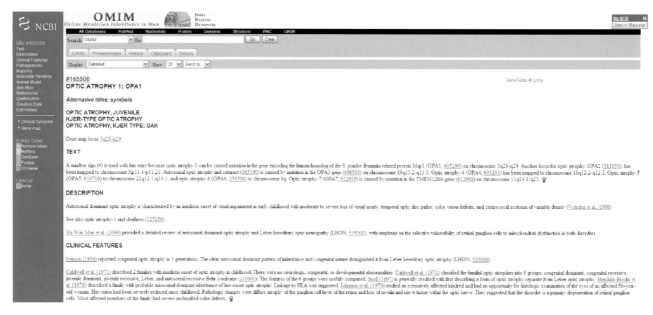

Fig. 19.3 OMIM disease-related article, after clicking on '#165500'. Clicking on the GeneTests link, if displayed in the top right of the page in OMIM, is a quick route to the relevant GeneReview.

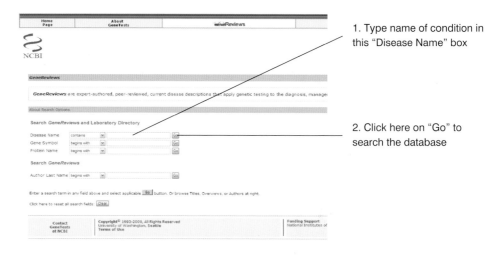

Fig. 19.4 GeneReviews search page.

provides basic information about the conditions, genes, gene families, mutations, inheritance, DNA, chromosomes, genetic testing and links to support groups and other organisations. It also includes a glossary of medical and genetic definitions.

Laboratories undertaking genetic testing

In the UK, the details of clinical laboratories offering diagnostic testing for a specific condition can be found from the UKGTN website (see Table 19.2, Fig. 19.7), and the diagnostic and research laboratories in Europe in general can be found on online databases such as ORPHANET. ORPHANET (which is funded by the French Ministry of Health and the European Commission and was recently redesigned) provides a directory of services for 7000 rare diseases in 35 countries. The European Directory of DNA Diagnostic Laboratories (EDDNAL) is also a useful searchable catalogue (Fig. 19.8).

The GeneTests website (which contains the GeneReviews mentioned above), funded by the US National Institutes of Health, provides a Laboratory Directory (Fig. 19.9) of the testing laboratories predominantly in the USA, together with information regarding the type of service they provide. More specialised websites have been established, such as that of the European Skeletal Dysplasia Network (ESDN), members of which provide expert diagnostic advice to specialists and, where appropriate, genetic testing, for specific skeletal dysplasia cases.

Patient information and support groups

Patients and their relatives often derive great benefit from making contact with appropriate support groups (see Table 19.3). These often have helpful and informative websites that provide local contact details. These websites may be found by

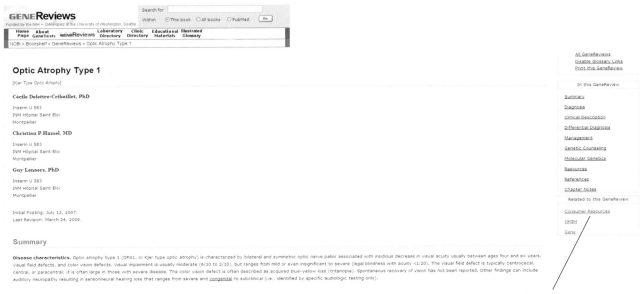

Fig. 19.5 GeneReviews article on the condition.

Click on "Consumer Resources" here, beneath the heading "Related to this GeneReview", to reach information regarding patient support groups (mainly in North America)

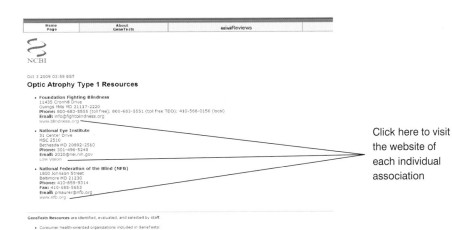

Fig. 19.6 GeneReviews list of 'Resources', such as patient support groups. This information can be reached by clicking on 'Consumer Resources' from the menu on the right side of the GeneReviews article.

Click here to visit the website of each individual association

Table 19.2 Directories of gene testing laboratories	
UKGTN (UK Genetic Testing Network)	http://www.ukgtn.nhs.uk/gtn/Home
GeneTests (particularly North America; select 'Laboratory Directory')	http://www.geneclinics.org/
ORPHANET (predominantly European)	http://www.orpha.net
EDDNAL (European)	http://www.eddnal.com
European Skeletal Dysplasia Network (ESDN)	http://www.esdn.org

using a general web search engine. However, most of the useful support groups are listed in online directories such as the CAF directory (UK), NORD (National Organization for Rare Disorders, Washington DC), Genetics Home Reference (USA, see above) and POSSUM (Australia) websites. Many families with members affected by a variety of chromosomal disorders benefit from contacting UNIQUE (Rare Chromosome Disorder Support Group). Many other valuable condition-specific websites exist, such as the Scottish Muscle Network, Cancer Research UK and Breakthrough Breast Cancer.

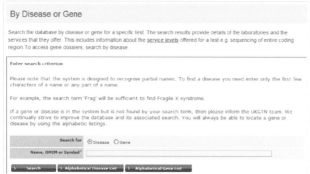

By Disease or Gene

Search the database by disease or gene for a specific test. The search results provide details of the laboratories and the services that they offer. This includes information about the service levels offered for a test e.g. sequencing of entire coding region. To access gene dossiers, search by disease.

Enter search criterion

Please note that the system is designed to recognise partial names. To find a disease you need enter only the first few characters of a name or any part of a name.

For example, the search term 'Frag' will be sufficient to find Fragile X syndrome.

If a gene or disease is in the system but is not found by your search term, then please inform the UKGTN team. We continually strive to improve the database and its associated search. You will always be able to locate a gene or disease by using the alphabetic listings.

Search for ⊙ Disease ○ Gene

Name, OMIM or Symbol*

> Search   > Alphabetical Disease List   > Alphabetical Gene List

Fig. 19.7 UKGTN search page (after clicking on 'Search' and 'By Disease or Gene' at the top of the home page). © UKGTN 2001–2010. All rights reserved.

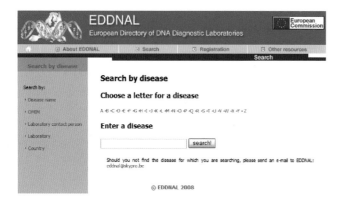

Fig. 19.8 EDDNAL search page (reached by clicking on 'Search' on the home page). © EDDNAL 2010.

Gene- and protein-specific sequence, structure, function and expression information

The DNA sequences for individual genes can be viewed and downloaded from several different websites, including the Ensembl and GeneCards databases described in this section, the NCBI website (which hosts the OMIM and PubMed databases) and the UCSC website that is discussed below (see Tables 19.4 and 19.5).

Fig. 19.9 GeneTests Laboratory Directory (reached from the GeneTests home page by clicking on 'Laboratory Directory').

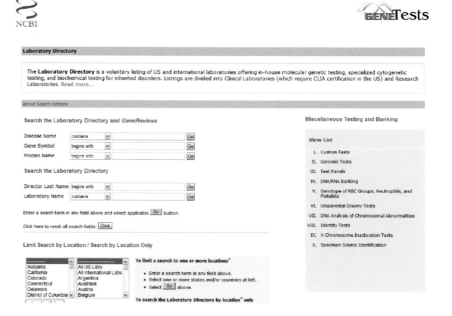

Table 19.3 Patient support directories

CAF directory (particularly useful for the UK)	http://www.cafamily.org.uk/index.php?section=861
Genetic Alliance UK (comprising over 130 patient organisations)	http://www.geneticalliance.org.uk/
Genetics Home Reference (via 'Patient Support' link)	http://ghr.nlm.nih.gov/
GeneReviews (via 'Resources' link)	http://www.geneclinics.org
NORD (National Organisation for Rare Disorders, Washington DC)	http://www.rarediseases.org/
POSSUM (based in Victoria, Australia)	http://www.possum.net.au/links/html
UNIQUE (Rare Chromosome Disorder Support Group)	http://www.rarechromo.co.uk/html/home.asp
Scottish Muscle Network (select 'Patient and carers' or 'Affiliations & links' from menu at top left of page)	http://www.gla.ac.uk/departments/ scottishmusclenetwork/
Cancer Research UK (in the 'Patient Information' section)	http://www.cruk.org/
Breakthrough Breast Cancer (in 'About breast cancer' section)	http://www.breakthrough.org.uk/

Table 19.4 Scientific information regarding genes and proteins

OMIM (Online Mendelian Inheritance in Man)	http://www.ncbi.nlm.nih.gov/omim/
GeneCards	http://www.genecards.org/
Ensembl (e.g. for exon/intron structure and location of known SNPs in a gene sequence)	http://www.ensembl.org/
UCSC (University of California, Santa Cruz) (e.g. for easy to use mapping and the microsatellite marker track)	http://genome.ucsc.edu/
NCBI (National Center for Biotechnology Information)	http://www.ncbi.nlm.nih.gov/
CEPH Genotype Database Browser	http://www.cephb.fr/en/cephdb/browser.php

Table 19.5 Tools for DNA or protein sequence analysis

BLAST (Basic Local Alignment Search Tool at NCBI)	http://blast.ncbi.nlm.nih.gov/Blast.cgi
BLAT /BLAST (at Ensembl)	http://www.ensembl.org/Multi/blastview
Pfam protein sequence analysis	http://pfam.sanger.ac.uk/
DNA or protein sequence alignment by ClustalW2	http://www.ebi.ac.uk/Tools/clustalw2/index.html
Restriction enzyme cutting site finder (New England Biolabs)	http://tools.neb.com/NEBcutter2/index.php

Ensembl database

Very clearly annotated sequence information (for several species) is available at the Ensembl genome browser (Table 19.4, Fig. 19.10), which is jointly provided by the EMBL-European Bioinformatics Institute and the Sanger Institute, and is primarily funded by the Wellcome Trust. It has recently been provided with a new user interface (as described here).

Finding one's way through Ensembl

Although a great deal of information is contained within the Ensembl database, navigation through its many pages to find the information being sought can sometimes appear slightly confusing at first. A summary flowchart of routes of navigation

to the pages described below is therefore provided in Fig. 19.11 to assist the user.

Coding sequences and transcripts

At Ensembl, it is possible to find a sequence by simply selecting the species and entering the gene (or disease) name (Fig. 19.10) and then, from the search results (Figs 19.12 and 19.13), clicking on 'Ensembl protein coding gene'. This will display the 'Ensembl Gene summary' page (Fig. 19.14) in which, for each gene, data regarding one or more associated transcripts is revealed. For each transcript, there is a 'Transcript summary' (Fig. 19.15) displaying the transcript length, number of exons and predicted protein length.

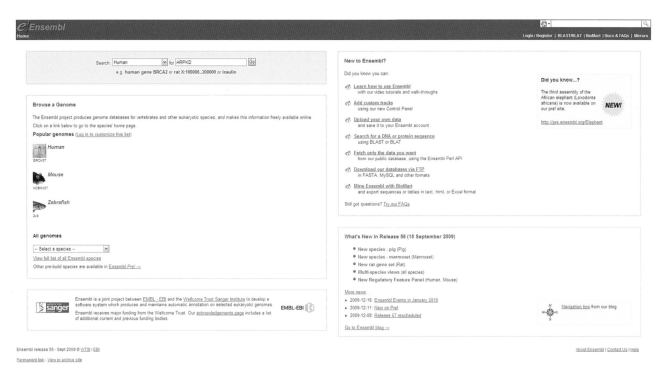

Fig. 19.10 Ensembl genome browser. Reproduced with kind permission of the Wellcome Trust Sanger Institute. See Flicek *et al.* (2010) in Further reading. Available from: http://www.ensembl.org/index.html.

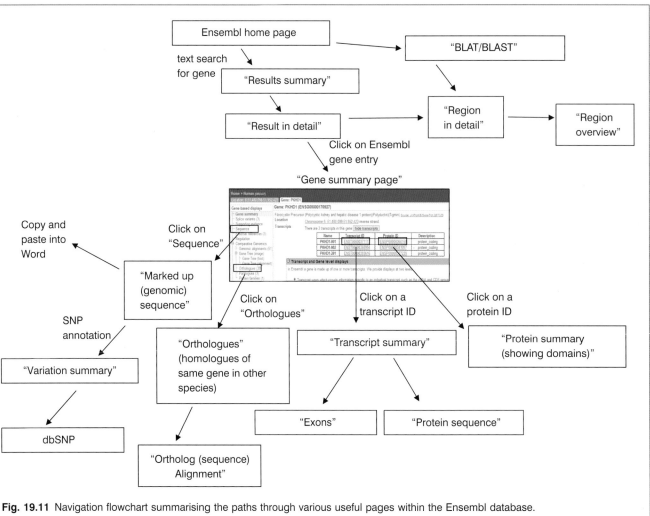

Fig. 19.11 Navigation flowchart summarising the paths through various useful pages within the Ensembl database.

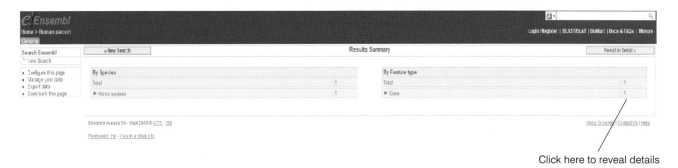

Click here to reveal details

Fig. 19.12 Ensembl Results Summary after selecting 'Human' from list and typing 'ARPKD' (for autosomal recessive polycystic kidney disease) into the search box at the top of the page. Reproduced with kind permission of the Wellcome Trust Sanger Institute. See Flicek *et al.* (2010) in Further reading.

Click here to reveal further details of the gene

Alternatively, click here to reveal "Region in detail" showing the chromosome region that contains the gene

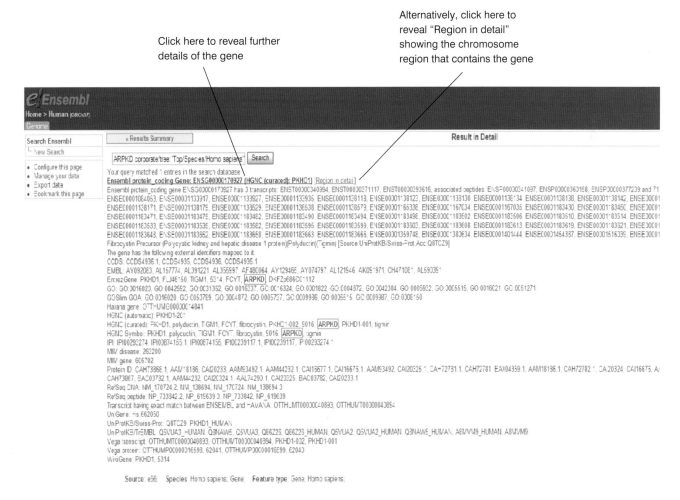

Fig. 19.13 Ensembl genome browser search 'Result in Detail'. The details shown may be more abbreviated than those shown here. Reproduced with permission of the Wellcome Trust Sanger Institute. See Flicek *et al.* (2010) in Further reading.

Protein domains

In addition, for each transcript there is also a 'Protein summary' (Fig. 19.16) containing coloured diagrams that show the various protein domains that have been identified automatically by several different domain-finding computer programs (such as Pfam).

When the 'Transcript summary' page is visible, clicking on 'Exons' beneath 'Sequence' at the extreme left of the page, reveals full sequence details of each exon together with surrounding intronic sequence (Fig. 19.17). By clicking on 'Configure this page', it is possible for more intronic sequence to be displayed. Alternatively, by clicking on 'Protein' in the same column, the amino acid sequence of the protein can be displayed (Fig. 19.18) with colours used (if desired) to differentiate the individual exons. This page can also be configured to display amino acid numbering and known variants.

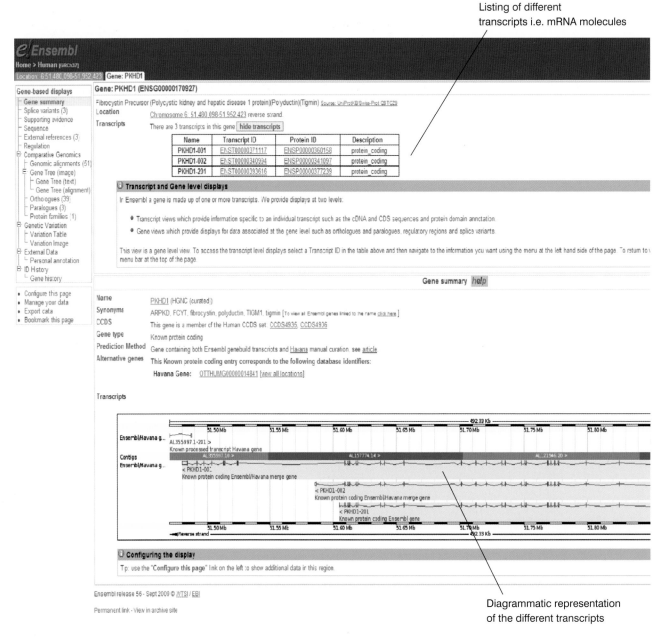

Fig. 19.14 Ensembl gene summary for *PKHD1*. Reproduced with permission of the Wellcome Trust Sanger Institute. See Flicek *et al.* (2010) in Further reading.

Particularly useful to those undertaking mutation analysis of a gene is the information that is revealed by selecting 'Sequence' from the list shown on the left side of the 'Ensembl Gene summary' page (Fig. 19.19). This displays the full sequence of the exons (in red) and introns, i.e. the genomic sequence of the gene.

Many other types of data and displays are accessible from the Ensembl website, which will become apparent as the website is browsed. For instance, from the 'Gene summary' page, by clicking on 'Orthologues' it is also possible to obtain a list of identified homologues of that specific gene in other species, showing the degree of identity with the 'query' gene (i.e. the originally selected gene) (Fig. 19.20) and to view each sequence alignment (Fig. 19.21). In addition, it may be useful to watch the video files describing the use of certain features, which can be viewed by clicking on the 'Help' hyperlinks.

BLAT/BLAST searches

As an alternative to searching for specific sequences in Ensembl using a gene name, it is possible to use a sequence similarity 'BLAST' search, searching for database sequences (nucleotide

Click on 'Gene' tab,
here, to return to
'Gene summary' page

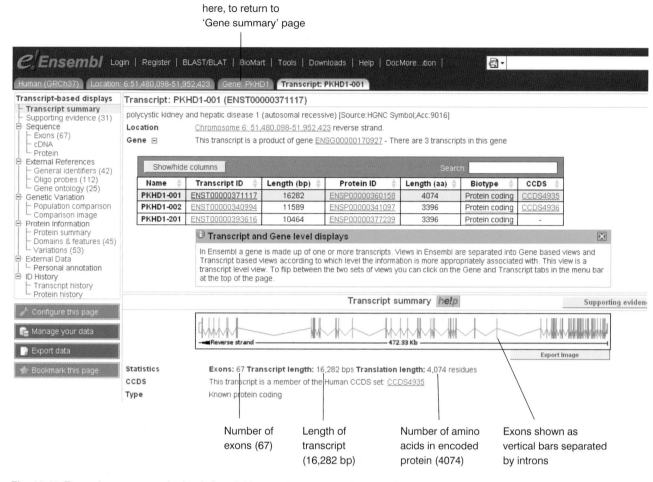

Fig. 19.15 Transcript summary, obtained after clicking on the transcript ID for the first transcript listed. Reproduced with permission of the Wellcome Trust Sanger Institute. See Flicek *et al.* (2010) in Further reading.

or peptide) that closely match your sequence of interest. To do this, click on BLAST in the top right corner of the Ensembl home page (at http://www.ensembl.org), or open the BLAST website directly (see Table 19.5), and then paste or type your sequence of interest into the box shown (Fig. 19.22). If desired, it is possible to change the species (human is currently the default) and the specific type of BLAST search. The default BLAST search, known as BLAT (or BLAST-like Alignment Tool), is an extremely rapid version that effectively searches non-overlapping sequences representing the assembled genome. In contrast, the slower, previously established BLAST algorithm searched enormous numbers of overlapping constituent database entries. After clicking on 'RUN', in the results ('BlastView') page, the positions of any similar sequences that have been found will be shown together with a summary table at the foot of the page (Fig. 19.23). In addition, clickable links to alignments are provided at the bottom left (with multiple selections possible by holding down the control key). For instance, clicking on the 'C' link will take

the user to the 'Region in detail' page (which was previously named 'ContigView', hence the name 'C' link) (Fig. 19.24). This 'Region in detail' page can also be reached by clicking on a 'Region in Detail' link from the 'Result in Detail' page, or by clicking on the Location tab at the top of the 'Gene summary' page.

GeneCards website

A fascinating variety of freely available detailed information about individual genes, the proteins they encode and links to specific data in many other databases is collated at the GeneCards website (Table 19.4, Figs 19.25–19.28) provided by the Weizmann Institute in Israel. Comprehensive hyperlinked data are summarised here in a single-page format, which is particularly helpful and easy to use for certain purposes. The information presented at GeneCards again includes alternative names, chromosomal and genomic locations, protein size, alternative transcript reference sequences or 'RefSeq mRNAs' and

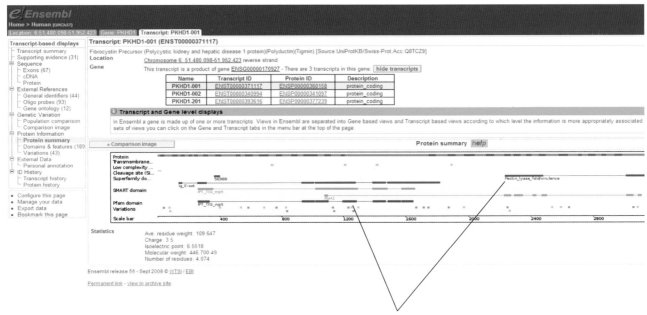

Indication of the types of functional domains and their locations within the protein. By convention, the amino (N) terminal is on the left with the carboxy (C) terminal on the right. The identification of domains differs slightly between different domain-finding algorithms named on the left (e.g. SMART and Pfam)

Fig. 19.16 Protein summary reached after clicking on the protein ID for the first transcript listed. Reproduced with kind permission of the Wellcome Trust Sanger Institute. See Flicek *et al.* (2010) in Further reading.

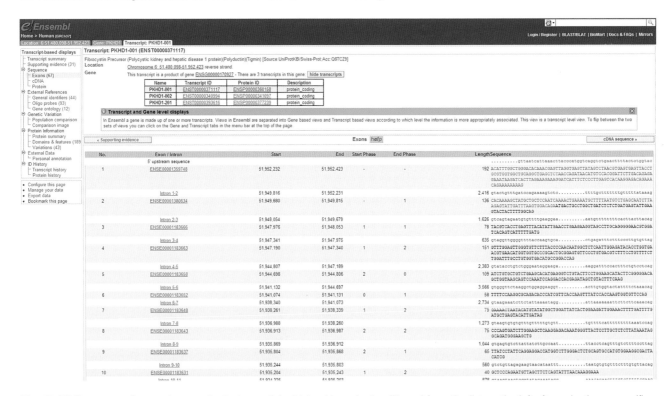

Fig. 19.17 Sequence of exons for a particular transcript, obtained by selecting 'Exons' from the list on the left after selecting a specific transcript ID to view. Reproduced with permission of the Wellcome Trust Sanger Institute. See Flicek *et al.* (2010) in Further reading.

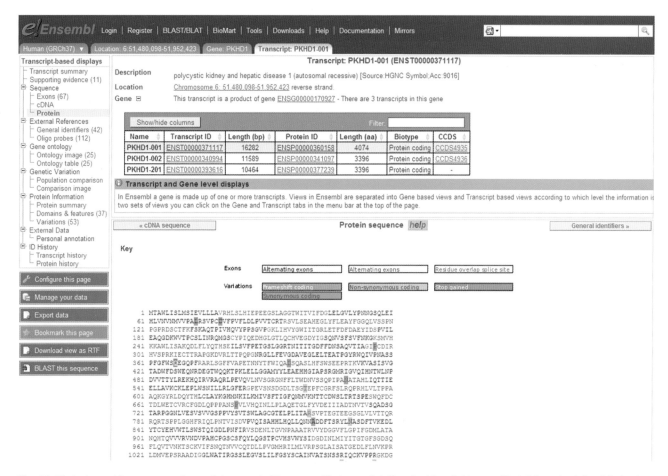

Fig. 19.18 Amino acid sequence of a protein encoded by a specific transcript. Reached by clicking on 'Protein' on the left, while in the Transcript Summary page. To display the features shown, it is then necessary to select 'Configure this page', switch on the display of numbering and variants and, finally, click on the 'save and close' tick in the top right. Reproduced with permission of the Wellcome Trust Sanger Institute. See Flicek *et al.* (2010) in Further reading.

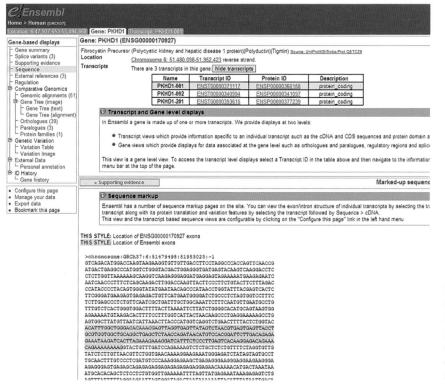

Fig. 19.19 Marked up genomic sequence, showing exons (in colour) and introns. Reached from the Gene summary page by clicking on 'Sequence' at its extreme left. Reproduced with permission of the Wellcome Trust Sanger Institute. See Flicek *et al.* (2010) in Further reading.

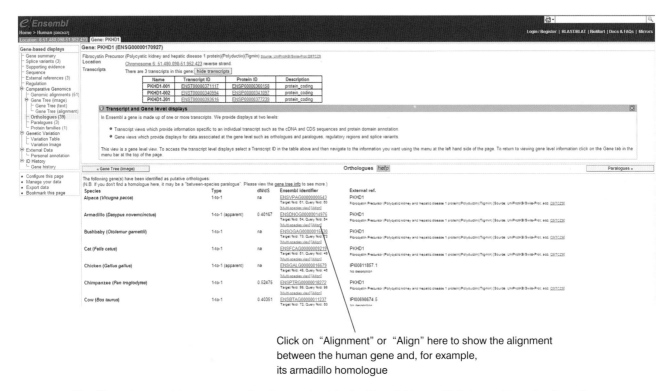

Click on "Alignment" or "Align" here to show the alignment between the human gene and, for example, its armadillo homologue

Fig. 19.20 List of homologues of the same gene in other species (obtained by clicking on 'Orthologues' from the Gene Summary page. Reproduced with permission of the Wellcome Trust Sanger Institute. See Flicek *et al.* (2010) in Further reading.

splicing patterns (in the 'Transcripts' section), disease relationships, mutations and single-nucleotide polymorphisms (SNPs) (with SNP types, frequencies and sequences, as well as a direct link to the Hapmap SNP haplotype database for the gene). A huge range of other interesting information is also available at GeneCards, including the identified protein domains (by clicking on 'Graphical view of domain structure' within the 'Protein domains' section), probable gene function (from beneath the UniProt/Swiss-Prot heading within the 'Gene function' section) and homologues in other species. Also presented is information regarding gene function and relevant research articles. Of particular interest to researchers will be the direct links to appropriate antibodies, recombinant proteins, clones, expression assays and RNA interference (RNAi) reagents.

Gene expression data

In addition, at the GeneCards website, helpful graphical summaries of the degree of expression of a gene in different tissues are presented (Fig. 19.28). Such data are obtained from microarray data following hybridisation with RNA from a variety of tissues, or are extrapolated, for example from the relative abundance of different expressed sequence fragments (i.e. 'electronic Northerns' or eNortherns).

CASE III

You wish to design oligonucleotide primers that will allow you to amplify each exon of a gene in turn and to sequence the exon and its exon/intron boundaries. Where on the internet could you find the following:

1. The relevant nucleotide sequence information.
2. Which mutations have already been identified within the gene and which ones are most frequently found (possible mutation hot-spots).
3. Software tools for automatic primer design for a single region or, alternatively, for an entire gene.
4. Tools to ensure that no SNP exists within your chosen primer sequences and to display the positions of known SNPs within a genomic sequence.
5. Algorithms to rapidly check that your chosen primer pairs will not inadvertently amplify any other sequence in the entire genome.

Answers are given in the following paragraphs.

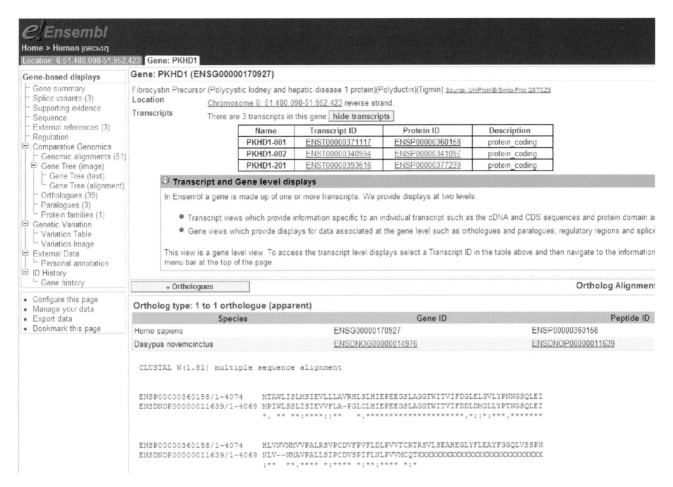

Fig. 19.21 Alignment between human and armadillo *PKHD1* gene sequences, (reached by clicking on 'Alignment' within the Ensembl Identifier column of the table of orthologues. Reproduced with permission of the Wellcome Trust Sanger Institute. See Flicek *et al.* (2010) in Further reading.

Nucleotide sequences and human mutations

When designing primers to amplify an exon, it is essential to have access to the DNA sequence for not only the exon, but also, of course, for its intronic flanking sequences. This can be easily obtained from Ensembl by viewing the 'Exon sequence' for a specific transcript of a gene or the 'Genomic sequence' links for a particular gene (as described in Table 19.4). The mutations that have already been identified may be listed in the 'Allelic variants' section within the gene-specific OMIM article, in individual review publications or in the Human Gene Mutation Database at Cardiff University (HGMD) or the Diagnostic Mutation Database at Manchester National Genetic Reference Laboratory (both requiring registration) (see Table 19.6). In addition, the mutations for many genes have been listed in disease-specific online databases such as the Breast Information Core (BIC) database of *BRCA1* and *BRCA2* mutations (again requiring registration), the database of HNPCC and FAP-related mutations freely accessible at the InSiGHT (International Society for Gastrointestinal Hereditary Tumours) website and the Leiden muscular dystrophy database (Table 19.6).

Automatic primer design tools

A popular primer design tool is the updated version of Primer3, which was originally designed by the Whitehead Institute in Massachusetts, USA. This version, Primer3Plus (Table 19.7, Fig. 19.29), now has a more user-friendly interface. This freely available online tool allows the user to paste in a nucleotide sequence and to specify which regions should be flanked by the primers. As the first 30 nucleotides of sequence generated by an automated sequencer are often unreliable and as the first few bases immediately adjacent to exons are important biologically for splicing efficiency and accuracy, it is usually preferable to instruct Primer3Plus to select potential primer sequences that are separated by at least 30 nucleotides from the exon in question. The software also permits the user to specify the minimum and maximum lengths of the primers and the required degree of similarity between the primers' annealing temperatures, in addition to many other parameters. It will provide a list of possible primer sequences, showing the predicted annealing temperatures and also an estimation of the likelihood of each primer forming unwanted secondary structure by base-paring internally.

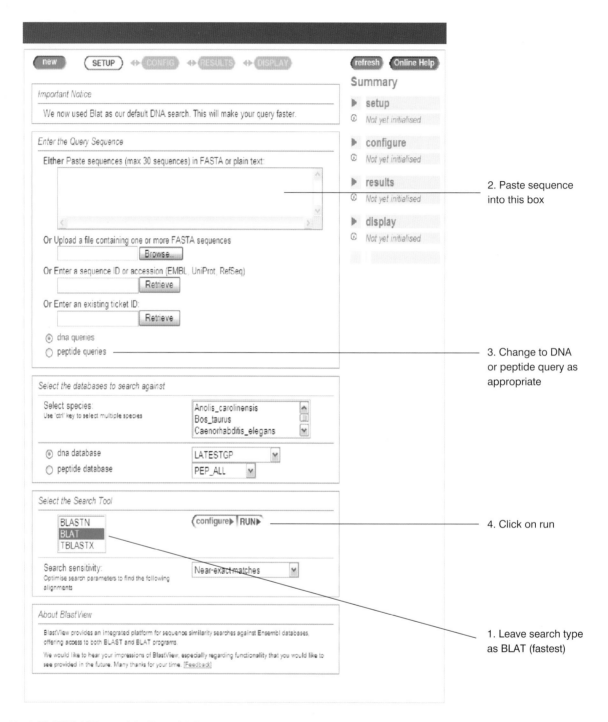

Fig. 19.22 BLAT/BLAST search in Ensembl. Reproduced with permission of the Wellcome Trust Sanger Institute. See Flicek *et al.* (2010) in Further reading.

Another website exists that not only automatically selects primer sequences but also does so for every exon in a gene automatically. This webpage (Fig. 19.30), which is based on Primer3 and is entitled 'Genomic Primers', is useful but requires as a reference file, a Genbank sequence file. The latter can be obtained by following the instructions obtained by clicking on the 'How to obtain a GenBank file' link on that page. The GenBank file must first be saved to disk and then

uploaded using the 'Browse' button in the Genomic Primers page.

Checking for SNPs

For each pair of apparently suitable primers that has been selected, it is worthwhile checking that neither of the primer sequences is located over a known SNP, as, if the

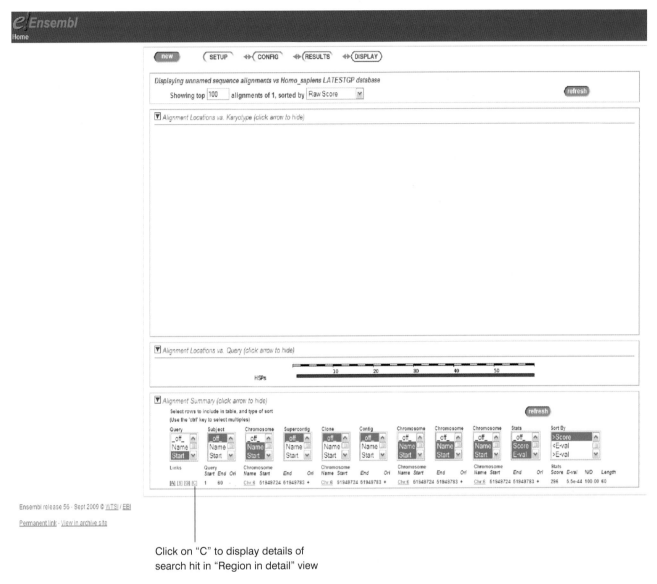

Click on "C" to display details of
search hit in "Region in detail" view

Fig. 19.23 Results of BLAT/BLAST search in Ensembl. Reproduced with permission of the Wellcome Trust Sanger Institute. See Flicek *et al.* (2010) in Further reading.

variant is present, allele drop-out could result in preferential amplification of a single allele. A useful web tool called SNPCheck (at the National Genetics Reference Laboratory in Manchester, UK; see Table 19.7) allows this to be checked in seconds.

Alternatively, the positions of the SNPs can be displayed in a genome browser, such as Ensembl. In the latter, one way of displaying the SNPs is as follows: from the 'Sequence display' reached from the 'Gene summary' page, click on 'Configure this page', activate 'Line numbering' and 'Show variations' (followed by 'Save and close') (Fig. 19.31). The genomic sequence of the gene will then be displayed together with the known SNP variations (in green). Moreover, for each SNP, the nucleotide position and precise change is displayed to the right of the sequence (Fig. 19.32), with embedded clickable

links to the associated 'Variation summary' page (Fig. 19.33), which contains further information regarding that variant, including a link to the specific dbSNP page (Fig. 19.34), which contains the population frequencies for the different alleles of that SNP, if known. Usefully, the genomic sequence together with the annotations to the right can be copied and pasted into a Microsoft Word document, although it will be necessary to select 'Landscape' orientation in 'Page setup' (from the File menu) within Word, in order to display the sequence correctly. The user can then annotate sections of the sequence (for instance, underlining chosen PCR primer sequences), save it and print it. The embedded links will usually also be retained within the Word document and can be opened individually by using a right-click followed by 'Open hyperlink'.

Position of "query" sequence that was used to initiate the BLAT search

Click here to zoom in or out on the region

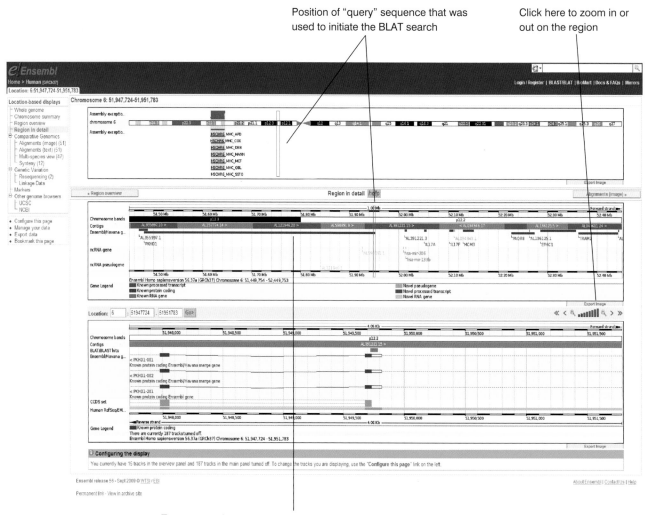

Target gene that contains a match to the query sequence

Fig. 19.24 Ensembl 'Region in detail' page (reached by clicking on the 'location' tab near the top of the 'Gene summary' page, or by clicking on the "C" link at the bottom left corner of the BLAT/BLAST results page. Reproduced with permission of the Wellcome Trust Sanger Institute. See Flicek *et al.* (2010) in Further reading.

Checking of primers for specificity

Another invaluable web page (at NCBI) is the Reverse e-PCR page (Table 19.7, Fig. 19.35) within which, the 'Table input' section is the most user-friendly. After selecting the *Homo sapiens* genome dataset and pasting one's primer sequences and predicted PCR product size into the appropriate boxes, it is best to reduce the stringency of the search by increasing the 'Allowed STS size deviation' to at least 100 and changing the 'Primer Alignment quality' to permit two mismatches and two gaps. The electronic genome search then automatically carries out a virtual PCR, displaying the precise chromosome locations and sizes of any predicted products. This should hopefully confirm that the chosen primer will amplify the desired sequence and, importantly, show whether any (undesired) products of a similar size could result from inexact sequence complementarity (i.e. slightly non-specific hybridisation) to any other regions in the genome.

CASE IV

You find the same mutation in two apparently unrelated families. You wish to compare the surrounding DNA sequence in the mutant alleles from the two families to try to find out whether the two apparently identical mutations have occurred independently or represent the same ancestral mutation. In order to do this, you wish to analyse nearby sequence polymorphisms. Where on the internet could you easily find out the following:

1. The position and identities of the intragenic $(CA)_n$ repeat microsatellite markers.
2. The approximate proportion of individuals found to be heterozygous at those markers.
3. The primer sequences that have already been found by others to successfully amplify those microsatellite markers by PCR.
4. The expected product sizes if those primers are used.

Answers are given in the following paragraphs.

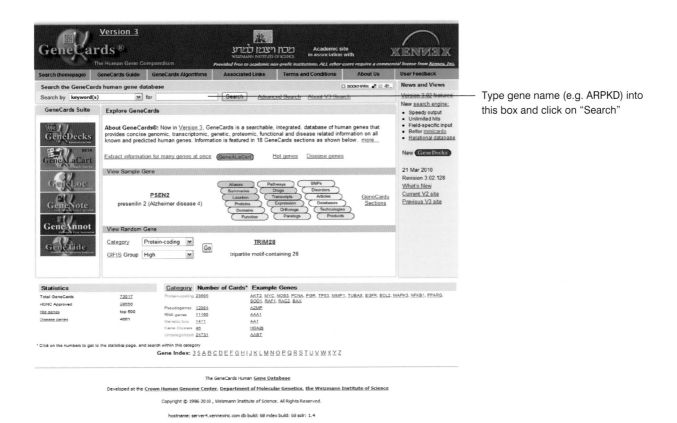

Type gene name (e.g. ARPKD) into this box and click on "Search"

Fig. 19.25 GeneCards homepage. With permission from the Weizmann Institute of Science.

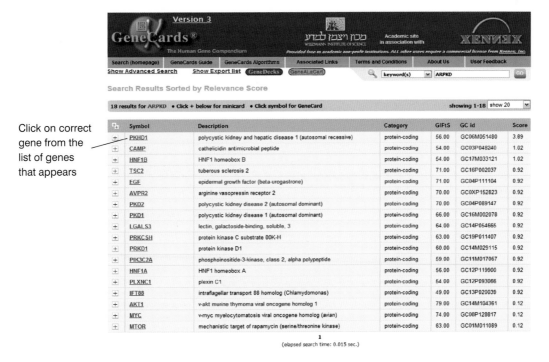

Click on correct gene from the list of genes that appears

Fig. 19.26 GeneCards search results. With permission from the Weizmann Institute of Science.

Fig. 19.27 First part of GeneCard for *PKHD1*, showing alternative names and the gene's chromosomal and genomic location. With permission from the Weizmann Institute of Science.

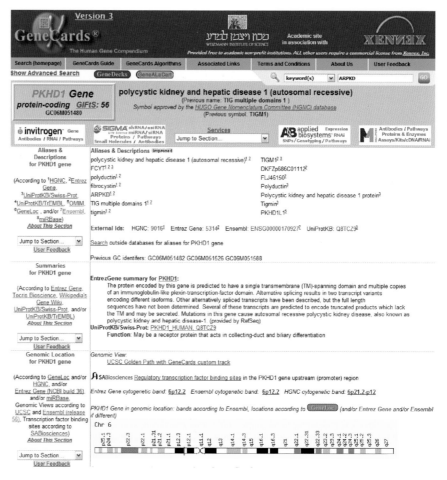

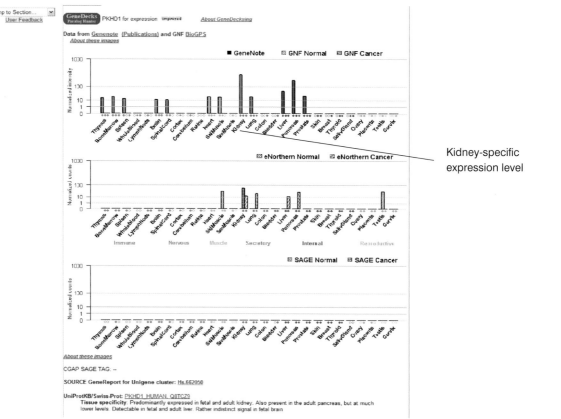

Kidney-specific expression level

Fig. 19.28 Expression data for *PKHD1* in GeneCards, obtained from microarray analysis (GeneNote and GNF) and electronic prediction (eNorthern). The relatively high level of expression in the kidney is visible. With permission from the Weizmann Institute of Science.

Table 19.6 Mutations and SNPs

HGMD (Human Gene Mutation Database at the Institute of Medical Genetics in Cardiff)	http://www.hgmd.cf.ac.uk
Breast Cancer Information Core (BIC) database (requires password)	http://research.nhgri.nih.gov/bic/
dbSNP (NCBI Single Nucleotide Polymorphism database)	http://www.ncbi.nlm.nih.gov/projects/SNP/
HapMap (International HapMap Project)	http://www.hapmap.org/
Human Genome Variation Society	http://www.hgvs.org/
Guidelines on lab reporting of unclassified variants (select Best Practice Guidelines, then Unclassified Variants)	http://www.cmgs.org
Diagnostic Mutation Database (at Manchester National Genetics Reference Laboratory)	http://www.ngrl.org.uk/Manchester/dmudb.html
InSiGHT (International Society for Gastrointestinal Hereditary Tumours)	http://www.insight-group.org/mutations/
Leiden muscular dystrophy database	http://www.dmd.nl/

Table 19.7 Websites useful when designing primers

Primer3Plus	http://www.bioinformatics.nl/cgi-bin/primer3plus/primer3plus.cgi
Genomic Primers (to obtain primers for multiple exons at once)	http://pcrsuite.cse.ucsc.edu/Genomic_Primers.html
DNA OligoCalculator (for calculating annealing temperatures)	http://www.sigma-genosys.com/calc/DNACalc.asp
SNPCheck (National Genetics Reference Lab at Manchester, UK)	https://ngrl.manchester.ac.uk/SNPCheckV2/snpcheck.htm
Reverse e-PCR (choose 'Table input') at NCBI	http://www.ncbi.nlm.nih.gov/sutils/e-pcr/reverse.cgi

If desired by laboratory, click here to set the GC clamp to 1 or 2 depending on preference

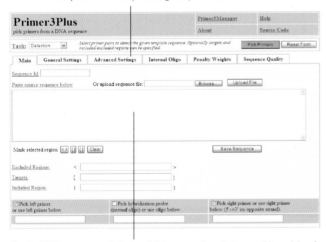

Paste DNA sequence in here. Add square brackets on either side of the exon to mark it as a target and then indicate the wider region to be flanked by primers by enclosing it within < and > symbols.

Fig. 19.29 Primer3Plus. © 2006, 2007 by Andreas Untergasser and Harm Nijveen.

Displaying map data for genes and markers

The UCSC genome browser

The UCSC Genome Browser at the University of California Santa Cruz (Table 19.4, Fig. 19.36) provides users with many similar features to those provided within the Ensembl website. Again, an enormous quantity of data is available. The presentation is different (with most display controls being present together, in the lower part of the browser page) and for certain tasks can be easier to use. For instance, some users find that showing all the markers of a specific type within and around a particular gene can be easier to perform at present in the UCSC browser. The user can link to the UCSC browser from Ensembl's 'Region in detail' page by clicking on the 'Other genome browser: UCSC' link at the left of the screen. Alternatively, one of many types of search term can be entered into the UCSC Genome Browser 'Gateway' search box before clicking on 'submit' (Fig. 19.36). Once the gene has been selected from the search results list (Fig. 19.37), the browser allows the user to zoom in or out by ×3 or ×10 (Fig. 19.38), to show as much or

Select and upload the saved
GenBank file by clicking on
this link

Obtain a GenBank file by
following the instructions
provided when you click on this
link. then save it to disk

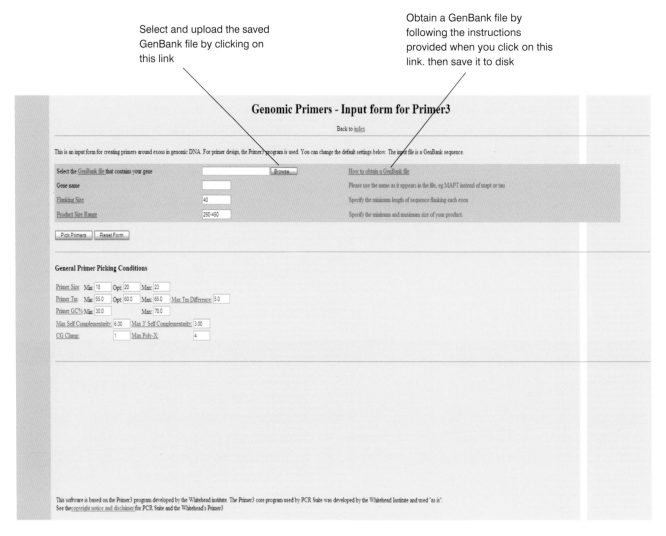

Fig. 19.30 Genomic Primers (for selection of multiple primer pairs). © 2003 Erasmus MC Rotterdam.

as little of the region as desired and to move the viewing window in the centromeric or telomeric direction.

Displaying microsatellite markers

The well-recognised Genethon set of polymorphic microsatellite $(CA)_n$ markers can be displayed beneath the idiogram in the UCSC browser showing their precise position and identity. This can be done by clicking on 'STS markers' from the 'Mapping and Sequencing Tracks' (Fig. 19.38), changing the display mode to 'full' and then clicking on 'refresh'. Subsequently, select the 'include' filter (Fig. 19.39) and 'Genethon' from the list of marker types (which is revealed by clicking on the grey vertical bar situated to the left of the 'STS markers' track), followed by 'submit'. Selecting one of these markers (Fig. 19.40) displays information regarding product size and suitable PCR primer sequences (Fig. 19.41). The proportion of individuals who are heterozygous for one of these markers can be obtained if desired by searching using the 'CEPH Genotype Database Browser' (Table 19.4).

CASE V

Mutation analysis of your gene of interest has revealed a previously unreported missense mutation (i.e. a nucleotide substitution that results in an amino acid substitution). The amino acid change may or may not be significant, as the chemical properties of the two residues are similar.

Which websites can be used to determine whether or not the substitution is likely to be significant?

Answers are given in the following paragraphs.

Online missense mutation analysis tools

There are now various websites that can be used to analyse a particular mutation of this type (see Table 19.8). The algorithms that they use take into account the chemical properties

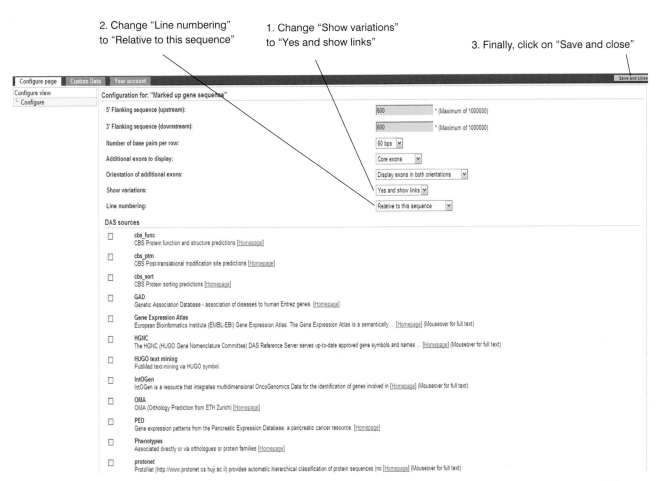

Fig. 19.31 Configuration page in Ensembl for 'Marked up gene sequence', in order to show SNPs. This page is reached by clicking on 'Configure this page', after clicking on 'Sequence' from the 'Gene summary' page. Reproduced with permission of the Wellcome Trust Sanger Institute. See Flicek *et al.* (2010) in Further reading.

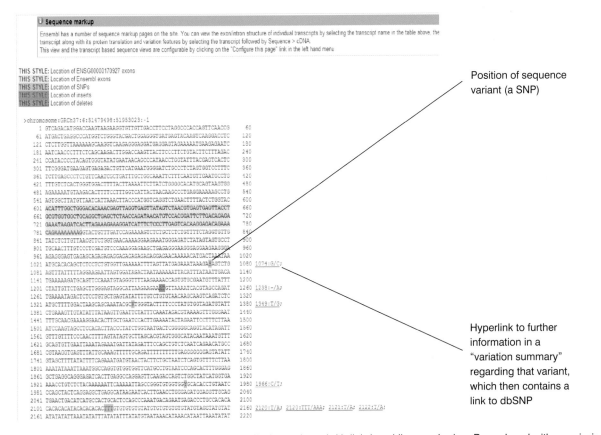

Fig. 19.32 Marked-up gene sequence, now configured to display variants (with links) and line numbering. Reproduced with permission of the Wellcome Trust Sanger Institute. See Flicek *et al.* (2010) in Further reading.

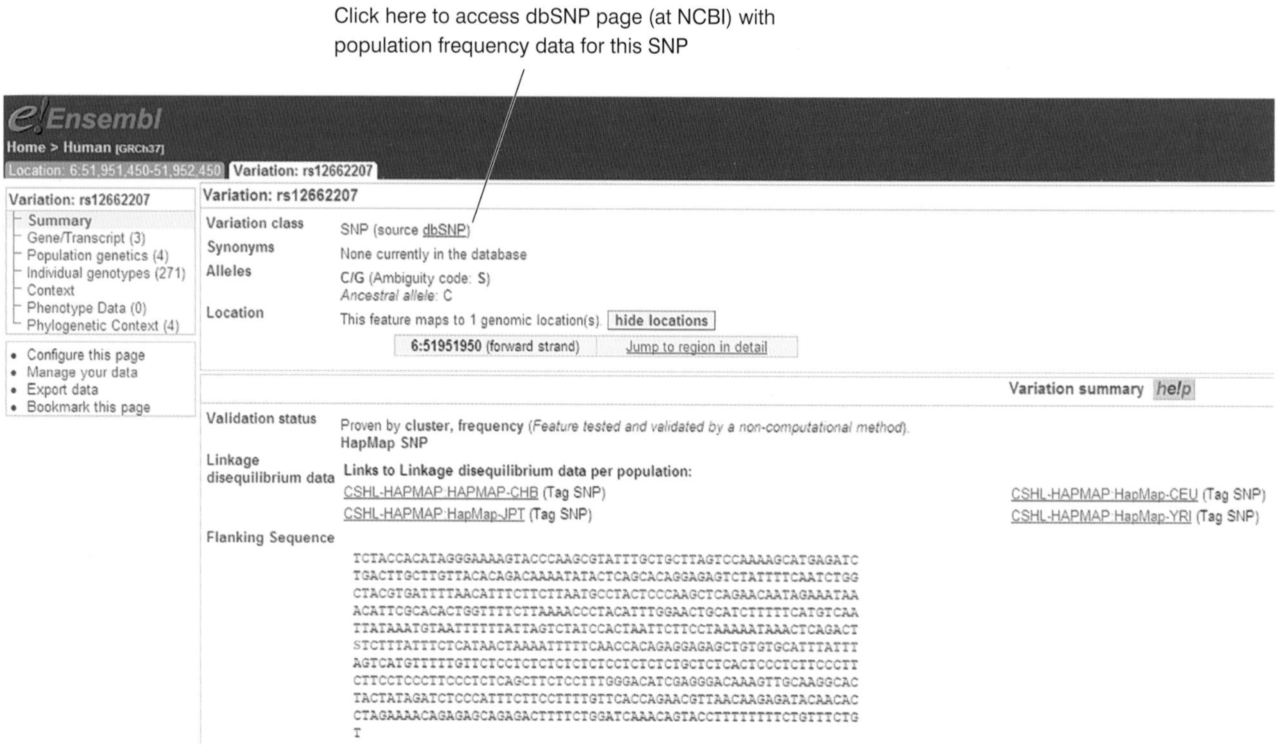

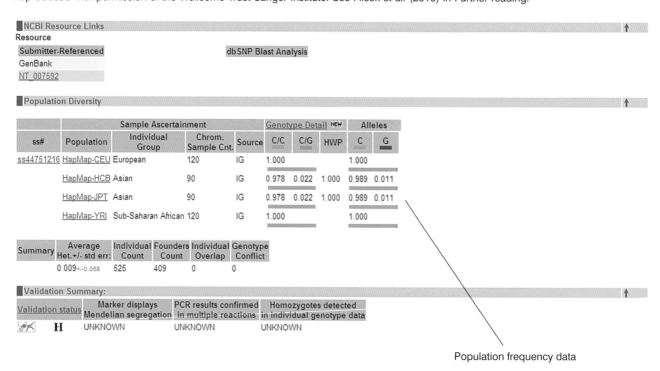

Fig. 19.33 'Variation summary' page reached by clicking on the hyperlink to the right of a SNP in 'Marked up gene sequence' view. Reproduced with permission of the Wellcome Trust Sanger Institute. See Flicek *et al.* (2010) in Further reading.

Fig. 19.34 Further information from dbSNP reached by clicking on the dbSNP link near the top of the 'Variation summary' page.

of the amino acid (e.g. the degree of water affinity, i.e. hydrophilicity or, conversely, hydrophobicity), as well as evolutionary conservation of that particular amino acid. For instance, in general, if there is considerable variation across species at that location within the protein, then a mutation causing an amino acid substitution at that position is less likely to be pathogenic, although the degree of change in the hydrophobicity of the residue caused by its substitution is also important. Websites that provide such analyses automatically include PolyPhen and SIFT. Both of these require a brief

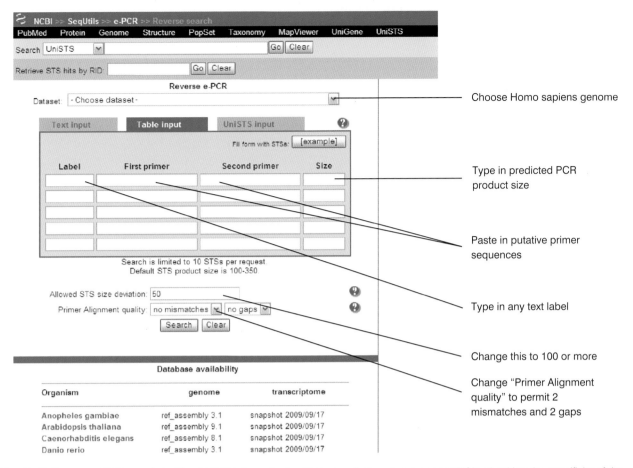

Choose Homo sapiens genome

Type in predicted PCR product size

Paste in putative primer sequences

Type in any text label

Change this to 100 or more

Change "Primer Alignment quality" to permit 2 mismatches and 2 gaps

Fig. 19.35 Reverse e-PCR search facility at NCBI (after selecting Table Input). It performs a virtual PCR, checking the specificity of the primer pair.

Type gene name or cytogenetic band in here (see examples at left of screen) and click on submit

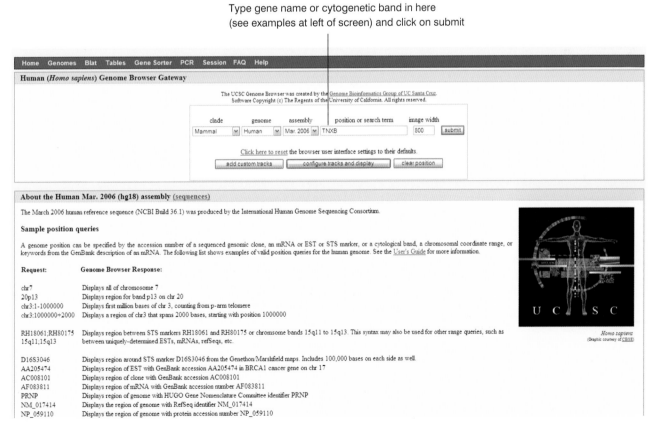

Fig. 19.36 UCSC Genome Browser 'Gateway'. This and following figures from http://genome.ucsc.edu/ (Kent WJ, et al., 2002. The human genome browser at UCSC. Genome Res. 2002 Jun;12(6):996–1006).

UCSC Genes

```
TNXB (uc010jbq.1) at chr6:32084175-32088778 - Homo sapiens tenascin XB, mRNA (cDNA clone IMAGE:40118876), complete cds.
TNXB (uc003sdo.2) at chr6_qbl_hap2:3223933-3268868 - tenascin XB isoform 1 precursor
TNXB (uc003sdm.1) at chr6_qbl_hap2:3223933-3229385 - tenascin XB isoform 2
TNXB (uc003sdl.1) at chr6_qbl_hap2:3223933-3228906 - tenascin XB isoform 2
TNXB (uc003rls.2) at chr6_cox_hap1:3416090-3484320 - tenascin XB isoform 1 precursor
TNXB (uc003rlp.1) at chr6_cox_hap1:3416090-3421542 - tenascin XB isoform 2
TNXB (uc003rlo.1) at chr6_cox_hap1:3416090-3421063 - tenascin XB isoform 2
TNXB (uc003nrl.2) at chr6:32116911-32185129 - tenascin XB isoform 1 precursor
TNXB (uc003nzh.1) at chr6:32116911-32122362 - tenascin XB isoform 2
TNXB (uc003nzg.1) at chr6:32116911-32121883 - tenascin XB isoform 2
TNR (uc009wvu.1) at chr1:173558558-173979375 - tenascin R
TNR (uc001gxp.1) at chr1:173858868-173642554 - tenascin R
```

From list of matches, click on appropriate gene name

RefSeq Genes

```
TNXB at chr6:32116911-32121883 - (NM_032470) tenascin XB isoform 2
TNXB at chr6_qbl_hap2:3223933-3228906 - (NM_032470) tenascin XB isoform 2
TNXB at chr6_cox_hap1:3416090-3421063 - (NM_032470) tenascin XB isoform 2
TNXB at chr6:32116911-32185129 - (NM_019105) tenascin XB isoform 1 precursor
TNXB at chr6_qbl_hap2:3223933-3268868 - (NM_019105) tenascin XB isoform 1 precursor
TNXB at chr6_cox_hap1:3416090-3484320 - (NM_019105) tenascin XB isoform 1 precursor
```

Non-Human RefSeq Genes

```
Tnxb at chr6_cox_hap1:3421258-3472057 - (NM_031176) tenascin XB
Tnxb at chr6_cox_hap1:3423308-3472240 - (NM_031176) tenascin XB
Tnxb at chr6_cox_hap1:3419942-3472243 - (NM_031176) tenascin XB
Tnxb at chr6_qbl_hap2:3229101-3267422 - (NM_031176) tenascin XB
Tnxb at chr6:32084369-32173926 - (NM_031176) tenascin XB
Tnxb at chr6_cox_hap1:3416284-3473117 - (NM_031176) tenascin XB
Tnxb at chr6:32117105-32173052 - (NM_031176) tenascin XB
Tnxb at chr6_qbl_hap2:3224127-3268867 - (NM_031176) tenascin XB
TNXB at chr6:32087908-32173052 - (NM_174703) tenascin XB
TNXB at chr6_qbl_hap2:3230528-3253155 - (NM_174703) tenascin XB
TNXB at chr6_qbl_hap2:3227941-3264373 - (NM_174703) tenascin XB
TNXB at chr6_cox_hap1:3421108-3472057 - (NM_174703) tenascin XB
TNXB at chr6:32123487-32172680 - (NM_174703) tenascin XB
TNXB at chr6:32117015-32173964 - (NM_174703) tenascin XB
TNXB at chr6:32125874-32173010 - (NM_174703) tenascin XB
TNXB at chr6_cox_hap1:3422622-3472201 - (NM_174703) tenascin XB
TNXB at chr6_cox_hap1:3423296-3472243 - (NM_174703) tenascin XB
TNXB at chr6_qbl_hap2:3224037-3268874 - (NM_174703) tenascin XB
TNXB at chr6_qbl_hap2:3232897-3267418 - (NM_174703) tenascin XB
TNXB at chr6_qbl_hap2:3232046-3267432 - (NM_174703) tenascin XB
TNXB at chr6_cox_hap1:3420048-3472150 - (NM_174703) tenascin XB
TNXB at chr6_qbl_hap2:3227559-3267421 - (NM_174703) tenascin XB
TNXB at chr6_cox_hap1:3430787-3471406 - (NM_174703) tenascin XB
TNXB at chr6_cox_hap1:3425054-3472243 - (NM_174703) tenascin XB
TNXB at chr6:32084279-32172866 - (NM_174703) tenascin XB
TNXB at chr6_cox_hap1:3427606-3472240 - (NM_174703) tenascin XB
TNXB at chr6_qbl_hap2:3228951-3265044 - (NM_174703) tenascin XB
TNXB at chr6_cox_hap1:3422863-3471778 - (NM_174703) tenascin XB
TNXB at chr6_cox_hap1:3416194-3473155 - (NM_174703) tenascin XB
TNXB at chr6_cox_hap1:3419942-3471871 - (NM_174703) tenascin XB
TNXB at chr6_qbl_hap2:3231236-3267418 - (NM_174703) tenascin XB
```

ENCODE Gencode Manual Gene Annotations (level 1+2) (Feb 2009) (wgEncodeGencodeManualRel2)

Fig. 19.37 Selection of gene from the list of search results in UCSC. Source: http://genome.ucsc.edu (Kent et al., 2002 in Further Reading).

description of the substitution using the single-letter code as well as a specific database protein identifier. It should be noted that if a sequence is to be inserted in, for instance, the PolyPhen website in FASTA format, then the sequence must not contain spaces and must be preceded by a header line that takes the form of '>sequencename', i.e. it must begin with a 'greater than' symbol. An alternative website, Align GVGD, is currently rather more difficult to use because of its requirement for a cross-species multiple sequence alignment to be created beforehand by the user. It is undergoing further development at present and is likely to become easier to use.

Unfortunately, it is not uncommon for these three websites to yield conflicting results for the same amino acid substitution in a specific protein. In practice, therefore, a thorough search of mutation databases and published reports must be undertaken to find any previous evidence of other families with that specific mutation or of any biological studies that have been carried out to verify the mutation's pathogenicity.

A database that is fascinating to browse is the RCSB Protein Data Bank website, which contains the atomic coordinates of many protein domains. This website allows the user to search for (Fig. 19.42) and view (Figs 19.43 and 19.44) impressive 3D representations of many protein regions and thus potentially identify the precise locations within the protein structure of specific amino acids of interest within the protein. However, the data, which have been obtained by structural biologists largely using X-ray crystallography and nuclear magnetic resonance spectroscopy, often do not cover entire protein molecules.

CASE VI

A child has been found to have mild developmental delay, unusually broad great toes and a head circumference that is more than two standard deviations below the mean. The karyotype has been found to be normal.

How could you use a computer database to identify a possible underlying syndrome diagnosis?

Answers are given in the following paragraphs.

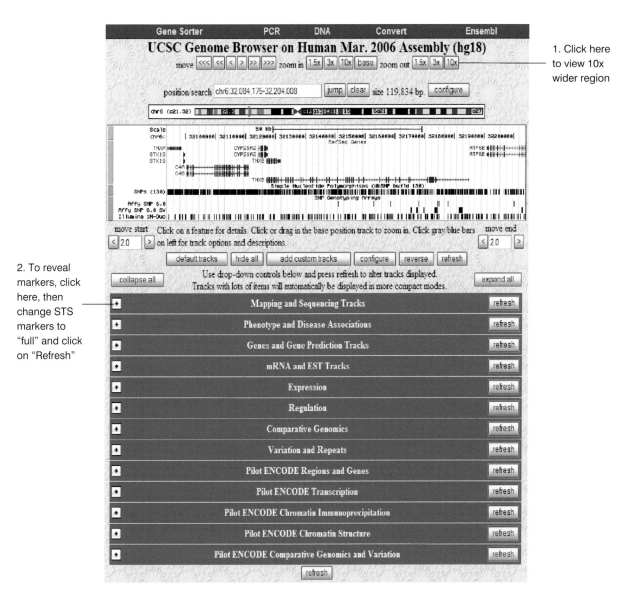

1. Click here to view 10x wider region

2. To reveal markers, click here, then change STS markers to "full" and click on "Refresh"

Fig. 19.38 UCSC Genome Browser window opened by clicking on 'Other genome browser: UCSC' (from menu at left of Ensembl's 'Region in detail' screen). It can also be reached by searching using the UCSC Genome Browser 'Gateway' and zooming out as shown. Source: http://genome.ucsc.edu (Kent et al., 2002 in Further Reading).

Computer-aided syndrome diagnosis

In this case, the use of commercial software is valuable, although it is not the only solution(see Table 19.9). If the Winter–Baraitser Dysmorphogy Database is available, then the 'Syndrome Feature Search' function can be used to search the database for possible underlying syndromes (Figs 19.45 and 19.46). Here, the search terms 'Broad hallux', 'Microcephaly' and 'Developmental delay' can be used to search for syndromes, as shown in Fig. 19.47. Search terms may be obtained from the expandable list on the right of the 'Search Syndrome on Features' display (Fig. 19.46) or can be obtained by directly searching for the term after clicking on the 'Find' button (Fig. 19.46). The list of possible syndromes that results is shown in Fig. 19.48. For each syndrome, clinical details, feature list and clinical photos can then be displayed.

Alternatively, if such a proprietary software package is not available for use, then the OMIM online database (described above; see Table 19.1) can often be used. or the new freely available Phenomizer database can be tried (see below). The same search terms can be typed into the box in the OMIM search page as shown in Fig. 19.49. The results are shown in Fig. 19.50. Selecting an individual syndrome (in the example shown, it is Rubinstein–Taybi syndrome) will result in the display of a detailed description (Fig. 19.51). In addition, a link (visible in blue at the top right corner of the page) is provided to the GeneTests database, which, as mentioned above, contains very clear reviews, with the relevant web pages shown in Figs 19.52 and 19.53.

The Phenomizer database (see Figs 19.54–19.56 and Köhler et al., 2009, in Further reading) allows the user to select clinical phenotypic features by searching for them directly or

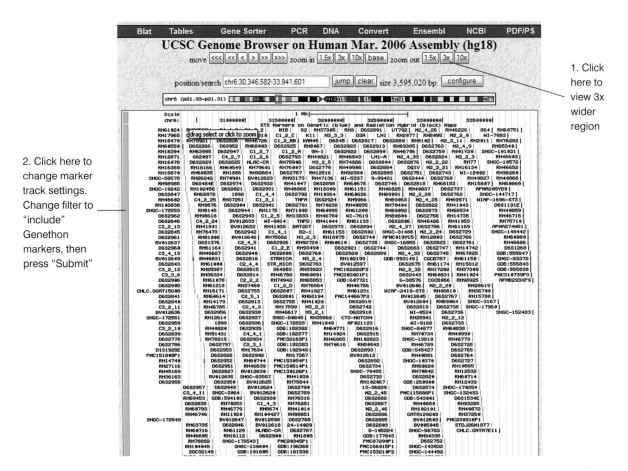

Fig. 19.39 UCSC Genome Browser window after clicking on 'zoom out ×10' to widen the genomic region viewed on screen. Source: http://genome.ucsc.edu (Kent et al., 2002 in Further Reading).

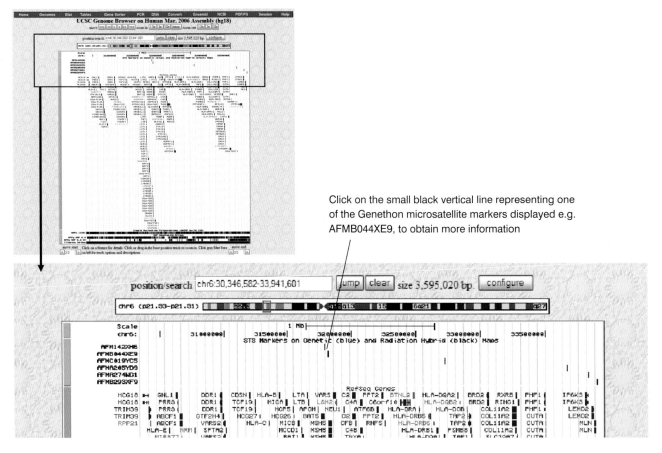

Fig. 19.40 UCSC Genome Browser window after choosing 'include' Genethon markers from the drop-down list and then clicking on 'submit'. Source: http://genome.ucsc.edu (Kent et al., 2002 in Further Reading).

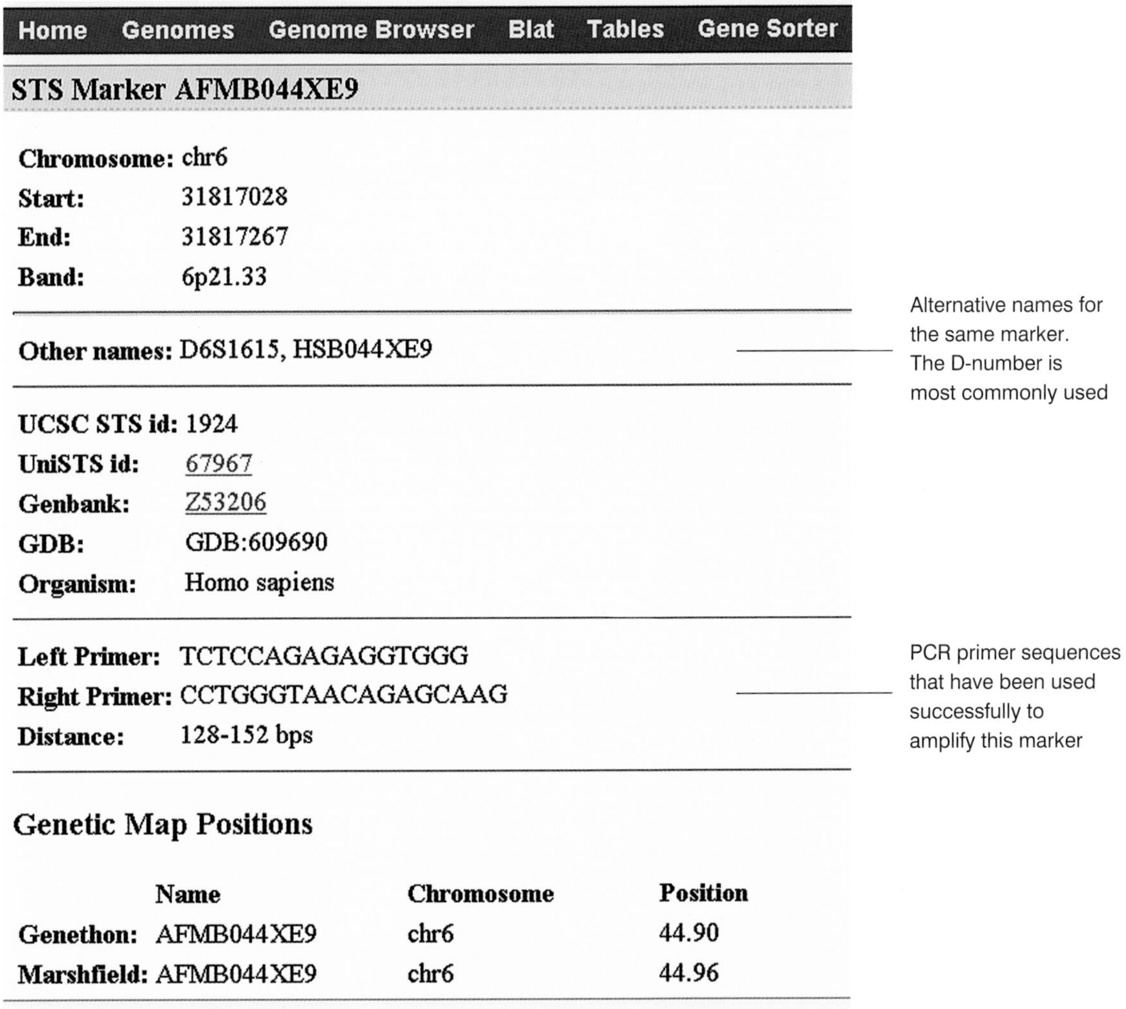

Home	Genomes	Genome Browser	Blat	Tables	Gene Sorter

STS Marker AFMB044XE9

Chromosome: chr6
Start: 31817028
End: 31817267
Band: 6p21.33

Other names: D6S1615, HSB044XE9 ———————— Alternative names for the same marker. The D-number is most commonly used

---

UCSC STS id: 1924
UniSTS id: 67967
Genbank: Z53206
GDB: GDB:609690
Organism: Homo sapiens

Left Primer: TCTCCAGAGAGGTGGG
Right Primer: CCTGGGTAACAGAGCAAG ———————— PCR primer sequences that have been used successfully to amplify this marker
Distance: 128-152 bps

Genetic Map Positions

	Name	Chromosome	Position
Genethon:	AFMB044XE9	chr6	44.90
Marshfield:	AFMB044XE9	chr6	44.96

Fig. 19.41 STS marker details in UCSC database, obtained after clicking on the small black vertical line (in the upper part of the window) representing, for example, STS Marker AFMB044XE9. Source: http://genome.ucsc.edu (Kent et al., 2002 in Further Reading).

Table 19.8 Websites providing analysis of possible functional significance of missense (amino acid substitution) mutations

PolyPhen (prediction of functional effect of human nsSNPs)	http://genetics.bwh.harvard.edu/pph/
SIFT BLink	http://sift.jcvi.org/www/SIFT_BLink_submit.html
Align GVGD	http://agvgd.iarc.fr/agvgd_input.php
RCSB Protein Data Bank	http://www.pdb.org/
Human splice site prediction tool (Berkeley Drosophila Genome Project)	http://www.fruitfly.org/seq_tools/splice.html
ESE Finder (to predict effects of mutations on any potential exonic splice enhancer sequences, necessary for splicing factor binding)	http://rulai.cshl.edu/cgi-bin/tools/ESE3/esefinder.cgi?process=home

from a hierarchical list. These features can, as in the Winter–Baraitser Dysmorphogy Database, be used in combination to search a syndrome database. The relationships between phenotypic features and clinical syndromes in this case are generated by computer, using automatic OMIM database analysis, rather than by experts in clinical dysmorphology. In addition, at present, there are no expert-curated syndrome summaries or carefully selected clinical photographs in the Phenomizer. For these reasons, therefore, the list of results obtained using the Phenomizer can in some cases be a little difficult to evaluate in practice. It may, nevertheless, prove to be a very useful additional diagnostic tool. Another free similar online

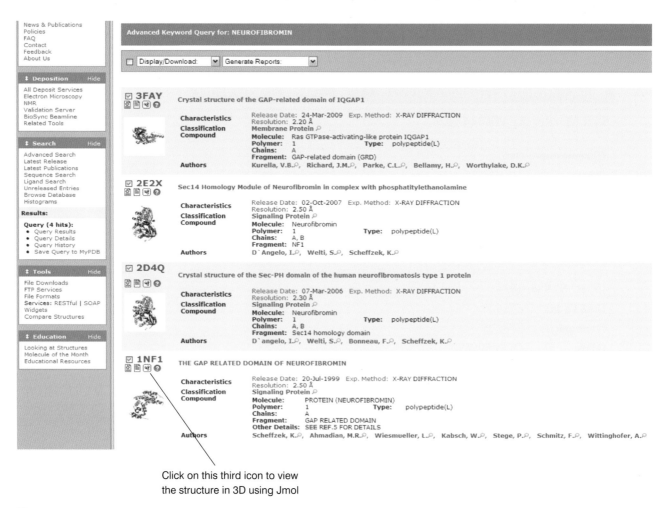

Click on this third icon to view
the structure in 3D using Jmol

Fig. 19.42 List of matching results after typing 'neurofibromin' into the search box at the top right of the PDB home page. Source: RCSB PDB (www.pdb.org); Scheffzek et al., 1998 in Further Reading.

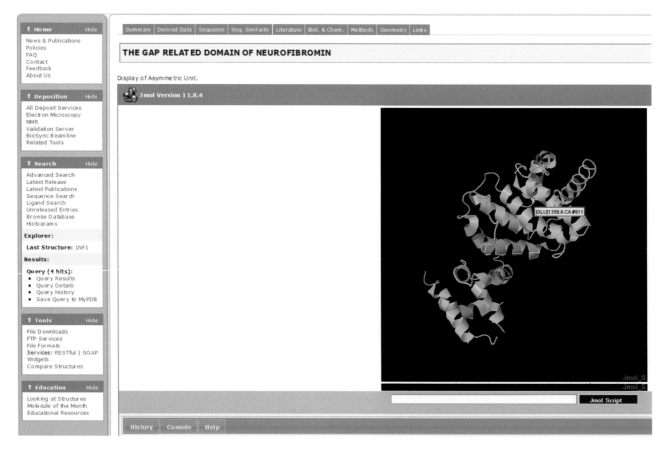

Fig. 19.43 The GAP-related domain of neurofibromin, viewed in 3D (and can be enlarged, rotated and annotated by right-clicking and selecting various options). Source: RCSB PDB (www.pdb.org). Scheffzek et al., 1998 in Further Reading.

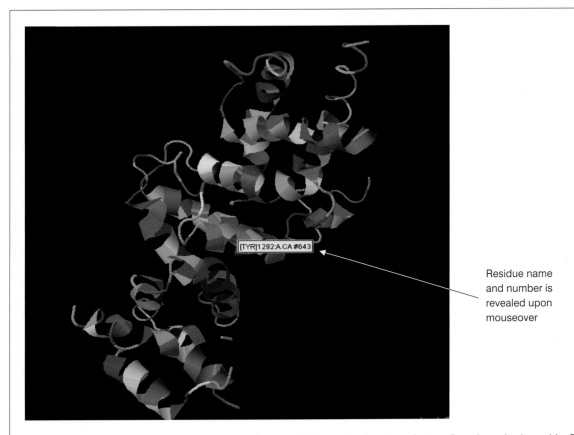

Residue name and number is revealed upon mouseover

Fig. 19.44 Coloured view obtained by selecting via right-clicking: colour/structures/cartoon/by-scheme/amino-acids. Source: RCSB PDB (www.pdb.org). Scheffzek et al., 1998 in Further Reading.

Table 19.9 Websites for computer-aided syndrome diagnosis	
OMIM (Online Mendelian Inheritance in Man)	http://www.ncbi.nlm.nih.gov/omim/
Phenomizer	http://compbio.charite.de/Phenomizer/Phenomizer.html
Winter–Baraitser Dysmorphogy Database (proprietary)	http://www.lmdatabases.com/
POSSUM Database (proprietary)	http://www.possum.net.au/
Orphanet: Search by clinical sign	http://www.orpha.net/

syndrome search is provided on the Orphanet website, although it currently appears to be unable to handle searches that generate a list of many possible syndromes.

CASE VII

You wish to find out more about genetics-related professional societies and governing bodies, as well as further details regarding the Human Genome Project and ethical issues.

Which are the useful websites from which to start looking for such information?

Answers are given in the following paragraphs.

Professional genetics societies

Table 19.10 lists the websites of several genetics societies, which may be interesting and useful from both a clinical and a research point of view. These provide information and links, for example to relevant ethical and governing bodies, that may not easily be found elsewhere.

The Human Genome Project: ethics and education

Table 19.11 gives details of websites that provide information about the Human Genome Project itself, such as the methods used, the data generated, the analyses, the benefits of the project to society and the ethical issues. Web-based sources of information for genetics-related education at a variety of levels are also included in the table.

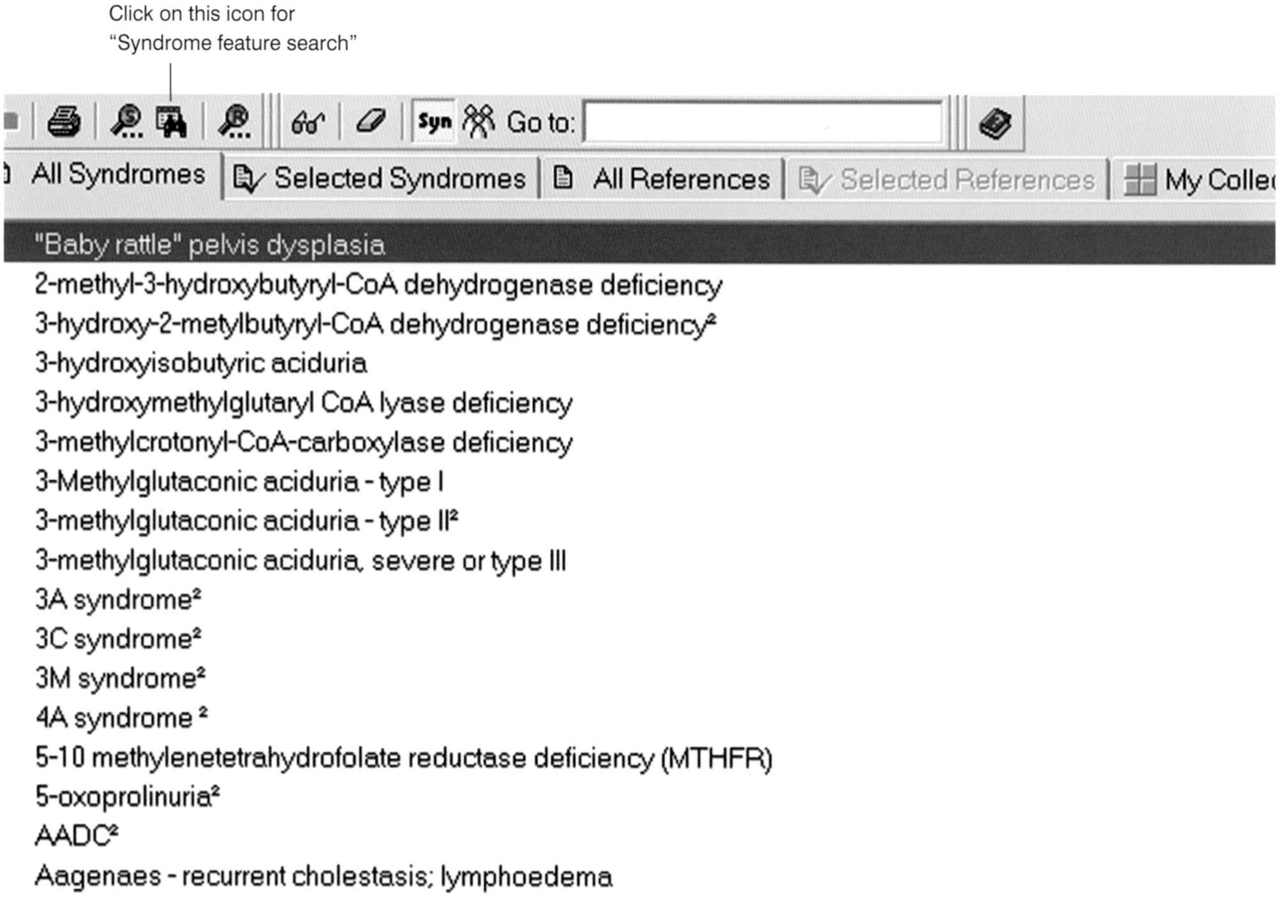

Click on this icon for
"Syndrome feature search"
Syn
Go to:
All Syndromes
Selected Syndromes
All References
Selected References
My Colle
"Baby rattle" pelvis dysplasia
2-methyl-3-hydroxybutyryl-CoA dehydrogenase deficiency
3-hydroxy-2-metylbutyryl-CoA dehydrogenase deficiency²
3-hydroxyisobutyric aciduria
3-hydroxymethylglutaryl CoA lyase deficiency
3-methylcrotonyl-CoA-carboxylase deficiency
3-Methylglutaconic aciduria - type I
3-methylglutaconic aciduria - type II²
3-methylglutaconic aciduria, severe or type III
3A syndrome²
3C syndrome²
3M syndrome²
4A syndrome ²
5-10 methylenetetrahydrofolate reductase deficiency (MTHFR)
5-oxoprolinuria²
AADC²
Aagenaes - recurrent cholestasis; lymphoedema

Fig. 19.45 Winter–Baraitser Dysmorphogy Database (London Medical Databases) software package. With permission from London Medical Databases.

Search Syndromes on Features
Criterion 1
Mandatory
Not
Criterion 2
Mandatory
Criterion 3
Mandatory
Criterion 4
Mandatory
ABDOMEN
PELVIS
GENITALIA
URINARY SYSTEM
UPPER LIMBS
HANDS
NAILS
LOWER LIMBS
FEET
Feet, general abnormalities
Hallux, general abnormalities
Absent or hypoplastic hallux
Broad hallux
Dorsi-flexed hallux
Long hallux
Polydactyly/bifid hallux
Short hallux
Hallux valgus
Hallux varus
Metatarsals, general abnormalities
Tarsals, general abnormalities
Toes, general abnormalities
Clear Criterion
Clear Feature
Add
Find
Details
Collapse Tree
Search
Close
Clear Search
Load
Save
Help
Find each clinical feature from this expandable list, then click and drag the feature to one of the "Criterion" boxes on the left
Alternatively, click on this "Find" button to access the direct feature "Search string" facility

Fig. 19.46 Finding clinical features within the 'Search Syndromes on Features' search window. With permission from London Medical Databases.

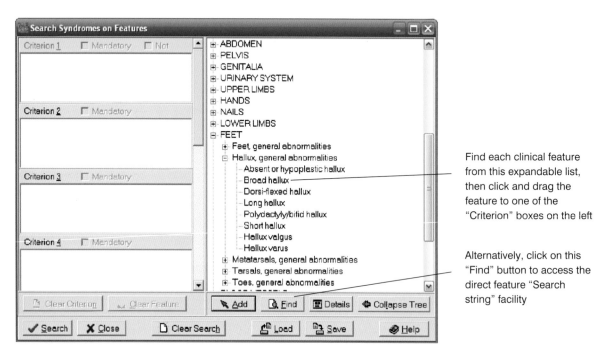

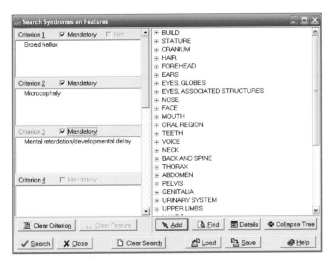

Fig. 19.47 Search window 'Search Syndromes on Features' within the Winter–Baraitser Dysmorphogy Database software package. With permission from London Medical Databases.

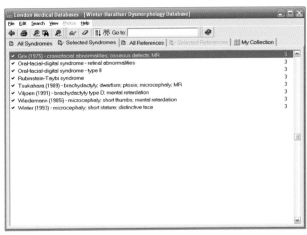

Fig. 19.48 Search results within the Winter–Baraitser Dysmorphogy Database software package. With permission from London Medical Databases.

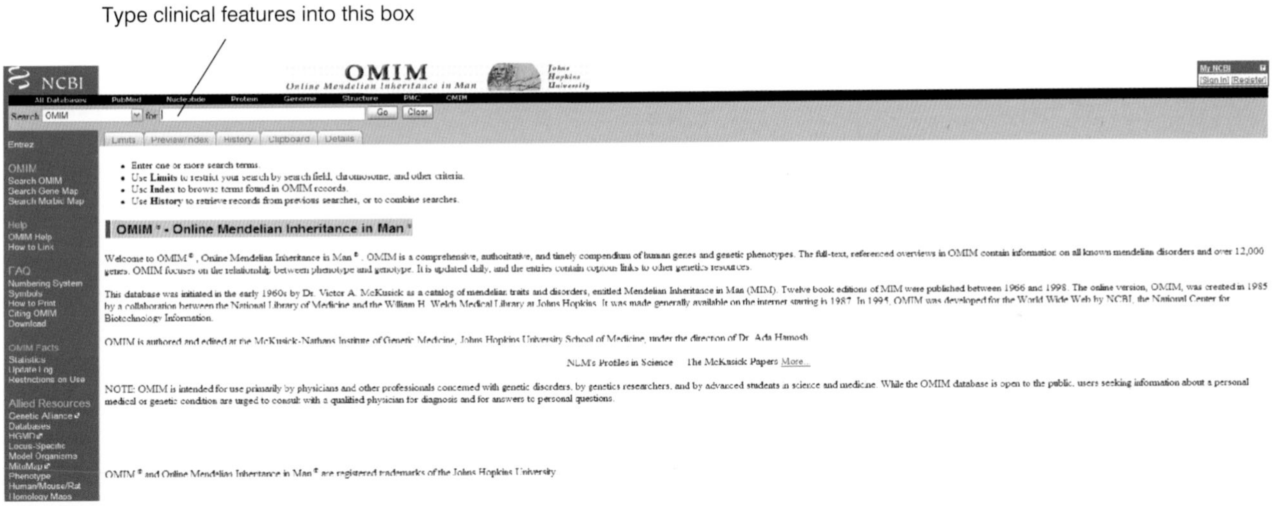

Type clinical features into this box

Fig. 19.49 OMIM home page.

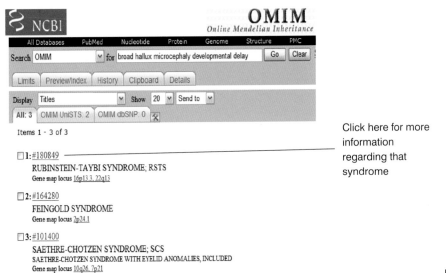

Click here for more information regarding that syndrome

Fig. 19.50 Search results using OMIM.

Click here to link to GeneTests in order to access a more readable review

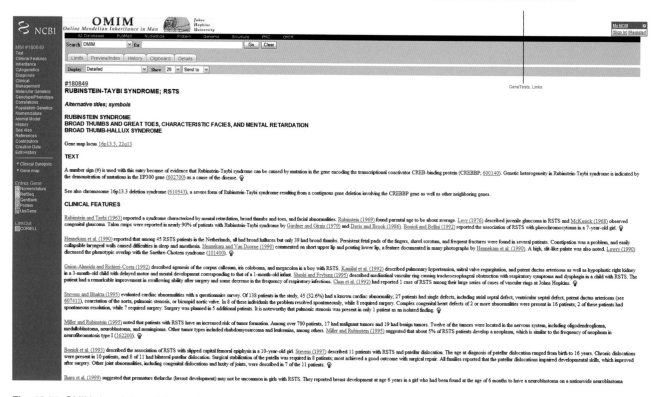

Fig. 19.51 OMIM description of the syndrome.

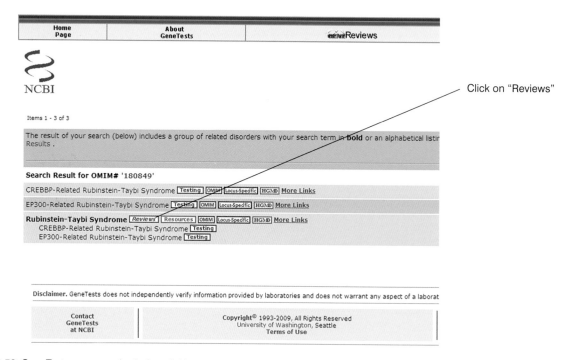

Click on "Reviews"

Fig. 19.52 GeneTests page reached after clicking on the blue 'Genetests' link at the top right of the page.

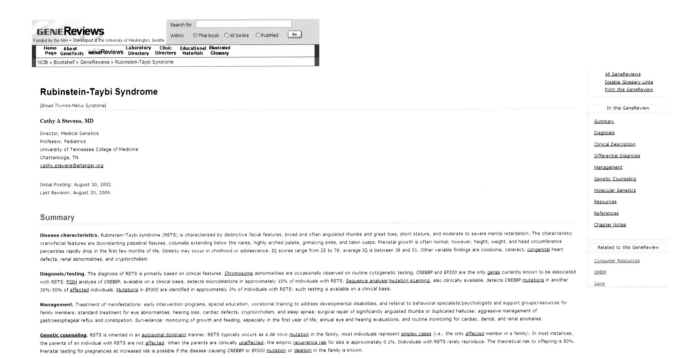

Fig. 19.53 GeneReview for genetic condition.

Enter observed clinical feature here,
then click on "search"

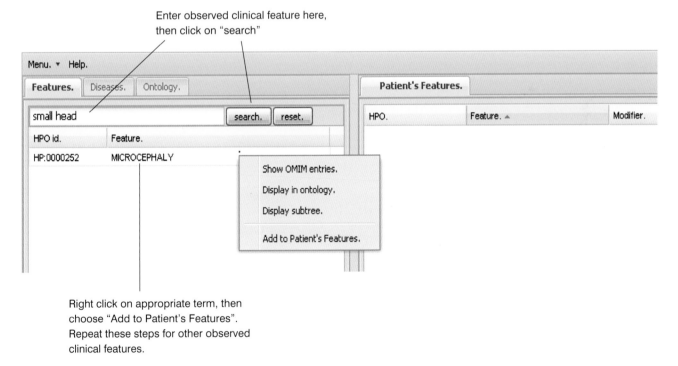

Right click on appropriate term, then
choose "Add to Patient's Features".
Repeat these steps for other observed
clinical features.

Fig. 19.54 Phenomizer online search. Selecting clinical features to add to the 'Patient's Features' list. Reproduced with kind permission of Sebastian Köhler from the Phenomizer website. See Köhler *et al.*, 2009, in Further reading.

Add other clinical features

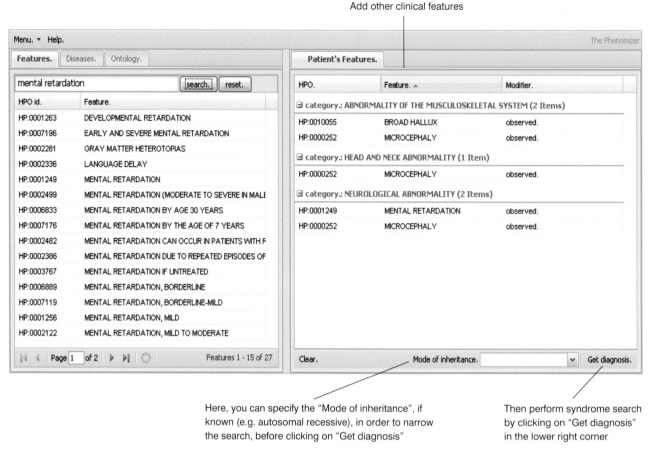

Here, you can specify the "Mode of inheritance", if known (e.g. autosomal recessive), in order to narrow the search, before clicking on "Get diagnosis"

Then perform syndrome search by clicking on "Get diagnosis" in the lower right corner

Fig. 19.55 Phenomizer online search page after adding specific clinical features to the Patient's Features list. Reproduced with kind permission of Sebastian Köhler from the Phenomizer website. See Köhler *et al.*, 2009, in Further reading.

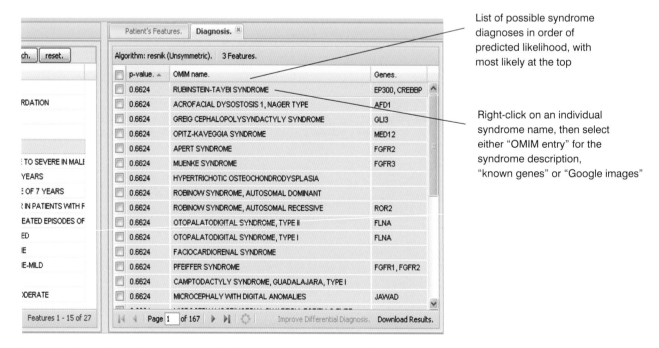

List of possible syndrome diagnoses in order of predicted likelihood, with most likely at the top

Right-click on an individual syndrome name, then select either "OMIM entry" for the syndrome description, "known genes" or "Google images"

Fig. 19.56 Phenomizer online search. Results list obtained after clicking on 'Get diagnosis'. Reproduced with kind permission of Sebastian Köhler from the Phenomizer website. See Köhler *et al.*, 2009, in Further reading.

Table 19.10 Genetics societies

British Society for Human Genetics	http://www.bshg.org.uk/
European Society of Human Genetics	http://www.eshg.org/
The American Society of Human Genetics	http://www.ashg.org/
The American College of Medical Genetics	http://www.acmg.net//AM/Template.cfm?Section=Home3
Human Genetics Society of Australasia	http://www.hgsa.com.au/
International Federation of Human Genetics Societies	http://www.ifhgs.org/

Table 19.11 Human Genome Project: ethics and education

US Human Genome Project Information (US Department of Energy & NIH)	http://www.ornl.gov/sci/techresources/Human_Genome/home.shtml
US National Human Genome Research Institute (of the NIH)	http://www.genome.gov/
Wellcome Trust Sanger Institute	http://www.sanger.ac.uk/ Cambridge/Sanger
The Human Genome Organisation	http://www.hugo-international.org/
The Geee! in Genome (developed by the Canadian Museum of Nature)	http://nature.ca/genome/index_e.cfm
ScotGEN (Scottish Genetics Education Network)	http://www.scotgen.org.uk/
Department of Medical Genetics, University of Glasgow	http://www.gla.ac.uk/departments/medgenetics/
Cambridge Resource Centre for Comparative Genomics	http://www.chromhome.org
Medical Genetics MSc Course at Glasgow University	http://www.gla.ac.uk/departments/medgenetics/mscinmedicalgenetics/

FURTHER READING

Flicek P, Aken BL, Ballester B, Beal K, Bragin E, Brent S, Chen Y, Clapham P, Coates G, *et al.* (2010) Ensembl's 10th year. *Nucleic Acids Res* **38** (Database issue):D557–62.

Kent WJ, Sugnet CW, Furey TS, Roskin KM, Pringle TH, Zahler AM, and Haussler D (2002) The human genome browser at UCSC. *Genome Res.* **12**(6):996–1006.

Köhler S, Schulz MH, Krawitz P, Bauer S, Dölken S, Ott CE, Mundlos C, Horn D, Mundlos S, Robinson PN (2009) Clinical diagnostics in human genetics with semantic similarity searches in ontologies. *Am J Hum Genet* **85**:457–64.

Scheffzek K, Ahmadian MR, Wiesmueller L, Kabsch W, Stege P, Schmitz F, and Wittinghofer A (1998) Structural analysis of the GAP-related domain from neurofibromin and its implications. *EMBO J.* **17**:4313–4327.

 Visit **www.wiley.com/go/tobias** for more resources on genetic databases.

Self-assessment

Using the appropriate internet databases described in this chapter, try to answer the following questions.

1. For the gene named CCNE1, which of the following ranges contains the correct number of its constituent exons?
A. 1–4
B. 5–9
C. 10–14
D. 15–19
E. 20–24

2. For the gene named FOXC1, which of the following describes the most likely function of the protein that it encodes?
A. Secreted hormone
B. Ion channel
C. Tyrosine kinase
D. Transcription factor
E. Nuclear membrane component

3. The number of RefSeq (i.e. reference) genes fully or partly contained within the chromosomal region at 7p15.1 is which of the following?
A. 1–5
B. 6–10
C. 11–15
D. 16–20
E. 21–25

4. For the RefSeq gene named CALCRL, find the alternative names, the PCR primer sequences and the predicted range of PCR product sizes for the (Genethon) intragenic $(CA)_n$ repeat microsatellite marker that is given in the appropriate section of the UCSC database.

5. According to the CEPH Genome Database Browser, the proportion of individuals who are heterozygous is highest for which of these neighbouring markers: AFM292WD1, AFMB297XC1 or AFMA057VG9?

Self-assessment – answers

Chapter 1

1. Answer: C. Introns are not present in the mitochondrial chromosome, which, in fact, contains very little non-coding DNA (see section entitled 'Mitochondrial disorders').

2. Answer: B. Only one of the cells of the embryo is removed and tested, at around the five- to ten-cell stage.

3. Answer: C. McCune–Albright syndrome is typically regarded as occurring as a result of a mutation in a single gene, *GNAS1*, although the condition is mosaic with the mutation occurring after fertilisation (i.e. the mutation is post-zygotic).

4. Answer: E. Enzyme replacement therapy is currently possible for Gaucher's disease and Fabry's disease. For FAP, bowel screening is appropriate, usually followed by bowel surgery for affected individuals.

5. Answer: D. Sir Alec Jeffreys is the individual associated with the development of the DNA fingerprinting technique (in 1984–1986). The first identification of a chromosomal abnormality, trisomy 21, was by Lejeune and colleagues, in 1959.

Chapter 2

1. Answer: False. The human genome contains approximately 3.2 thousand million (3.2×10^9) base pairs.

2. Answer: True.

3. Answer: False. Only approximately 1.1% of the human genome actually codes for proteins.

4. Answer: True. Several RNA gene classes have now been defined, including so-called microRNAs (miRNAs). These short single-stranded RNA molecules can regulate the expression of other genes by binding to their mRNAs.

5. Answer: False. The human genome was sequenced using a non-radioactive method in which the nucleotides within the DNA molecules that are analysed are labelled with four different fluorescent dyes, corresponding to the four different bases (A, C, G and T).

6. Answer: False. The number of genes per autosome varies enormously and generally progressively decreases from the largest, chromosome 1, to the smallest, chromosomes 21 and 22.

7. Answer: C. Several types of RNA molecules are present in the cytoplasm, including ribosomal RNA (rRNA), transfer RNA (tRNA), small cytoplasmic RNA (scRNA) and microRNA (miRNA).

Chapter 3

1. Answer: False. The pyrimidine bases are cytosine and thymine whilst adenine and guanine are the purine bases.

2. Answer: True.

3. Answer: False. C pairs with G and A pairs with T (in DNA) or with U (in RNA).

4. Answer: True.

5. Answer: E. The spliceosome, which contains RNA molecules and proteins, functions in splicing of the primary transcript, i.e. after transcription has been carried out.

6. Answer: E. *MutYH*-associated polyposis is caused by a type of base excision repair defect, while xeroderma pigmentosum is due to defective nucleotide excision repair. Hereditary colon cancer can be caused by a mismatch repair defect and Huntington disease is associated with an abnormally increased number of CAG trinucleotide repeats within the Huntington disease coding sequence.

7. Answer: D. A single-nucleotide substitution of this type well within an exon may cause an amino acid substitution but would not usually affect the amount or length of the encoded protein. A T to C substitution will not generate a translation termination (stop) codon or cause a frameshift. The insertion or deletion of a number of bases that is not a multiple of three will result in a frameshift. A frameshift close to the start of the protein will be likely to result in a premature translational termination codon and thus truncation of the protein. Methylation of the cytosines in the promoter often results in transcriptional silencing.

8. Answer: B. Polyadenylation occurs at the 3′ end of a primary transcript, after transcription but prior to translation.

Chapter 4

1. Answer: A, C, D. A thermostable DNA (not RNA) polymerase is required. The time taken to perform PCR is generally 2–3 hours (rather than days).

2. Answer: A, C, D. They would not be useful for the detection of very large duplications or deletions as it is difficult to amplify regions of over 10 kb using PCR. Standard cytogenetic analysis would be the current method of choice for detecting a centric fusion translocation.

3. Answer: A, B, E. TP-PCR is used to detect large triplet repeat expansions in myotonic dystrophy and Friedreich's ataxia. MLPA is used to detect deletions or duplications that are generally much larger than could easily be detected by DNA sequencing. Neither technique would be followed by DNA sequencing.

4. Answer: A, B, E. The existence of different causative genes (locus heterogeneity) or the presence of a pseudogene makes indirect mutant gene tracking more difficult as the wrong locus may be tracked inadvertently.

5. Answer: A, C, D, E. A DNA-binding filter or membrane is necessary instead for Southern blotting, to immobilise the (electrophoretically separated) DNA fragments, which can then be incubated with a specific probe to permit hybridisation and subsequent detection.

6. Answer: Suspect 1.

7. Answer: F2 is the father.

Chapter 5
1. Answer: A, C, E. Acetylation of various amino acids in histone tails is associated with an increased level of gene transcription. Those chromosomal regions that have reduced levels of gene transcription tend to replicate late rather than early in S phase.

2. Answer: B.

3. Answer: A, B, C, D, E.

4. Answer: B, D, E. The mitochondrial chromosomes are double-stranded but, unlike chromosomes in the nucleus, they are circular rather than linear. There are no introns in mitochondrial chromosomes.

Chapter 6
1. Answer: A, E. In meiosis, DNA replication only occurs once, before the first meiotic cell division. Meiosis results in chromosomes that do consist of a pair of chromatids but the latter are not identical, on account of crossing over, thus increasing genetic variation. Pairing occurs between homologous chromosomes during zygotene. The X and Y chromosomes, however, pair with each other only at the distal ends of their short arms at the so-called pseudoautosomal regions.

2. Answer: A, B, C, D, E.

3. Answer: E. Following the birth of a child with Turner syndrome, there does not appear to be a significantly increased chance of the next pregnancy being affected by Turner syndrome.

4. Answer: A, B, E. The *SRY* gene, the master-switch TDF in humans, is believed to encode a transcription factor that causes activation of genes such as *SOX9*. The *SOX9* gene is active in male sex determination but it is located on an autosome (chromosome 17) rather than the Y chromosome.

5. Answer: A, B, D. *XIST* regulates X chromosome inactivation but not autosomal genomic imprinting. Prader–Willi syndrome may result from maternal (not paternal) uniparental disomy, as the copies of the Prader–Willi syndrome genes at 15q11–13 that are normally active are paternal rather than maternal.

Chapter 7
1. Answer: B, C, E. Generally, light microscopes can detect deletions of at least 4–5 Mb in size. Polyploidy is the situation in which the total number of chromosomes is an exact multiple of the haploid number and also exceeds the diploid number.

2. Answer: A, B, C, D. The distribution of chromosomal breaks is not random.

3. Answer: B. Carriers of a balanced translocation are usually clinically normal. Translocations can affect the X chromosome, resulting in X-autosome translocations. For some translocations, viable offspring can result from a three-to-one separation of the quadrivalents.

4. Answer: A, E. The breaks that result in Robertsonian translocations most often occur just above the centromere such that one of the products is a single chromosome with two centromeres (dicentric). Carriers of Robertsonian translocations typically have a total of 45 not 46 chromosomes, as two of the acrocentric chromosomes will have become fused into one chromosome. During gametogenesis, in carriers of Robertsonian translocations, a trivalent forms at meiosis.

5. Answer: A, C, D. DNA sequencing is not a reliable method to detect chromosomal submicroscopic deletions (microdeletions), as normal sequence may be obtained from the normal chromosome. Duplications are actually more common than deletions, although deletions tend to be more harmful.

6. Answer: A, C, E. Uniparental disomy results in a total of 46, not 47, chromosomes. Uniparental isodisomy refers to the situation where both chromosomal homologues originated in the same grandparent and can thus result in an autosomal recessive condition even when just one parent is a carrier.

7. Answer: This QF-PCR result shows either trisomic diallelic (two peaks with a 2 : 1 size ratio) or triallelic patterns for the microsatellite markers on all three chromosomes tested, i.e. 13, 18 and 21. This pregnancy is most likely to be affected by triploidy.

Chapter 8

1. Answer: A, B. Metabolic enzyme defects and parental consanguinity are common in autosomal recessive but not autosomal dominant conditions. An increased paternal (not maternal) age is associated with an increased frequency of new mutations.

2. Answer: B. This, of course, is also true for each of their children.

3. Answer: D.

4. Answer: C.

5. Answer: A.

6. Answer: D.

7. Answer: B.

8. Answer: A, E. Females are usually unaffected but may be mildly affected. Males pass on their Y chromosome but not their X chromosome to their sons, so male-to-male transmission of an X-linked condition is not observed.

9. Answer: A, B, C, D, E.

10. Answer: A, B, E. X-linked ichthyosis, as well as both haemophilia A and B, are X-linked recessively inherited.

Chapter 9

1. Answer: A, B, C, E. Although Friedreich ataxia is most commonly caused by a trinucleotide repeat expansion (in intron 1 of the *FXN* gene), the condition is autosomal recessive and genetic anticipation is thus not typically observed (as the condition usually occurs in just one generation of a family).

2. Answer: C. These conditions are all associated with genes located on the X chromosome. Of these conditions, however, only Léri–Weill dyschondrosteosis is known to

be caused by a gene located within the pseudo-autosomal regions (PARs) of the X chromosomes (the regions at the tips of the Xp and Xq arms within which recombination can occur with the Y chromosomes).

3. Answer: A, D, E. In pseudodominant inheritance, as in autosomal recessive inheritance, both alleles must be abnormal for the individual to be affected. The inheritance may, however, appear to be dominant on account of the high carrier frequency (and the consequence that the unrelated partner of an affected individual may be a carrier). Crigler–Najjar syndrome type 1 is inherited in an autosomal recessive fashion and is rare. It is caused by mutations in the same gene (*UGT1A1*) that is associated with Gilbert syndrome. In Gilbert syndrome, however, the genetic abnormality is much more frequent (particularly in the European North American population) and is located in the promoter of the gene. In Crigler–Najjar syndrome type 1, the mutations lie within the gene's coding region.

4. Answer: A, D, E. Vitamin D-resistant rickets (or X-linked hypophosphatemia) is an X-linked dominant condition but it does not usually exhibit male lethality. Haemophilia B (factor IX deficiency or Christmas disease) is an X-linked recessive (not dominant) condition.

5. Answer: C, D, E. On account of parent-specific imprinting, Prader–Willi syndrome and Angelman syndrome may result from *maternal* and *paternal* UPD of chromosome 15, respectively. Uniparental isodisomy of chromosome 7 is a recognised (although rare) cause of CF.

Chapter 10

1. Answer: D. Cystic fibrosis is regarded as a single-gene disorder as only one gene (*CFTR*) strongly determines whether or not an individual is affected by this condition. Blood pressure, weight and head circumference are multifactorial but are continuous traits.

2. Answer: A, B, E. Cleft lip and neural tube defects are discontinuous multifactorial traits.

3. Answer: B, D, E. Only around 75% of monozygous twins share a single chorion. Dizygotic twins result from the fertilisation of two ova by two spermatozoa.

4. Answer: A, E. Fatal infantile cardioencephalomyopathy is the result of mutations in the gene on (nuclear) chromosome 22 that is necessary for (mitochondrial) cytochrome *c* oxidase function. Progressive external ophthalmoplegia may be mitochondrially inherited or may be autosomal dominantly inherited due to an autosomal (chromosome 15) *POLG* mutation. In contrast,

LHON, MELAS and MERRF are mitochondrially inherited conditions.

5. Answer: D (i.e. 1/8 or 12.5%).

Chapter 11

1. Answer: A, B, C, E. An increase in the population size should not, by itself, affect the disorder's prevalence.

2. Answer: A, B, D, E. Individual SNPs are commonly located in blocks of linkage disequilibrium, resulting in several SNPs being closely associated with each other

3. Answer: A, C, D, E. Polymorphic markers could help determine which members of a family possess a mutation in a specific gene, but the detection of the mutation itself would require a technique such as DNA sequencing.

Chapter 12

1. Answer: D. The finding of apparent 46,XX/46,XY mosaicism on fetal karyotyping following amniocentesis almost always represents maternal cell contamination, with a male fetus.

2. Answer: D. This risk is commonly overestimated. It may, however, be significantly greater than 5%, of course, if there is a family history of a genetic condition or if there is previous consanguinity.

3. Answer: A, B, C, E. QF-PCR is not useful for the detection of a balanced chromosome translocation if the breakpoints have not previously been identified. This is because it is not possible to design specific oligonucleotide PCR primers without knowing the sequence of the flanking DNA.

4. Answer: E.

5. Answer: A, B, D. There is currently no useful DNA-based diagnostic test for renal agenesis or anencephaly.

Chapter 13

1. Answer: E. Proto-oncogenes are normal cellular genes that are involved, for instance, in growth factor response pathways and are expressed in many non-malignant tissues. Activating mutations in a single allele of such genes (resulting in so-called 'oncogenes') are often found in tumours. The *MLH1* gene is a tumour suppressor gene.

2. Answer: A, E. TSGs encode proteins that may, when functioning normally, promote apoptosis or inhibit mitosis. The *c-MYC* gene is a proto-oncogene.

3. Answer: B. The p53 protein is an intracellular transcription factor and is not a kinase.

4. Answer: C. The *NF1* gene is associated with neurofibromatosis type 1, the *APC* gene with familial adenomatous polyposis, the *RB1* gene with retinoblastoma and the *MUTYH* gene with autosomal recessive colorectal cancer (see Tables 13.1 and 13.2).

5. Answer: D. Her risk of inheriting the mutation is 50% (assuming that her mother possessed it; see below) and her risk of developing breast cancer, if she possesses the mutation, is around 80%. Her current risk is therefore: 50% (0.5) multiplied by 80% (0.8), i.e. 40% (0.4).

6. Answer: B, C. Familial breast cancer is more commonly caused by a *BRCA1* or *BRCA2* mutation than by *TP53* mutation. BRCA1 and BRCA2 proteins are involved in the homologous recombination form of DNA repair. Pancreatic cancer and malignant melanoma are tumours that are more commonly associated with inherited *BRCA2* mutations than with *BRCA1* mutations.

7. Answer: D. See Tables 13.1 and 13.2, and the Colorectal cancer section.

8. Answer: E. See Tables 13.1 and 13.2.

9. Answer: C. Regular colonoscopy rather than sigmoidoscopy is required. CHRPE is associated with FAP. Unlike FAP and AFAP (both autosomal dominant), MAP is autosomal recessively inherited. Microsatellite instability is a feature of a defect in mismatch repair.

Chapter 14

1. Answer: B. Male-to-male transmission excludes X-linked inheritance. Inheritance of the condition from a male makes mitochondrial inheritance very unlikely.

2. Answer: D. Type 1 and type 2 diabetes are not inherited in a Mendelian fashion. Donohue syndrome, which involves severe insulin resistance, is an autosomal recessively inherited condition. CADASIL is autosomal dominant but is a form of familial dementia rather than diabetes.

3. Answer: A, C, E. The risk to any future offspring of individuals III:1 and III:3 of being affected is 50% for each child. In the situation described in C (i.e. with a mitochondrial mutation as the underlying cause), the risk to the future offspring of II:1 would be low as such mutations are not transmitted from a male. Such mitochondrial mutations are, however, transmitted by a mother to all of her children, although the age of onset and severity of phenotype can vary significantly.

4. Answer: E. The likelihood that the condition is being inherited in an autosomal dominant fashion in this family is low, as the ages of the affected individuals would not be regarded as being typical of early-onset Alzheimer disease. For this reason, together with the fact that Billy is a second-degree relative of the affected individual, the risk of Billy developing the condition before the age of 65 is low. In the UK, *APOE* genotyping is not currently regarded as appropriate in the genetics clinic. The *APOE* ε4 allele-associated risks are complex and do not allow a precise risk to be calculated. Moreover, in late-onset dementia cases, susceptibility is most likely to be a combination of environmental and several known and unknown genetic factors.

5. **Answer: C, D, E.** Genetic susceptibility variants of small effect contribute to most cases of common adult-onset disorders. The risks are similar for siblings and offspring in most cases of common adult-onset disorders. The risk of repeat tract expansion is significantly greater during transmission from the father than from the mother. Presymptomatic testing is possible but requires careful genetic counselling according to established protocols.

6. **Answer: B.** The repeat lies within an exon and encodes a tract of glutamine amino acids.

Chapter 15

1. **Answer: B.** She is not affected by cystic fibrosis and therefore does not possess the mutant/mutant genotype. This leaves two carrier genotypes out of three possible genotypes (i.e. normal/normal, normal/mutant or mutant/normal) with a consequent carrier risk of 67%.

2. **Answer: C.** If Linda's partner's niece is affected, then his chance of being a carrier is 1/2. This is because, as his niece's parents will both be carriers, one of his own parents must also be a carrier. He will have had a 50% chance of having inherited the mutation from that parent. As Linda's partner's chance of being a carrier is 1/2, the chance of the couple both being carriers is 1/2 multiplied by 2/3, i.e. 2/6 or 1/3. Where a couple are both carriers, the chance of having an affected child is 1/4. Therefore, in this case, where the chance of the couple being carriers is only 1/3, the chance of having an affected child is 1/3 multiplied by 1/4, i.e. 1 in 12.

3. **Answer: D.** As the parents of the affected child are almost certainly carriers, one of the maternal grandparents (I:1 or I:2) must be a carrier. Therefore, the affected boy's maternal uncle (II:3) has a 50% chance of being a carrier and his daughter (III:5) will have a 25% chance of being a carrier (plus a much smaller chance of inheriting a mutation from her mother, II:4). Mutation analysis would, of course, be helpful in assessing the carrier risks with more precision.

4. **Answer: II:2 and therefore also 1:2.**

5. **Answer: B.** Helen's chance of being a carrier is 1 in 2 (since her mother is an obligate carrier). The chance of the child being male and affected is therefore ½ x ½ x ½ i.e. 1 in 8.

6. **Answer: A.** Lucille's chance of being a carrier is ¼ (since her maternal grandmother is an obligate carrier and Lucille's mother has a 1 in 2 chance of being a carrier). Therefore the chance of Lucille's child being male and affected is ¼ x ½ x ½ i.e. 1 in 16.

7. **Answer: C.** Phaeochromocytoma was reported in only 1% of 96 adult cases of NF1 studied by Huson et al. 1989 and around 2% of those cases reported by Ferner et al., 2007.

Chapter 16

1. **Answer: B, D, E.** Identification of the pathogenic gene alteration would normally be undertaken by PCR, by triplet repeat-primed PCR or by Southern blotting. Fetal DNA analysis permits prenatal diagnosis but prediction of the phenotypic severity in the future child is unreliable, although most congenitally affected infants have more than 1000 repeats when tested prenatally.

2. **Answer: C, D.** Even though she is phenotypically normal, there is a significant chance of her having an affected child. In this situation, it is likely that her mother possessed a premutation that expanded at meiosis. Carol herself is a carrier of a large premutation that is sufficiently large to be likely to expand to a full mutation if she were to pass it on to a child. If she were to have a son, there would be an approximately 50% chance of him being affected and a daughter would have a 50% chance of being a carrier (and a 25% chance of being affected, albeit generally more mildly than an affected male). Determination of the size of a full mutation in female carriers cannot predict the severity of the phenotype in those individuals, which is largely dependent upon the pattern of X chromosome inactivation established in the fetus.

3. **Answer: B.** As the condition is the result of a mitochondrial DNA mutation, it is maternally inherited. All the children of Arthur's mother (and of Arthur's sister) are therefore at risk of developing the condition, but those of Arthur's father's second marriage are not at risk. Although prenatal diagnosis is possible, it is difficult to predict the disease severity or age of onset, as the proportion of mitochondrial DNA molecules that contain the mutation in the amniocytes and chorionic villi will most likely differ from the proportion present subsequently in the adult tissues. The m.11778G>A

mutation is the commonest LHON mutation. In LHON, males are four times more likely to be affected than females but, as mentioned above, the inheritance of the mutation is maternal, as for other mitochondrial conditions. The mutation rate in mitochondrial DNA is higher than in nuclear DNA.

4. **Answer: A, C, E.** The UPD is maternal in origin in Prader–Willi syndrome and paternal in Angelman syndrome. The recurrence risk following the birth of a child with Prader–Willi syndrome is very low if the child has a cytogenetically visible deletion, or UPD, at the Prader–Willi syndrome/Angelman syndrome region of chromosome 15q and the parents have normal karyotypes. Imprinting centre microdeletions, however, although relatively rare in Prader–Willi syndrome/Angelman syndrome, can be present in an unaffected parent and can thus confer a recurrence risk of 50%. They interfere with the normal parent-specific imprinting that takes place in gametogenesis (see Fig. 16.9). In particular, they block the reprogramming process by which appropriate alleles would normally have become active. This can therefore result in Prader–Willi syndrome (where a paternal chromosome 15 has a maternal type imprint that results in the Prader–Willi syndrome-associated genes being unusually inactive) or Angelman syndrome (where a maternal chromosome 15 has a paternal type imprint, resulting in the Angelman syndrome genes being inactive). In Angelman syndrome, high recurrence risks also apply if there is an inherited *UBE3A* mutation, if there is paternal UPD with (unusually) a predisposing parental translocation or if there is an inherited cytogenetic abnormality.

5. **Answer: A, C, D, E.** Apparently balanced translocations generally do not affect the health or lifespan of the carrier. The t(11;22)(q23;q11) translocation is, in fact, the most common constitutional non-Robertsonian translocation in humans and is believed to arise through recombination between Alu repeats on chromosomes 11 and 22. Balanced carriers are, however, at risk of having affected offspring with the resulting derivative 22, or 'der(22)', syndrome being due to a 3 : 1 meiotic non-disjunction event. Clinical features of the der(22) syndrome include mental retardation, craniofacial abnormalities and congenital heart defects.

Chapter 17
1. **Answer: A, B, D.** The biochemical marker levels are affected by maternal weight, ethnicity, cigarette smoking, diabetic status and gestation. Such factors are therefore taken into account in the interpretation of the results. There *is* a possibility of detecting a chromosome abnormality that is unrelated to that for which the test was being undertaken. This needs to be mentioned beforehand.

2. **Answer: B, E.** A single raised IRT result is not a reliable indicator that a child is affected by CF (as ΔF508 mutation carriers may also give positive IRT results). It would normally be followed by further testing, such as a repeat IRT test, *CFTR* mutation analysis if that repeat test is raised and, if a diagnosis of CF is suspected on subsequent tests, sweat testing. The ΔF508 *CFTR* mutation is a deletion of 3 bp, resulting in the loss of a single amino acid, phenylalanine, at position 508 in the CFTR protein, and does not affect the reading frame. Phenylalanine is abbreviated to F in the single-letter amino acid code, as P is used to represent proline. The ΔF508 mutation results in impaired protein folding after translation. This, in turn, leads to failure of the protein to insert properly into the plasma membrane and to subsequent protein breakdown in the intracellular organelles known as proteasomes.

3. **Answer: A, C.** Carriers of β-thalassaemia typically show an increased proportion of HbA_2 on haemoglobin electrophoresis. Mutation analysis, when performed, can detect a mutation in most carriers. It is facilitated by the ability to selectively test for the small number of known mutations that are particularly prevalent within each population at risk. This can be undertaken, for instance, by allele-specific PCR (see Chapter 4), followed, if negative, by DNA sequencing. Unlike in α-thalassaemia, large gene deletions are very uncommon in β-thalassaemia. In this condition, most mutations are instead single-nucleotide substitutions, deletions or insertions.

4. **Answer: A.** Death usually occurs prior to the age of 4. Unfortunately, enzyme replacement therapy is not currently available (in contrast to Gaucher's disease). The carrier frequency is approximately ten times higher in Ashkenazi Jews (e.g. Jews of central and eastern European ancestry) than in Sephardic Jews (e.g. those with ancestry in Spain and North Africa) and non-Jews. The neuronal damage responsible for the clinical effects results from GM_2 accumulation in the lysosomes.

5. **Answer: C, D, E.** His risk of being a carrier is not 2/3 but 1/2, as, despite his normal health, we cannot at this stage rule out the possibility that he is homozygous for the mutation (as might have been possible if he were a healthy adult with a brother who had cystic fibrosis – see Chapter 15). Although he has a 25% chance of being homozygous for the C282Y mutation, his chances of developing the condition are considerably less, on account of incomplete penetrance. William's son will have a 1 in 20 chance of inheriting two *HFE* mutations as he will receive one from his father and has a 1 in 20 chance of receiving one from his mother.

Chapter 18

1. Answer: B, C, D, E. Talipes represents a congenital deformation rather than a malformation.

2. Answer: A, B. The presence of the additional chromosome number 21 is most likely to have been due to non-disjunction during meisosis, and is maternal in origin in around 90% of cases. The chance of recurrence is small, around just 1% given her age, and is not increased by the presence of mosaicism in the fetus.

3. Answer: D. Spina bifida is usually multifactorial but occasionally occurs, together with other congenital malformations, in trisomy 18. Trisomies 13, 18 and 21 usually occur as a result of the inheritance of an extra *maternal* chromosome.

4. Answer: E. The child would be a second-degree relative of the affected individual, with a risk of approximately 1 in 70 of being affected by an NTD.

5. Answer: D. Valproate is a known teratogen (rather than a mutagen) causing a variable phenotype but including the typical facial appearance described above (see Table 18.11). This is known as fetal valproate syndrome. Effects of this drug on gene expression have in fact been observed, including altered *Hox* gene expression in mice. A high-penetrance autosomal dominant condition is not likely in this situation, given the history of maternal sodium valproate medication and the absence of the condition in any family member other than the two children. Gonadal mosaicism for an autosomal dominant condition in one of the parents is a theoretical possibility, although less likely here. The chromosomes of the children could be checked to exclude an abnormality resulting, for instance, from a balanced chromosomal translocation in one parent, although again this is less likely.

6. Answer: B, D, E. The deletion is only present in a parent in 6% of cases, but both parents should be offered testing for it. Gonadal mosaicism is a possibility when neither parent carries the deletion, with the result that recurrence in a sibling could occur.

7. Answer: D.

Chapter 19

1. Answer: C. After searching for the gene in the Ensembl database, it can be seen from the genomic sequence and from the longest transcripts that the gene itself has a total of 12 exons (although the third transcript listed contains only ten of the exons).

2. Answer: D. A search of the GeneCards database reveals that the gene encodes a protein that contains a DNA-binding forkhead domain and is currently regarded as a member of the so-called forkhead transcription factor family, although its precise function is not known for certain.

3. Answer: A. Searching the latest version of the UCSC genome browser after entering '7p15.1' into the search box shows that the RefSeq genes that are fully or partly located within that cytogenetic band are *JAZF1* and *CREB5*. The display of the 'RefSeq genes' can be activated at the foot of the web page (within the 'Genes and Gene Prediction Tracks' section of controls).

4. Answer: The alternative names of the single microsatellite Genethon marker that is located within this gene (according to the current version of the UCSC database) are: AFM207XG1, D2S152, 207XG1, GC378-D2S152, RH15228, RH9538 and HS207XG1. The primer sequences that can be used to carry out PCR across this marker are: AGCTGCTGGTATATATTATCTTCCA and TAATGAAATTATTTAATGCATCTCC. The predicted PCR product size range (shown as 'distance') is 269–285 bp. To find this information, follow the instructions provided under the subheading 'Displaying microsatellite markers' in the text of this chapter.

5. Answer: AFMB297XC1. The heterozygosity of each of these markers, obtained easily from the CEPH Genome Database Browser that is mentioned in the text and in Table 19.4, is as follows: AFM292WD1: 42.86%, AFMB297XC1: 75.00% and AFMA057VG9: 64.29%.

APPENDIX 1
Odds, probabilities and applications of Bayes' theorem

The probability of an event is the *proportion* of times the event occurs in a long series of experiments. Conventionally, this is expressed as a fraction or decimal in the range 0 (event never happens) to 1 (event always happens). For example, if a coin is tossed, the probability of heads is 1/2, and similarly the probability of tails is 1/2. In this example, the outcome is either heads or tails (not both) and so these are *mutually exclusive events*. For mutually exclusive events, the probability of either one outcome *or* the other outcome is the *sum* of their individual probabilities and, as there must be an outcome, the sum of the probabilities of all possible outcomes is 1. Thus, for example, with one throw of a dice the probability of a 5 or a 6 is 1/3 (i.e. 1/6 + 1/6).

In contrast, *independent events* are such that the outcome of one event has no influence whatsoever on the outcome of the other event. So, for example, if two coins are tossed and the first comes down heads, the prediction about the outcome of the second coin is unchanged. For two independent events, the probability of a specified outcome of the first *and* a specified outcome of the second is the *product* of their individual probabilities. Thus, the probability that a toss of two coins will produce two heads is 1/4 (i.e. $1/2 \times 1/2$).

Thus, for a couple who are both carriers of an autosomal recessive trait such as cystic fibrosis, the chance of a recessive homozygous child represents one of the four possible outcomes (see Fig. 8.8). Their chance of having an unaffected child is 3/4 (representing the sum of two mutually exclusive events: a 1 in 4 chance of having a homozygous normal child plus a 2 in 4 chance of having a heterozygous child).

In contrast, for a non-consanguineous Caucasian couple with no relevant family history, the chance of having a child with cystic fibrosis is approximately 1 in 1600, which represents the combination by multiplication of three independent events: the father's carrier risk (approximately $1/20$) × the mother's carrier risk (approximately $1/20$) × the chance (if both parents are carriers) of them both transmitting their mutant allele to the child (1/4).

Bayes' theorem is used in genetic counselling to combine other information with pedigree data in the assessment of an individual's chance of being a carrier.

For example, Fig. A1.1 shows the pedigree of a family with Duchenne muscular dystrophy. In this family, I:2 is an obligate carrier as she has two affected sons. Thus, her daughter II:3 has a 1 in 2 chance of also being a carrier. If the daughter is a carrier, then half of her sons would be affected. She has four normal sons and thus she is either a carrier who has been lucky or, more likely, she is not a carrier. Bayes' theorem combines this conditional information (the normal sons) with the prior risk of 1 in 2 to produce a final risk (Table A1.1). In the

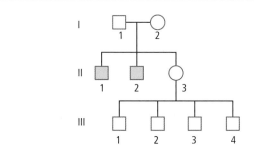

Fig. A1.1 Pedigree of a family with Duchenne muscular dystrophy.

Table A1.1 Bayes' calculation – 1

	II:3 carrier	II:3 not a carrier
Prior risk (Fig. A1.1)	1/2	1/2
Conditional information (four normal sons)	$(1/2)^4 = 1/16$	$1^4 = 1$
Joint odds (product of first two entries)*	1/32	1/2 (= 16/32)
Final risk (each joint odds divided by the sum of the joint odds)	(1/32)/(17/32) = 1/17	(16/32)/(17/32) = 16/17

*Using the same denominator in the joint entry simplifies the last calculation as it becomes each numerator over the sum of the numerators.

Essential Medical Genetics, 6th edition. © Edward S. Tobias, Michael Connor and Malcolm Ferguson-Smith. Published 2011 by Blackwell Published Ltd.

Table A1.2 Bayes' calculation – 2

	II:3 carrier	II:3 not a carrier
Prior risk	1/2	1/2
Conditional information (four normal sons and normal CK)	$(1/2)^4 \times 1/3 = 1/48$	$1^4 \times 1 = 1$
Joint odds	1/96	1/2 (= 48/96)
Final risk	1/49	48/49

second line of the table, '$(1/2)^4$' is the chance that, if II:3 were a carrier, she would have had four normal sons (i.e. $1/2 \times 1/2 \times 1/2 \times 1/2$), Similarly, the next entry in the second line, '1^4', is the chance of having four normal sons if she were not a carrier.

Thus, the final risk that II:3 is a carrier is 1 in 17, a substantial reduction from the prior risk of 1 in 2.

A normal level of creatine kinase (CK) will also reduce the risk of II:3 being a carrier. For example, if her median CK was 50 IU/l, then from Fig. 8.12 the risk of being a carrier is 1 in 3 (from the relative heights of the two curves at this point). The conditional information (the CK level) is again combined with the pedigree risk using Bayes' theorem (Table A1.2). Her final risk of being a carrier is thus 1 in 49.

APPENDIX 2
Calculation of the coefficients of relationship and inbreeding

The coefficient of relationship (r) is the proportion of all genes in *two* individuals that are identical by descent. Calculation of this may be helpful in providing a recurrence risk for an autosomal recessive trait for members of an inbred family.

The coefficient is calculated from the formula:

$$r = (1/2)^n$$

where n is the number of steps apart on the pedigree for the two individuals via the common ancestor. If there is more than one common ancestor, then their contributions are added to give a final r value.

For example, in Fig. A2.1, first cousins have an r value of:

$$r = (1/2)^4 + (1/2)^4 \text{ or } 1/8$$

Thus, on average, 1 in 8 of the genes of first cousins are identical by descent.

The coefficient of inbreeding (F) is the proportion of loci at which *one* individual is homozygous by descent. Thus, if first cousins married, their child's proportion of loci that would be homozygous by descent would be on average half of the proportion of parental genes identical by descent or $r/2$. Thus:

$$F = r/2$$

In Fig. A2.2, a man by his first wife has a child with an autosomal recessive disorder. The man then marries his first cousin. What is the risk of recurrence?

He is an obligate heterozygote. As r for first cousins is 1 in 8, the chance that his wife has the same recessive allele from a common ancestor is 1 in 8. For two heterozygotes, the risk of recurrence is 1 in 4. Thus, the final risk is the product of these probabilities:

$$1 \text{ (i.e. his carrier risk)} \times 1/8 \text{ (i.e. her carrier risk)} \times 1/4 = 1/32$$

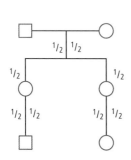

Fig. A2.1 Pedigree example of calculation of coefficient of relationship.

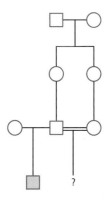

Fig. A2.2 Consanguineous pedigree with a single-gene disorder.

Essential Medical Genetics, 6th edition. © Edward S. Tobias, Michael Connor and Malcolm Ferguson-Smith. Published 2011 by Blackwell Published Ltd.

APPENDIX 3
Population genetics of single-gene disorders

Maintenance of gene frequencies

In a population, the relative frequencies of different alleles tend to be kept constant from one generation to the next. This can be demonstrated mathematically and helps to explain why dominant traits do not automatically increase at the expense of recessive traits.

Consider one autosomal locus with two alternative alleles, A and a. If the frequency of the allele A is p and the frequency of the allele a is q, then the sum of these allele frequencies must be 1, or 100%. Therefore:

$$p + q = 1$$

Table A3.1 shows the frequencies of each genotype at this locus.

In the production of the next generation, each of the three types of paternal genotype may mate with each of the three types of maternal genotype (Table A3.2). Table A3.3 indicates the genotypes of the offspring for each mating type, and as can be seen, the relative frequency of each remains unchanged and the population is said to be in genetic equilibrium. Although the actual numbers of individuals with each genotype may have increased, the relative proportions of each genotype (and allele)

Table A3.1 Allele and genotype frequencies at a locus with two alleles, A and a

Maternal gametes	Paternal gametes	
	A (p)	a (q)
A (p)	AA (p^2)	Aa (pq)
a (q)	Aa (pq)	aa (q^2)

Table A3.2 Frequencies of different parental genotypes at reproduction

Maternal genotypes	Paternal genotypes		
	AA (p^2)	Aa ($2pq$)	Aa (q^2)
AA (p^2)	AA × AA (p^4)	AA × Aa ($2p^3q$)	AA × aa (p^2q^2)
Aa ($2pq$)	Aa × AA ($2p^3q$)	Aa × Aa ($4p^2q^2$)	Aa × aa ($2pq^3$)
aa (q^2)	aa × AA (p^2q^2)	aa × Aa ($2pq^3$)	aa × aa (q^4)

Table A3.3 Frequencies of different types of offspring after reproduction

Mating type	Frequency (from Table A3.2)	Offspring		
		AA	Aa	aa
AA × AA	p^4	p^4		
AA × Aa	$4p^3q$	$2p^3q$	$2p^3q$	
AA × aa	$2p^2q^2$		$2p^2q^2$	
Aa × Aa	$4p^2q^2$	p^2q^2	$2p^2q^2$	p^2q^2
Aa × aa	$4pq^3$		$2pq^3$	$2pq^3$
aa × aa	q^4			q^4

AA offspring = $p^4 + 2p^3q + p^2q^2 = p^2(p^2 + 2pq + q^2) = p^2(p + q)^2 = p^2(1)^2 = p^2$
Aa offspring = $2p^3q + 4p^2q^2 + 2pq^3 = 2pq(p^2 + 2pq + q^2) = 2pq$
aa offspring = $p^2q^2 + 2pq^3 + q^4 = q^2(p^2 + 2pq + q^2) = q^2$

Essential Medical Genetics, 6th edition. © Edward S. Tobias, Michael Connor and Malcolm Ferguson-Smith.
Published 2011 by Blackwell Published Ltd.

have remained constant (AA at p^2, Aa at $2pq$ and aa at q^2). This principle is called the Hardy–Weinberg law.

The most important application of this law is the calculation of carrier frequencies for autosomal recessive traits.

For any autosomal recessive trait, if q is the frequency of the mutant allele and p the frequency of the normal allele, then the frequency of the recessive homozygote *genotype* is equal to the square of the mutant *allele* frequency (q^2), or the disease frequency (for a condition with childhood onset). Thus, for cystic fibrosis: recessive homozygote frequency, $q^2 = 1/1600$. Therefore, $q = \sqrt{(1/1600)} = 1/40$. Consequently, as above, $p = 1 - q = 39/40$. The heterozygote (carrier genotype) frequency is $2pq$, i.e. $2 \times 39/40 \times 1/40$ or approximately 1/20. Generally, for a rare autosomal recessive disorder, the carrier frequency is approximately twice the square root of the disease frequency.

APPENDIX 4
Legal aspects

Genetic counselling

In the UK, under the Congenital Disabilities (Civil Liability) Act 1976 (as amended; see Further Reading), which applies in England, Wales and Northern Ireland, legal action can be brought against a person whose breach of duty to parents results in a child being born disabled, abnormal or unhealthy. In both the UK and the USA, there has been an escalation of litigation concerning genetic disease. Most cases concern physician errors of omission, and it is important for all doctors who provide genetic advice to ensure that such information is valid and up to date. Thus, failure (whether from ignorance or religious objections) to take a family history and to follow up with appropriate tests or referrals and failure to give correct genetic advice may constitute medical negligence. The claim would be likely to fail if at any time both parents knew and accepted the risk that the child might be abnormal.

Prenatal diagnosis

Prenatal diagnosis with selective termination of pregnancy became a reality in the UK with the Abortion Act 1967 (as amended; see Further Reading). Under this Act, which applies throughout the UK, one ground for termination of pregnancy is '… a substantial risk that if the child were born it would suffer from such physical or mental abnormalities as to be seriously handicapped'. The legal position in other countries varies from total prohibition of abortion for fetal abnormality to relative liberality. Prenatal diagnostic tests need informed consent, and parents should be reminded that no single test excludes all known fetal abnormalities, and that occasionally the test fails to give a result.

Consanguinity

Almost all human societies in existence prohibit the mating of first-degree relatives (incest). Marriage between relatives less close than siblings or parents and offspring is not necessarily outlawed, but the dividing line between legal and illegal varies somewhat between countries. Thus, in about half of the USA, uncle–niece, aunt–nephew and first-cousin matings are forbidden by law, and in most African societies consanguineous marriage is not allowed. In contrast, in parts of the Middle East, Pakistan and India, marriage between relatives is common, and up to 20% of marriages are consanguineous. The marriage of double first cousins (both sets of grandparents in common) is the closest legal union in the UK.

Paternity testing

Historically, disputed paternity was tested using a series of polymorphic blood groups and enzymes. With a combination of these markers, paternity could be excluded in at least 95% of cases but could never be proven, only excluded. This area has been transformed by the use of variation at the DNA level and in particular by DNA fingerprinting. The polymerase chain reaction (PCR) is used by commercial agencies to identify multiple (e.g. 16 or more) dispersed sequences of variable size named short tandem repeats and the pattern produced is characteristic for an individual. The hypervariability of size of each product is such that the chance of two unrelated individuals having an identical pattern is extremely low. A child's pattern is a combination of that from each parent, and a putative father can be either excluded or positively identified with a quoted certainty of at least 99.999%. The DNA fingerprints are identical in monozygotic twins and this approach is also employed to resolve family relationships in immigration disputes and for forensic testing of DNA from semen or dried blood spots (see Chapter 4).

FURTHER READING

Congenital Disabilities (Civil Liability) Act 1976. The UK Statute Law Database. Office of Public Sector Information. http://www.statutelaw.gov.uk/content.aspx?activeTextDocId=1242382

Abortion Act 1967. The UK Statute Law Database. Office of Public Sector Information. http://www.statutelaw.gov.uk/content.aspx?activeTextDocId=1181037

Glossary

Acrocentric — a chromosome with the centromere near one end, i.e. chromosomes 13, 14, 15, 21, 22 and Y

Alleles — alternative forms of a gene at the same locus

Alternative splicing — the formation of diverse mRNAs through differential splicing of an RNA precursor

Amniocentesis — aspiration of amniotic fluid

Aneuploid — any chromosome number that is not an exact multiple of the haploid number

Anticipation — the apparent tendency for some diseases to begin at an earlier age and to increase in severity with each succeeding generation

Antisense RNA — non-functional RNA that is complementary to an individual mRNA strand

Array comparative genomic hybridisation (aCGH) — a method for the detection of duplications or deletions of DNA regions by competitive hybridisation of fluorescently labelled control and test DNA to a microarray of known mapped sequences

Ascertainment — identification of families with an inherited condition

Association — a non-random combination of two or more structural defects that are not due to a single localised defect of embryogenesis

Assortative mating — the preferential selection of a spouse with a particular genotype

Assortment — random distribution of non-homologous chromosomes to daughter cells in meiosis

Autosome — any chromosome other than the sex chromosomes

Bivalent — a pair of homologous chromosomes as seen following synapsis prior to the first meiotic division

Burden — consultant's perception of the cost (emotional, physical and financial) of a genetic disorder

Carrier — a recessive heterozygote

Centimorgan — a length of DNA within which there is a 1% chance of recombination, i.e. one cross-over per 100 gametes, with (very approximately) 1 cM per megabase

Centromere — the heterochromatic region within a chromosome by which the chromatids are held together

Chiasma — the crossing of chromatid strands between homologous chromosomes during meiosis as a result of meiotic recombination

Chimaera — an individual whose cells are derived from more than one zygote

Chorionic villus sampling (CVS) — a technique for prenatal diagnosis which biopsies chorionic villi

Chromatid — newly formed replicated DNA (a single DNA double helix) prior to separation from its sister chromatid. During cell division the chromosomes consist of two chromatids (joined at the centromere) rather than just one

Chromatin — the complex of DNA and associated proteins that represents the normal state of genes in the nucleus

Chromosomal aberration — any abnormality of chromosome number or structure visible under the microscope

Cis — location of two genes on the same chromosome

Clone — a cell line derived by mitosis from a single diploid cell or gene sequences that are propagated through recombinant techniques from an identical parent gene

Co-dominant — both alleles of a pair are expressed in the heterozygote

Codon — three consecutive bases in DNA or RNA which specify an amino acid

Coefficient of inbreeding (F) — the proportion of loci at which an individual is homozygous by descent

Coefficient of relationship (r) — the proportion of all genes in two individuals that are identical by descent

Complementarity — two single-stranded nucleic acid molecules are complementary when they form a succession of perfectly matched A : T and G : C base pairs in antiparallel (adjacent but opposite) orientation

Essential Medical Genetics, 6th edition. © Edward S. Tobias, Michael Connor and Malcolm Ferguson-Smith. Published 2011 by Blackwell Published Ltd.

Complementary DNA   a single-stranded DNA fragment that is synthesised from the mRNA strand by reverse transcriptase

Compound heterozygote   an individual with two different mutant alleles at the same locus. Note that if the two mutant alleles are at different loci, then the individual is termed a **double heterozygote**

Concordant   both members of a twin pair showing the trait

Congenital   present at birth

Consanguineous   mating between individuals who share at least one common ancestor

Consensus sequence   an idealised nucleotide sequence in which each position represents the base most often found when many sequences with similar function in several different genes are compared

Conserved sequence   DNA sequences that are present in multiple, related members of a gene family and can be conserved between tissues or among species

Constitutive gene   genes whose expression is controlled only by basal promoter activity (usually no developmental or hormonal regulation and expressed at a constant level in most cells – see **housekeeping genes**)

Construct   the assembly of a given set of DNA fragments in an appropriate vector using recombinant techniques

Consultand   any person requesting genetic counselling

Cosmid   synthetic cloning vector which can accommodate large fragments of foreign DNA

CpG island   a region of DNA often found close to the 5′ end of housekeeping genes that is relatively rich in 5′-CG-3′ oligonucleotide sequences where the C is often not methylated

Cross-over   exchange of genetic material between homologous chromosomes during meiosis

Deformation   alteration in shape of an organ due to unusual mechanical forces

Denaturation   the separation of complementary DNA and/or RNA strands by exposure to alkali or elevated temperature

Dicentric   a structurally abnormal chromosome with two centromeres

Diploid   the chromosome number of somatic cells

Discordant   only one member of a twin pair showing a trait

Disomy, uniparental (UPD)   inheritance of both homologues of a chromosome from one parent, with loss of the corresponding homologue from the other parent

Disruption   a morphological defect due to breakdown of a previously normal organ or tissue

Distal elements   nucleic acid sequences that are located toward the 3′ end from a reference point

Domain   a segment of protein that is responsible for a specialised structure or function

Dominant negative   a mutation that prevents the normal functioning of not only the encoded protein but also the functioning of the protein encoded by a normal allele (e.g. via dimerisation)

Dominant   a trait expressed in the heterozygote

Downstream   refers to sequences that are distal or 3′ of the reference point

Empiric risk   recurrence risk based on experience rather than calculation

Enhancer   the region or regions of a gene that bind specific gene regulatory proteins and thus help to determine the level and cell type of gene expression

Epigenetic   refers to changes in the methylation or chromatin structure (without changing the DNA sequence) that result in altered gene expression levels. These can be passed on from cell to daughter cell.

Euchromatin   the majority of nuclear DNA that remains relatively unfolded during most of the cell cycle and is therefore accessible to transcriptional machinery

Exon   the segments of a gene that remain after splicing of the primary RNA transcript (5′ untranslated sequences, coding sequences and 3′ untranslated sequences)

Exonic splice enhancer (ESE)   short DNA sequence that assists splicing by acting as a binding site for a splicing accessory protein

Expressed sequence tag (EST)   partial sequence of an expressed gene usually representing its 3′ end

Expressivity   variation in the severity of a genetic trait

Familial   refers to any condition that is commoner in relatives of an affected individual than in the general population

Flanking markers   markers on either side of a disease locus

Flanking region   the DNA sequences that are upstream (5′) of the transcriptional start site and downstream (3′) of the transcription termination signal

Flow karyotype   a histogram of chromosome DNA measurements generated by a fluorescence-activated cell sorter

Fluorescence *in situ* hybridisation (FISH)   hybridisation using a probe (usually fluorescently labelled DNA) to bind to specific regions of chromosomes

Frameshift mutation   an insertion or deletion of a number of bases that is not a multiple of three and which therefore changes the triplet reading frame

Gain of function   a mutation that results in the encoded protein acquiring increased or new functional activity

Gene amplification   the presence of additional copies of a gene present on a chromosome (e.g. the *NMYC* gene in neuroblastoma)

Gene conversion   a process whereby two homologous portions of paired duplex DNA molecules become identical in sequence during recombination. In contrast to normal recombination, there is a unidirectional flow rather than an exchange of genetic information

Gene expression   production of the gene product (usually a protein, but occasionally a functional RNA such as a microRNA)

Gene pool   all the genes present at a given locus in the population

Gene   a linear collection of DNA sequences required to produce a functional RNA molecule

Genetic counselling   the communication of information and advice about inherited disorders

Genetic engineering   the artificial production of new combinations of heritable material

Genetic epidemiology   study of the role of genetic factors and their interaction with environmental factors in the distribution and determination of disease

Genetic heterogeneity   when a single phenotype can result from different genetic causes

Genetic lethal   a genetic disorder in which affected individuals fail to reproduce

Genetics   the scientific study of variation and heredity

Genomic imprinting   parent-specific expression or repression of genes or chromosomes in offspring

Genotype   the genetic constitution of the organism

Haploid   the chromosome number in gametes

Haploinsufficiency   when a phenotypic effect results from the loss of function of one of the two alleles

Haplotype   a group of closely linked alleles that are inherited together as a unit

Heredity   the transmission of characteristics to descendants

Heritability   the fraction of the phenotypic variance due to genetic effects

Heterochromatin   chromosomal regions that remain tightly folded during the entire cell cycle. These regions replicate late during S phase and do not contain actively transcribed genes

Heterozygote   an individual with one normal and one mutant allele at a given locus on a pair of homologous chromosomes

Holandric   Y-linked inheritance

Homologous   matched

Homozygote   an individual with a pair of identical alleles at a given locus on homologous chromosomes

Housekeeping genes   genes that are constitutively expressed in most or all cells because they provide basic functions

Hybridisation   the binding of nucleic acid sequences through complementary base pairing

Idiogram   a diagram of the chromosome complement

Imprinting   where the parental origin of a gene determines the level of its expression

Inbreeding   the mating of closely related individuals

Intron   a segment of a gene that is transcribed into the primary RNA transcript but which is excised during exon splicing

Isochromosome   an abnormal chromosome in which there is loss of one arm and two identical copies of the other

Isodisomy, uniparental   inheritance of two copies of one homologue of a chromosome from one parent, with loss of the corresponding homologue from the other parent

Isolate   a genetically separate population

Karyotype   the classified chromosome complement of an individual or cell

Kilobase (kb)   a unit of length with 1000 bases in DNA or RNA

Kindred an extended family

Library a collection of DNA fragments that have been inserted into vector molecules

Linkage disequilibrium the association of two linked alleles more frequently than would be expected by chance

Linkage linked genes have their loci within measurable distance of one another on the same chromosome

Locus the precise location of a gene on a chromosome

Lod score logarithm of the odds score for the likelihood of two loci being within a measurable distance of each other

LOH loss of heterozygosity. This is the apparent homozygosity, in tumour DNA, at a DNA polymorphism that shows heterozygosity in the normal DNA of that patient. It is often caused by a large deletion affecting one chromosome and may, if it occurs frequently, indicate the presence of a tumour suppressor gene within that chromosomal region

Loss of function a mutation that causes reduced activity of the encoded protein

Malformation a primary error of normal development or morphogenesis of an organ or tissue

Megabase 1×10^6 bp of DNA

Meiosis reduction cell division, which occurs in gamete production

Microdeletion chromosomal deletion too small to be clearly visualised with the light microscope (less than 4–5 Mb)

Micronuclei separate small nuclei containing chromosomes or chromosomal fragments that are not participating in normal mitosis

Microsatellite a type of polymorphic DNA sequence consisting of a repeated unit of 1–6 nucleotides. Dinucleotide repeats (e.g. CACACA …) have proved very useful polymorphic markers for linkage analysis.

Microsatellite instability the generation of new microsatellite allele sizes in the DNA of tumours that are deficient in mismatch repair

MicroRNA (miRNA) short RNA molecules of 21–22 bp that can regulate gene expression and which are encoded by sequences in normal genomes

Mismatch repair the normal repair mechanism for the nucleotides that can be wrongly incorporated during DNA replication

Missense mutation a base-pair substitution that leads to an altered amino acid specification (cf. **silent** and **nonsense mutations**)

Mitosis somatic cell division

Monosomy one of a chromosome pair is missing

Mosaic an individual derived from a single zygote with cells of two or more different genotypes

Multifactorial inheritance due to multiple genes at different loci, which summate and interact with environmental factors

Multiplex ligation-dependent probe amplification (MLPA) a method of testing for copy number changes in DNA, such as deletion or duplication of exons

Mutation a change in the genetic material

Non-disjunction failure of two members of a chromosome pair to disjoin during anaphase

Nonsense-mediated decay (NMD) a process which degrades mRNA molecules that contain a premature stop codon which is at least 50 nt upstream of the last splice junction

Nonsense mutation a base-pair substitution that results in the replacement of an amino acid codon with a termination (stop) codon (UGA, UAA or UAG)

Northern blotting filter transfer of RNA separated by size in gel electrophoresis

Nucleotide a purine or pyrimidine base attached to a sugar and phosphate group

Oligonucleotide a short single-stranded DNA molecule (e.g. 20 nt), used e.g. as a PCR primer

Oncogene a gene sequence capable of causing transformation and tumorigenesis

Open reading frame series of triplet codons within a DNA sequence that does not include any stop or nonsense codons

Palindrome a stretch of DNA in which identical base sequences run in opposite directions

Pseudoautosomal region (PAR) region at the tip at each end of the X and Y chromosomes, containing homologous genes. X/Y recombination occurs here, resulting in an apparently autosomal mechanism of inheritance is observed for alleles in these regions.

Penetrance the frequency of phenotypic expression of the genotype

Pharmacogenetics the study of genetically controlled variation of response to drugs

Phenocopy an environmentally induced mimic of a genetic disease

Phenotype the outward appearance of an individual

Plasmid extrachromosomal closed circular DNA molecule found in bacteria

Polygenic effect determined by multiple genes at different loci each with a small but additive effect

Polymerase chain reaction (PCR) a technique for the exponential amplification of a target segment of DNA

Polymorphism any sequence variant that is present in at least 1% of the population or that is known to be non-pathogenic

Polyploid an abnormal chromosomal complement that exceeds the diploid number and is an exact multiple of the haploid number

Probability the ratio of the number of occurrences of a specified event to the total number of possible events

Proband the individual who draws medical attention to the family

Probe a labelled DNA or RNA fragment used to identify complementary sequence(s) by molecular hybridisation

Prokaryote a simple unicellular organism that lacks a nuclear membrane

Promoter the region of a gene that determines where RNA polymerase binds and initiates transcription

Pseudodominance the direct transmission, generation to generation, of a recessive trait if the gene is frequent or if inbreeding is intense, or the carrier frequency is high

Pseudogene a non-functional replica of a functional gene

Quantitative PCR (qPCR) methods (usually involving real-time measurements of PCR product accumulation) that permit accurate quantification of the amount of template DNA or, in qRT-PCR (quantitative reverse transcriptase PCR), mRNA.

Race a group of historically related individuals who share a gene pool

Random mating selection of a mate without regard to genotype

Recessive a trait that is expressed only in homozygotes

Recombinant an individual in a linkage study in whom the marker and disease loci have assorted at parental meiosis

Recombination the process whereby two homologous duplex DNA molecules exchange information by crossing over

Restriction enzyme an enzyme that cleaves DNA at sequence-specific sites (the recognition site)

Restriction fragment length polymorphism (RFLP) a recognition site for a restriction enzyme, which may or may not be present

Reverse transcriptase an enzyme that can make complementary DNA from mRNA

Reverse transcriptase polymerase chain reaction (RT-PCR) a method commonly used to study mRNA levels. The RNA is converted by the enzyme, reverse transcriptase, into cDNA, prior to PCR

RNA editing modification of the mRNA sequence during processing so that it is no longer complementary to the original DNA template (e.g. production of two apolipoproteins, apoB48 and apoB100, from the same gene)

Satellite DNA Highly repetitive DNA (generally repeat lengths of less than 5–10 bp) that is often found in heterochromatin and can be separated from the majority of genomic DNA by density-gradient centrifugation

Secondary structure the proposed structural domains of a protein on the basis of its amino acid sequence (primary structure)

Segregation the separation of allelic genes at meiosis

Sequence a series of abnormalities causally related to a primary malformation

Sex-limited a trait expressed in only one sex

Sex-linked inheritance of a gene carried on a sex chromosome

Sibling a brother or sister

Sibship a group of brothers and/or sisters

Silent mutation a base-pair substitution that alters a codon but does not result in an altered amino acid due to degeneracy of the genetic code (e.g. GGA and GGU both code for glycine)

Single-copy DNA DNA that is present in one copy per set of haploid chromosomes (represents about 45% of the total)

Sister chromatid exchange exchange of DNA by sister chromatids

Site-directed mutagenesis the production of specific mutations in a DNA fragment

Single-nucleotide polymorphism (SNP) a position in the genome at which two (or sometimes three) alternative nucleotides are common in the population

Southern blotting filter transfer of DNA fragments separated by size in gel electrophoresis

Species a set of individuals who can interbreed and have fertile progeny

Sporadic occurring in just one individual in a family

Synapsis pairing of homologous chromosomes during prophase of the first meiotic division

Syndrome a non-random combination of features

Synteny loci on the same chromosome, which may or may not be linked

Teratogen any agent that causes congenital malformations

Tertiary structure refers to the three-dimensional structure of a protein

Trait any gene-determined characteristic

Trans location of two genes on opposite chromosomes of a pair

Transcription factors DNA-binding proteins required for the initiation of RNA synthesis by RNA polymerase

Transcription production of mRNA from the DNA template

Transgenic where synthetic DNA has been introduced into the genome of an animal in order to change its genotype

Translation the process whereby protein is synthesised from a mRNA sequence

Translocation the transfer of chromosomal material between chromosomes

Triploid a cell with three times the haploid number of chromosomes

Trisomy three copies of a given chromosome per cell

Truncating mutation a mutation causing shortening of the protein, such as a frameshift or nonsense mutation

Tumour suppressor gene a gene in which inactivating mutations, affecting both alleles, lead to tumorigenesis

Untranslated region the portion of a gene that is transcribed into mRNA but not translated into protein. By definition, untranslated regions are found in exons

Upstream refers to sequences located in the opposite direction to transcription

Vector a plasmid, phage or cosmid into which foreign DNA may be inserted for cloning

Western blotting filter transfer of proteins separated by size in gel electrophoresis

YAC yeast artificial chromosome used for cloning of large sections of DNA

Zygote the fertilised ovum

Index

Note: page numbers in *italics* refer to figures; those in **bold** to tables.

Essential Medical Genetics, 6th edition. © Edward S. Tobias, Michael Connor and Malcolm Ferguson-Smith.
Published 2011 by Blackwell Published Ltd.